Pregnancy, Childbirth and Maternal Health

Pregnancy, Childbirth and Maternal Health

Editor: Katie Beckett

AMERICAN
MEDICAL PUBLISHERS
www.americanmedicalpublishers.com

AMERICAN
MEDICAL PUBLISHERS
www.americanmedicalpublishers.com

Cataloging-in-Publication Data

Pregnancy, childbirth and maternal health / edited by Katie Beckett.
p. cm.
Includes bibliographical references and index.
ISBN 978-1-63927-164-1
1. Pregnancy. 2. Childbirth. 3. Maternal health services. 4. Obstetrics. I. Beckett, Katie.
RG551 .P74 2022
618.2--dc23

American Medical Publishers,
41 Flatbush Avenue,
1st Floor, New York,
NY 11217, USA

ISBN 978-1-63927-164-1 (Hardback)

Contents

Preface

The main aim of this book is to educate learners and enhance their research focus by presenting diverse topics covering this vast field. This is an advanced book which compiles significant studies by distinguished experts in the area of analysis. This book addresses successive solutions to the challenges arising in the area of application, along with it; the book provides scope for future developments.

Pregnancy or gestation refers to the time when one or more offspring are developed inside a woman's womb. It can occur by sexual intercourse or using reproductive technology. Childbirth generally occurs in 40 weeks or 9 months from the start of the last menstrual period. Some of the symptoms of pregnancy are missed periods, tender breasts, hunger, frequent urination, and nausea and vomiting. It can be diagnosed by doing physical tests, using biomarkers and obstetric ultrasonography. Maternal health is managed by taking proper prenatal care, managing nutrition, and intake of multivitamins and pharmaceutical drugs. This book unfolds the innovative aspects of pregnancy, childbirth and maternal health which will be crucial for the progress of these fields in the future. The extensive content of this book provides the readers with a thorough understanding of the subjects. It presents researches and studies performed by experts across the globe.

It was a great honour to edit this book, though there were challenges, as it involved a lot of communication and networking between me and the editorial team. However, the end result was this all-inclusive book covering diverse themes in the field.

Finally, it is important to acknowledge the efforts of the contributors for their excellent chapters, through which a wide variety of issues have been addressed. I would also like to thank my colleagues for their valuable feedback during the making of this book.

Editor

1

The effect of twin-to-twin delivery time intervals on neonatal outcome for second twins

L. Lindroos[1*], A. Elfvin[2], L. Ladfors[1] and U.-B. Wennerholm[1]

Abstract

Background: The objective was to examine the effect of twin-to-twin delivery intervals on neonatal outcome for second twins.

Methods: This was a retrospective, hospital-based study, performed at a university teaching hospital in Western Sweden. Twin deliveries between 2008 and 2014 at ≥32 + 0 weeks of gestation, where the first twin was delivered vaginally, were included. Primary outcome was a composite outcome of metabolic acidosis, Apgar < 4 at 5 min or peri/neonatal mortality in the second twin. Secondary outcome was a composite outcome of neonatal morbidity.

Results: A total of 527 twin deliveries were included. The median twin-to-twin delivery interval time was 19 min (range 2–399 min) and 68% of all second twins were delivered within 30 min. Primary outcome occurred in 2.6% of the second twins. Median twin-to-twin delivery interval was 34 min (8–78 min) for the second twin with a primary outcome, and 19 min (2–399 min) for the second twin with no primary outcome ($p = 0.028$). Second twins delivered within a twin-to-twin interval of 0–30 min had a higher pH in umbilical artery blood gas than those delivered after 30 min (pH 7.23 and pH 7.20, $p < 0.0001$). Secondary outcome was not associated with twin-to-twin delivery interval time. The combined vaginal-cesarean delivery rate was 6.6% ($n = 35$) and the rate was higher with twin-to-twin delivery interval > 30 min ($p < 0.0001$).

Conclusions: An association, but not necessarily a causality, between twin-to-twin delivery interval and primary outcome was seen. An upper time limit on twin-to-twin delivery time intervals may be justified. However, the optimal time interval needs further studies.

Keywords: Second twin, Delivery time interval, Birth order, Cesarean section, Obstetric methods*, Neonatal, Outcome*, Pregnancy, Apgar score, Asphyxia Neonatorum

Background

Twin gestations are increasing worldwide as a result of higher maternal age and conceptions resulting from assisted reproductive technologies (ART) [1]. These pregnancies and deliveries are a challenge in obstetric practice. Twin gestations increase the risk of morbidity and mortality of both children, mainly due to preterm labor, intrauterine growth restriction and circumstances unique to twin pregnancies such as twin-twin transfusion syndrome (TTTS) and umbilical cord complications [2–4].

* Correspondence: linnea.lindroos@vgregion.se
[1]Department of Obstetrics and Gynecology, Institute of Clinical Sciences at Sahlgrenska Academy, Gothenburg University, Diagnosvägen 15, 416 85 Gothenburg, Sweden

It is not only the pregnancy itself but also the delivery that constitutes a greater risk to twins than singletons. Kiely showed that normal sized twins (birthweight > 3000 g) had a 70% increased risk of perinatal mortality and a threefold increased risk of intrapartum death compared to singletons [5]. The second twin is at higher risk than the first twin [6, 7] mainly due to the second twin being more difficult to monitor and also because complications such as cord prolapse, premature placental separation and fetal distress during labor are more common in the second twin than in the first one [8–10].

Several studies over the years have resulted in quite a clear understanding of how to deliver twins with regard to their presentation and gestation. Vaginal delivery is advocated if the first twin is in cephalic presentation, both twins are normal sized (1500–4000 g) and the second twin is not substantially larger than the first [7]. There is however no consensus as to whether the time between deliveries of the first twin and the second twin affects the neonatal outcome for the second twin. Some studies show that the risks mentioned above increase with a prolonged twin-to-twin time interval > 30 min [9, 11] as well as the risk of a combined vaginal-cesarean delivery [3, 4]. A correlation between longer twin-to-twin delivery intervals and decreasing pH in umbilical arterial blood gas, as well as a reduction of Apgar scores in the second twin, have been found in several previous studies [11, 12]. It has been suggested that the time interval should be kept short, ideally below 30 min. However, there are also a few studies showing that this is not of clinical significance and that there is no need for an upper time limit [9, 13, 14]. Recent guidelines as those from The American College of Obstetricians and Gynecologists offer no guideline regarding the optimal delivery time interval [15].

The aim of the current study was to investigate the relation between twin-to-twin time interval and the neonatal outcome for the second twin, considering both metabolic acidosis and Apgar score at birth, as well as neonatal mortality and morbidity within the first 28 days of life. The study was conducted at an obstetric unit where active management of the delivery of the second twin is not advocated.

Methods

After ethical approval from the Ethical committee at University of Gothenburg, Sweden, information regarding all twin deliveries at Sahlgrenska University Hospital, Gothenburg, Sweden, between 2008 and 2014 was retrieved from Obstetrix, a computerized obstetric medical record system. This university teaching hospital is the largest obstetric unit in Sweden and has an average annual delivery rate of 10,000 deliveries. A total of 527 twin deliveries were studied after exclusion of the following deliveries:

- delivery before 32 weeks of gestation
- the first twin delivered by cesarean section (CS)
- intrauterine death of one or both twins before onset of labor
- known fetal malformations or chromosome aberrations in one or both twins
- monoamniotic twin gestations

Because of its possible impact on neonatal outcome, information regarding maternal age, body mass index (BMI), smoking, parity, previous CS, maternal chronic hypertension, gestational hypertension, preeclampsia, diabetes mellitus type 1 or 2, gestational diabetes, gestational age, chorionicity, induction of labor, regional anesthesia, presentation, mode of delivery, time of delivery of both twins and birthweight was collected. From this information twin-to-twin time interval, large for gestational age (LGA), small for gestational age (SGA) and inter-twin birthweight discordance was calculated. LGA and SGA was defined as a birthweight of greater than + 2 standard deviations (SD) or less than − 2 SD, respectively, according to the Swedish reference value for singletons, with adjustment for gestational age and sex [16]. We used the reference values for singletons since there are no reference values available for twins. Inter-twin birthweight discordance was calculated as 100 × (birthweight of the largest twin minus birthweight of the smallest twin)/ birthweight of the largest twin, and was defined as a difference ≥ 25% [17]. Chorionicity was determined by ultrasonography in the first or second trimester.

Information regarding umbilical blood gas analysis including pH and base excess (BE), Apgar score, perinatal mortality and morbidity was retrieved from the obstetric computerized medical records system as well as from the Swedish neonatal quality register (SNQ), a national perinatal computerized medical record system in which all perinatal units in Sweden register their patients. After this it was possible to link the information from Obstetrix and SNQ to each other by means of the mother's 10-digit social security number.

The twin-to-twin time interval was defined and calculated as the time interval between the delivery of the first twin and the second twin. In order to examine trends of pH, Apgar and neonatal outcome over time, the time interval was divided into periods of 15 min (1–15, 16–30, 31–45, 46–60 and > 60 min). Analyses of twin-to-twin time intervals < 30 min and > 30 min were also performed since some previous studies suggested an upper time limit of 30 min.

Gestational age was based on a routine ultrasound examination, usually made in the second trimester by an expert midwife or obstetrician in ultrasound. Gestational age is calculated in days but presented in weeks + days as this is the most common and generally accepted method.

Primary outcome was defined as a composite measure consisting of any of the following factors:

- severe metabolic acidosis in umbilical arterial blood gas with pH < 7.05 and BE < − 12 or pH < 7.00
- if no blood gas was available; Apgar < 4 at 5 min
- perinatal mortality defined as death after onset of labor and within 7 days after birth
- neonatal mortality as death within 28 days after birth

Secondary outcome was defined as a composite measure consisting of any of the following factors:

- Apgar < 7 at 5 min
- acidosis in umbilical arterial blood gas with pH < 7.10
- interventricular hemorrhage (IVH) verified by ultrasonography and/or magnetic resonance imaging (MRI) within 28 days after birth
- hypoxic ischemic encephalopathy I-III (HIE)
- seizure within 7 days after birth
- septicemia confirmed by positive blood culture within 28 days after birth
- necrotizing enterocolitis (NEC) within 28 days after birth
- infant respiratory distress syndrome (IRDS) and transient tachypnea of the newborn (TTN)
- need for assisted ventilation – continuous positive air pressure (CPAP), ventilation by mask or mechanical ventilation
- If gestational age ≥ 34 weeks; admittance to neonatal intensive care unit (NICU) > 7 days

The intrapartum management of all twin deliveries followed the department's protocol. All twin pregnancies with the first twin in cephalic presentation were planned for vaginal delivery. Regional anesthesia was not mandatory. Continuous cardiotocography (CTG) was applied during active labor, predominately with fetal scalp registration on the first twin and external transducer for the second twin. A specialist in obstetrics and often resident in training as well as two midwives, at least one with experience, were present at delivery. If oxytocin was used it was paused immediately after the delivery of the first twin. Fetal presentation and heartrate of the second twin was examined with digital examination, ultrasonography and CTG. Amniotomy could be performed to enhance contractions if the second twin was engaged. If the second twin was in transverse lie an attempt of external version, to either cephalic or breech presentation, was performed - if needed with intravenous terbutaline or nitroglycerin for uterus relaxation. If lack of effective spontaneous contractions, oxytocin was started and spontaneous vaginal delivery, in head or breech presentation, was preferred. If this failed an internal version and breech extraction were to be considered. Otherwise CS was performed. There was no upper time limit for twin-to-twin time interval and if no complications occurred expectant management was applied. All twin deliveries were conducted at a special delivery ward which has an operating theatre where the CS were performed.

Statistical analysis

For comparison between two groups independent T-tests were used for continuous variables with normal distributions, Mann-Whitney U-test for continuous variables with non-normal distributions and Fisher's exact test for dichotomous variables. Logistic regression with calculation of odds ratio (OR) with 95% confidence interval (CI) and adjustment for gestational age was performed. Subgroup analysis was performed for chorionicity, presentation of the second twin and for twin pregnancies with vaginal deliveries of the second twin excluding cesarean deliveries of the second twin. Spearman's rho was used for analysis of correlation between umbilical cord arterial pH and twin-to-twin delivery time interval. Statistical calculations were performed using SPSS Statistics 22. All significance tests were two-sided and conducted at the 5% significance level.

Results

A total of 527 twin deliveries (1054 infants) met the inclusion criteria between January 2008 and December 2014. During this time period there were 71,908 deliveries at the obstetric unit with 1.6% (1123/71908) being twin deliveries between 22 + 1 to 41 + 2 weeks of gestation and with 23.9% (268/1123) elective CS before onset of labour.

The baseline maternal characteristics are described in Table 1. There were 501 twin gestations with known chorionicity, 386 (77%) were dichorionic and 115 (23%) were monochorionic.

In 463 (87.9%) deliveries the first twin had a spontaneous delivery in cephalic presentation, 61 (11.6%) had an assisted vaginal delivery (vacuum extraction/forceps) and although CS is advocated when the first twin is in breech there were three (0.6%) spontaneous vaginal breech deliveries. A total of 35 (6.6%) of the deliveries were combined vaginal/cesarean deliveries. In 411 (78.0%) deliveries the second twin had a spontaneous delivery in cephalic or breech presentation, in 72 (13.7%) an assisted vaginal delivery and in nine cases (1.7%) a breech extraction was performed.

Neonatal characteristics for the first and second twins are shown in Table 2. The median gestational age was 262 days (range 225–286 days) with 200/527 (38.0%) of the deliveries being preterm.

The median twin-to-twin time interval was 19 min (range 2–399) with 217 (41.2%) of the second twins being born within 15 min, 143 (27.1%) second twins were born within 16–30 min, 70 (13.3%) within 31–45 min, 37 (7%) within 46–60 min and 60 (11.4%) after 60 min.

Composite primary outcome occurred in 2.7% (14/527) in the second twins (Table 3). Of the 14 s twins with a composite primary outcome there were two cases of perinatal mortality. One was a case of intrapartum death after breech extraction at 34 weeks of gestation, where the obstetrician was unable to deliver the head (twin-to-twin time interval 29 min) and one was a second twin born at

Table 1 Baseline characteristics in women with twin deliveries after 32 completed gestational weeks and with vaginal delivery of the first twin

	Twin deliveries *N* = 527
Maternal age, years, mean (SD) median (range)	32.5 (4.8), 32.7 (17.5–51.4)
≥35 years	145 (27.5)
Nulliparous	202 (38.3)
Previous cesarean section	22 (4.2)
Body Mass Index, mean (SD) median (range)	24.2 (4.2) 23.4 (16–43) *n* = 452
Body Mass Index ≥35[a]	13/452 (2.8)
Smoking at first antenatal visit[a]	20/436 (4.6)
Chronic hypertension	2 (0.4)
Gestational hypertension	2 (0.4)
Preeclampsia	46 (8.7)
Diabetes mellitus type 1 or 2	1 (0.2)
Gestational diabetes mellitus	6 (1.1)
Dichoriotic/diamniotic twin gestations[b]	386/501 (77.0)
Monochoriotic/diamniotic twin gestations[b]	115/501 (23.0)
Pregnancies with twin-twin transfusion syndrome	2 (0.4)
Mode of delivery of the second twin	
Spontaneous cephalic	288 (54.6)
Spontaneous breech	123 (23.3)
Breech extraction	9 (1.7)
Vacuum extraction	72 (13.7)
Cesarean section	35 (6.6)

Values are n (%), unless otherwise stated
[a]There were missing values on Body Mass Index, smoking
[b]Chorionicity was unknown in 26 deliveries

33 weeks of gestation (twin-to-twin time interval eight minutes) who developed NEC at four days of age, underwent major surgery and died shortly thereafter. The remaining 12 s twins with composite primary outcomes had severe metabolic acidosis. One of these neonates, born at 38 weeks of gestation, was admitted to NICU for five days because of transient tachypnea of the newborn (TTN).The other 11 recovered within 15 min.

There were two pregnancies diagnosed with TTTS included in the study. They delivered at 35 + 5 and 37 + 0 weeks of gestation with twin-to-twin time interval of 14 min and 11 min, respectively. The twin delivered at 35 + 5 weeks of gestations was admitted to NICU for 7 days because of suspected infection and seizures, both of which could not be confirmed. No other complications occurred.

Twin-to-twin time interval had a significant impact on the composite primary outcome for the second twin

Table 2 Neonatal characteristics in the first and second twins in twin deliveries after 32 completed gestational weeks and with vaginal delivery of the first twin

	First twin N = 527	Second twin N = 527	*p*-value
Gestational age, days, mean (SD), median (range)	262 (13.7) 262 (225–286)		
≥ 37 + 0 weeks	327 (62)		
34 + 0–36 + 6 weeks	168 (31.9)		
32 + 0–33 + 6 weeks	32 (6.1)		
Fetal sex			
Female	263 (49.9)	260 (49.3)	0.90
Male	264 (50.1)	267 (50.7)	
Birthweight			
Birthweight, g, mean, (SD), median (range)	2695 (488) 2723 (1285–4350)	2673 (496) 2690 (1230–4065)	0.46
< 2500 g	187 (35.5)	193 (36.6)	0.75
< 1500 g	3 (0.6)	3 (0.6)	
SGA (< −21%)	113 (21.4)	140 (26.6)	0.06
LGA (> + 21%)	2 (0.4)	1 (0.2)	
Weight difference, %, mean (SD), median (range)	−12.1 (11.1) − 12.2 (− 54.4 – + 25.6)	− 12.8 (11.9) − 12.5 (− 56 – + 26.8)	0.31
Inter-twin birthweight discordance ≥25%	27 (5.1)		
First twin larger than second twin	16/27 (59.3)		

Values are n (%), unless otherwise stated
SGA Small for Gestational Age, *LGA* Large for Gestational Age, *SD* standard deviation

(Table 4). Median twin-to-twin time interval was 34 (8–78) min for the second twin with a composite primary outcome and 19 (2–399) min for the second twin without a composite primary outcome ($p = 0.028$). Lower mean birth weight was associated with a higher rate of primary outcome ($p = 0.028$) (Table 4).

The composite secondary outcome occurred in 17.4% (92/527) in the second twin. This was mainly due to pH < 7.10 or the need for assisted ventilation (Table 3).

Median twin-to-twin time interval, 21 (3–331) min vs. 18 (2–399) min ($p = 0.13$), had no significant impact on the composite secondary outcome for the second twin. Factors associated with secondary outcomes were lower mean birthweight ($p < 0.0001$), lower gestational age ($p < 0.0001$) and inter-twin birthweight discordance ≥25% ($p = 0.036$) (Table 4).

Composite primary and secondary outcomes are shown in relation to the stratified twin-to-twin time intervals in Fig. 1.

When twin-to-twin time intervals were divided into groups of 0 to 30 min and > 30 min, a significant difference could be seen in composite primary outcome ($p =$

Table 3 Neonatal morbidity in first and second twins in twin deliveries after 32 completed gestational weeks and with vaginal delivery of the first twin

	First twin N = 527	Second twin N = 527	*p*-value
Composite primary outcome[a]	4 (0.7)	14 (2.7)	0.029
Apgar score < 4, 5 min[b]	0	2 (0.4)	1.0
pH < 7.05 and BE< −12 or pH < 7.00[c]	4 (1.0)	12 (2.8)	0.08
Perinatal mortality < 7 days	0	2 (0.4)	0.50
Neonatal mortality < 28 days	0	0	1.0
Composite secondary outcome[a]	68 (12.9)	92 (17.4)	0.048
Apgar score < 7, 5 min	4 (0.8)	9 (1.7)	0.46
pH < 7.10	5 (1.2)	40 (9.4)	< 0.0001
Admitted to NICU	129 (24.5)	123 (23.3)	0.72
NICU, mean (SD), median, (range) days	11 (7.3) 10 (1–35)	11 (7.0) 10 (1–37)	1.0
NICU > 7 days	81 (15.4)	76 (14.4)	0.90
IRDS	1 (0.2)	5 (0.9)	0.23
TTN	8 (1.5)	10 (1.9)	0.81
IVH	0	0	1.0
Septicemia	3 (0.6)	2 (0.4)	1.0
NEC	0	1 (0.2)	1.0
Convulsions	0	0	1.0
HIE	0	0	1.0
Assisted ventilation	26 (4.9)	30 (5.7)	0.68

Values are n (%), unless otherwise stated
BE Base Excess, *NICU* Neonatal Intensive Care Unit, *IRDS* Infant Respiratory Distress Syndrome, *TTN* Transient Tachypnea of the Newborn, *IVH* Intraventricular Hemorrhage, *NEC* Necrotizing Enterocolitis, *HIE* Hypoxic Ischemic Encephalopathy
[a]as defined in Material and Methods
[b]There were missing Apgar score in first twin (n = 5) and second twin (n = 3)
[c]There was missing pH values in first twin (*n* = 121) and second twin (*n* = 101)

0.016), severe metabolic acidosis ($p = 0.002$), mean arterial ($p < 0.0001$) and mean venous umbilical cord pH ($p =$ 0.016). The outcome was more adverse when the second twin was delivered > 30 min after the first twin (Table 5). The odds ratio (OR) for a composite primary outcome for the second twin delivered > 30 min vs ≤ 30 min was 4.0 (95% CI 1.3–12.2) and 4.1 (95% CI 1.4–12.6) after adjustment for gestational age. Also, when restricting the analysis to twins with a vaginal delivery ($n = 492$) a higher rate of the composite primary outcome occurred in twins delivered > 30 min after the first twin ($p =$ 0.007), OR 5.3 (95% CI 1.6–17.9) and OR 5.6 (95% CI 1.6–18.9) after adjustment for gestational age.

Stratified into chorionicity, the composite primary outcome occurred in 0/87 monochorionic twins delivered within 0 to 30 min and in 3.6% (1/28) delivered > 30 min after the first twin ($p = 0.243$). Composite secondary outcome occurred in 16.1% (14/87) and 21.4% (6/28) monochorionic twins delivered within 0–30 min and > 30 min after the first twin, respectively ($p = 0.569$). The composite primary outcome occurred in 1.6% (4/256) and 6.2% (8/130) dichorionic twins delivered within 0–30 min and > 30 min after the first twin, respectively ($p = 0.025$). There was no significant difference in composite secondary outcome for dichorionic twins delivered within 30 min or > 30 min after the first twin.

There was no difference in composite primary or secondary outcomes according to presentation (cephalic or breech) and intertwin delivery interval.

Figure 2 shows the correlation between arterial umbilical pH and twin-to-twin interval time.

Most of the CS to deliver the second twin occurred in the group with a twin-to-twin time interval > 30 min 28/35 vs. 7/35 ≤ 30 min, $p < 0.0001$). The indications for CS to deliver the second twin were fetal distress ($n = 15$), malpresentation ($n = 9$), uterine inertia ($n = 5$), cord prolapse ($n = 3$), placental separation ($n = 1$), failed internal version ($n = 1$) and failed external version ($n = 1$). The mode of delivery for the second twin in relation to twin-to-twin time interval is shown in Fig. 3.

Discussion

This study reaffirms previous evidence that the second twin is at greater risk of metabolic acidosis and neonatal morbidity than the first twin [3, 6, 12, 18]. We were able to confirm that there is an association, but not a clear causality, with the twin-to-twin time interval [11, 12]. Only 14 of the second twins had a composite primary outcome but they had significantly longer median twin-to-twin time intervals than second twins without a composite primary outcome. Second twins with a twin-to-twin time interval of more than 30 min had higher rates of primary composite outcomes than second twins born within 30 min. No differences were seen in composite secondary outcomes that related to twin-to-twin time intervals.

Previous studies have come to varying results on the possible impact of twin-to-twin time interval on neonatal outcome for the second twin [9, 11, 13]. Most studies imply that considering the fact that umbilical cord pH decreases with longer duration of the delivery of the second twin, it is important to apply active management to keep the twin-to-twin time interval as short as possible, ideally below 30 min. Leung found that pH deteriorates faster in the second twin than in the first twin [19], and recommend a fast delivery of the second twin. In this study we found a significantly higher rate of metabolic acidosis and lower mean arterial pH in second twins born after a twin-to-twin time interval of 30 min than in second twins born within 30 min. However, there was no difference in Apgar score, the differences in pH were small and most of the second twins with

Table 4 Composite primary ($n = 14$) and secondary outcome [a] ($n = 92$) in the second twin ($n = 527$) in relation to birth characteristics

	Primary outcome $N = 14$	No primary outcome $N = 513$	Primary outcome vs no primary outcome *p*-value	Secondary outcome $N = 92$	No secondary outcome $N = 435$	Secondary outcome vs no secondary outcome *p*-value
Twin-to-twin time interval, min, mean (SD) median (range)	37 (21) 34 (8–78)	30 (36) 19 (2–399)	0.028	37 (49) 21 (3–331)	29 (31) 18 (2–399)	0.13
Gestational age, days, mean (SD) median (range)	256 (14) 257 (226–279)	262 (13.7) 263 (225–286)	0.13	252 (14.1) 249 (226–281)	264 (12.6) 265 (225–286)	< 0.0001
Birthweight, g, mean (SD) median (range)	2384 (462) 2515 (1230–2905)	2680 (495) 2690 (1240–4065)	0.028	2365 (523) 2325 (1560–4050)	2737 (466) 2750 (1230–4065)	< 0.0001
Birthweight difference[b] mean (SD) median (range)	−17.7 (14.7) − 17.4 (− 40.1–4)	− 12.7 (11.8) − 12.5 (− 56–26.8)	0.12	−14.9 (13.3) − 15.1 (− 46.8–26.8)	−12.4 (11.6) − 12.2 (− 56–20.8)	0.07
Small for gestational age (<− 21%)	6 (42.9)	134 (25.5)	0.23	29 (31.5)	111 (25.6)	0.24
Inter-twin birthweight discordance ≥25%	1 (7.1)	26 (5.1)	0.53	9 (9.8)	18 (4.1)	0.036
Monochoriotic twins	1 (7.1)	26 (5.1)	0.53	20 (21.7)	95 (21)	1.0
Assisted vaginal delivery	2 (14.2)	70 (13.7)	1.0	13 (13.5)	59 (13.7)	0.87
Spontaneous breech delivery	7 (50.0)	125 (24.4)	0.053	25 (27.2)	107 (24.7)	0.60
Breech extraction, including internal version	1 (7.1)	8 (1.6)	0.22	3 (3.3)	6 (1.4)	0.20
Cesarean section, emergency	2 (14.3)	20 (3.9)	0.11	6 (6.5)	16 (3.7)	0.25
Cesarean section, urgent[c]	0	13 (2.5)	1.0	5 (5.4) ·	8 (1.8)	0.06

Values are n (%) unless otherwise stated
[a]as defined in Methods
[b]according to Marsal et al. [16]
[c]urgent cesarean section is an emergency cesarean section performed without any delay and in general anesthesia without routine antiseptic cleaning

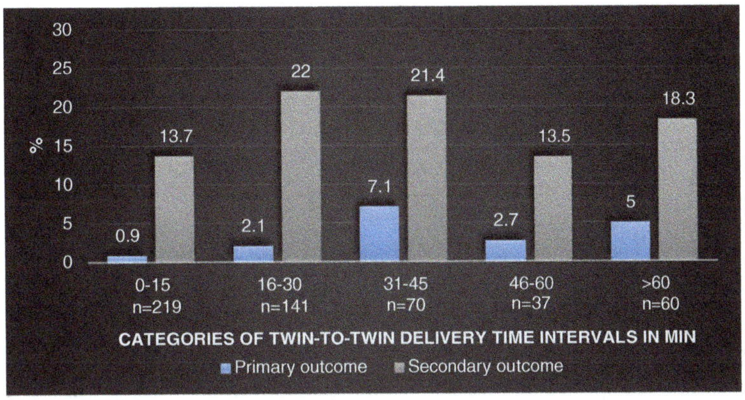

Fig. 1 Composite primary* and secondary** outcome in the second twin according to twin-to-twin delivery time interval in minutes

metabolic acidosis recovered quickly. The two cases of perinatal mortality occurred in second twins born within 30 min. Furthermore, there was no difference in neonatal morbidity, and admission to NICU was not associated with twin-to-twin time interval.

Table 5 Composite primary and secondary outcomes* and mean umbilical cord arterial and venous pH values in the second twin according to twin-to-twin time interval ≤ 30 min or > 30 min

	0–30 min *N* = 360	> 30 min *N* = 167	*p*-value
Primary composite outcome	5 (1.4)	9 (5.4)	0.016
pH < 7.05 and BE < −12 or pH < 7.00	3/290 (1)	9/136 (6.6)	0.002
Apgar score < 4 at 5 min	2/357 (0.6)	0	1.0
Perinatal mortality	2 (0.6)	0	1.0
Neonatal mortality	0	0	1.0
Secondary composite outcome	61 (16.9)	31 (18.6)	0.71
Apgar < 7 at 5 min	8 (2.2)	1 (0.6)	0.28
pH < 7.10	18/290	22/136	0.002
Admitted to NICU	88/360	35/167	0.44
NICU, mean (SD), median, (range) days	11 (7.2) 10 (1–35)	12 (7.7) 9 (2–37)	0.26
NICU > 7 days	54/88	22/35	1.0
IRDS	4/360	1/167	1.0
TTN	6/360	4/167	0.73
Septicemia	2/360	0/167	1.0
NEC	1/360	0/167	1.0
Assisted ventilation	21/360	9/167	1.0
Mean a-pH (SD)	7.23 (0.08) *N* = 290	7.20 (0.09) *N* = 136	< 0.0001
Mean v-pH (SD)	7.29 (0.08) *N* = 284	7.27 (0.09) *N* = 140	0.016

Values are n (%) unless otherwise stated
BE Base Excess, *NICU* Neonatal Intensive Care Unit, *IRDS* Infant Respiratory Distress Syndrome, *TTN* Transient Tachypnea of the Newborn, *NEC* Necrotizing Enterocolitis, *a-pH* umbilical cord arterial pH, *v-pH* umbilical cord venous pH, *BE* Base Excess, *SD* standard deviation
[a]as defined in Methods

Although the small difference in pH-levels in umbilical blood gas (7.23 vs. 7.20) for second twins delivered within or after 30 min may not have a clinical impact, other findings may justify an upper time limit on the interval between twin-to-twin deliveries. In this study there was a combined vaginal-cesarean delivery in 35 cases (6.6%), a rate consistent with other findings [20]. Cesarean delivery of the second twin is considered to be the least desirable mode of delivery and should be avoided [4, 6] due to possible complications for both mother and child. Studies have shown a worsened outcome, with increased physical and psychological maternal morbidity [18, 21] as well as higher neonatal morbidity [4, 6]. Twenty eight of these 35 combined vaginal-cesarean deliveries occurred in the twin-to-twin time interval of more than 30 min, 17 in the interval of more than 60 min. This is in agreement with previous studies that have found a six-fold increased risk of combined vaginal-cesarean delivery after 30 min and an eight-fold increased risk after 60 min [4]. Our study does not show any differences in primary and secondary neonatal outcome related to CS. However, maternal physical and psychological morbidity was not analyzed.

The fact that most combined deliveries occurred in the group where the twin-to-twin delivery time interval was more than 30 min, is in itself not surprising. If the second twin is not spontaneously delivered, the risk of assisted delivery increases over time. Previous studies have found that combined vaginal-cesarean twin delivery can be avoided with active management in the second stage of delivery of the second twin [22]. Active management is generally considered to be internal podalic version (IPV) followed by breech extraction of the non-vertex and the unengaged vertex second twin. Previous findings suggest that IPV may be more successful than external version when it comes to vaginal delivery, and with better neonatal outcome [1, 22–24]. External version has been found to be associated with complications

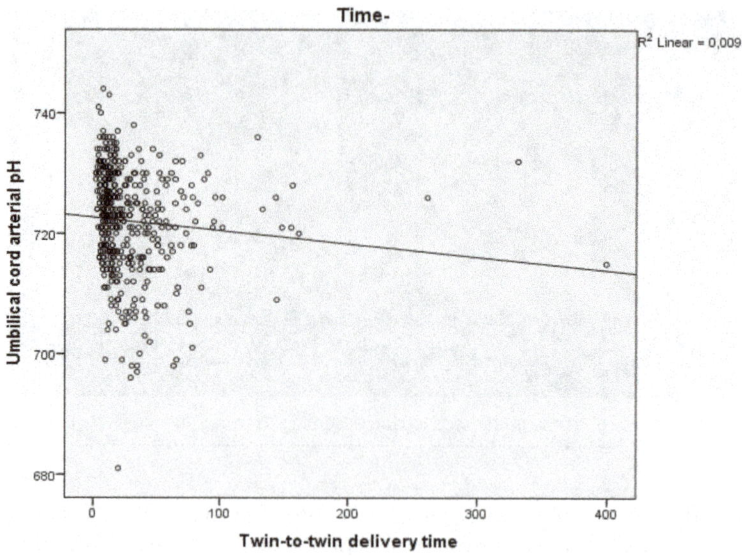

Fig. 2 Umbilical cord arterial pH in the second twin related to twin-to-twin delivery time interval in minutes

such as fetal distress, cord prolapse and compound presentations [25]. However, this maneuver was only performed in 10 cases, of which nine were successful. Active management is not praxis at our unit and unfortunately the IPV maneuver is therefore seldom taught to junior obstetricians. A decreasing rate of IPV and breech extraction, and an increased rate of CS, has also been seen in recent years in several other countries around the world [24]. In the Danish register study a better neonatal outcome was seen for the second twin after IPV and extraction than after a CS [24]. If an upper time limit is to be advocated, the management of the delivery of the second twin would need to be more active than what is recommended at our unit today. This may lead to an increase in use of oxytocin, instrumental deliveries (VE/forceps), breech extraction of a second non vertex twin and IPV and breech extraction of a second vertex non-engaged twin. Without adequate knowledge of, and training in, active management the clinical outcome of such a change in strategy is unknown.

Our unit is able to monitor both twins simultaneously and continuously. We also have 24-h in-house pediatric and anesthesia coverage and immediate availability for performing emergency CS. This may partly explain the few primary outcomes. Because of this the results of this study cannot be extrapolated to other units with other preconditions. It is important for every unit delivering twins to look at their results and from this stipulate guidelines that are in accordance with their preconditions. Factors such as the level of experience of the obstetrician in charge at the delivery, the skill of intrauterine manipulation and the wish of the women giving birth, may all influence the twin-to-twin delivery time interval. Results from the Twin Birth Study showed

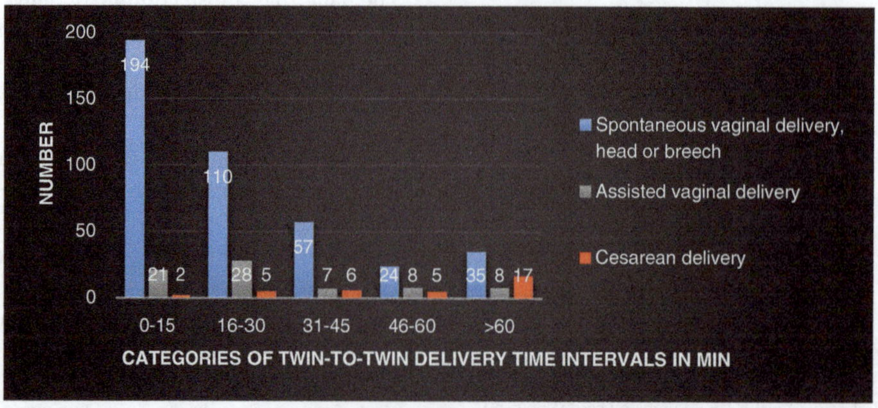

Fig. 3 Mode of delivery of the second twin according to twin-to-twin delivery time interval in minutes

that the maternal preference is for vaginal birth, therefore skills need to be maintained [26].

The limitations of the study are, as in all retrospective studies, that we have no control over available information. A rather large number of the twins had missing pH values (23% in the first twin and 19.2% in the second twin). However, analysis was made of complete data on more than 400 twins in each group. Despite a relatively large sample size there were few primary outcomes and regression analysis could not be performed for all potential confounders. The results are to be analyzed in the light of the relatively high gestational age of the sample. Twin gestations delivered before 32 + 0 weeks of gestation are complicated per see and excluding them may result in a selected sample. Including them might on the other hand result in morbidity outcomes that are not related to twin-to-twin delivery interval but prematurity in itself. There may also be other important confounders that we did not have information on. A randomized controlled trial with different twin-to-twin time intervals would be the optimal study design, but would probably be impossible to perform. Further, in this study we have not addressed the impact on maternal morbidity as postpartum hemorrhage and length of hospital stay etc.

Conclusions

An association, but not necessarily causality, between lengths of twin-to-twin time intervals and primary outcome in second twins, was found. Based on the findings of this study an upper time limit for twin-to-twin time intervals may be justified, due to the increased rate of metabolic acidosis and combined vaginal-cesarean deliveries associated with prolonged intervals between deliveries. However, the optimal twin-to-twin time interval needs further study before any recommendation can be made. Furthermore, active second stage management of the second twin needs an obstetrician with skills in the requisite maneuvers, so adequate training of the next generation of obstetricians is therefore necessary.

Abbreviations

BE: Base excess; BMI: Body mass index; CPAP: Continuous positive air pressure; CS: Cesarean section; HIE: Hypoxic ischemic encephalopathy; IPV: Internal podalic version; IRDS: Irregular respiratory distress syndrome; IVH: Intraventricular hemorrhage; LGA: Large for gestational; MRI: Magnetic resonance imaging; NEC: Necrotizing enterocolitis; NICU: Neonatal intensive care unit; OR: Odds ratio; SD: Standard deviation; SGA: Small for gestational age; SNQ: Swedish neonatal quality register; TTN: Transient tachypnea of the newborn; TTTS: Twin-twin transfusion syndrome

Acknowledgements

We thank Nils-Gunnar Pehrsson for statistical advice and Gwyneth Olofsson for language revision.

Funding

Financial support was received from the Health & Medical Care Committee of the Regional Executive Board, Region Västra Götaland (VGFOUREG) and through an agreement concerning research and the education of doctors (ALFGBG-70940). Funding bodies had no role in the design of the study and collection, analysis, interpretation of data and in writing the manuscript.

Authors' contributions

All authors (LLi, AE, LLa and UBW) have contributed to study conception, design, analysis and interpretation of data. LLa collected all data from the medical records. LLi wrote the manuscript in collaboration with AE, LLa and UBW. All authors have revised the manuscript and approved the final version of the article.

Competing interests

The authors declare that they have no competing interests.

Author details

[1]Department of Obstetrics and Gynecology, Institute of Clinical Sciences at Sahlgrenska Academy, Gothenburg University, Diagnosvägen 15, 416 85 Gothenburg, Sweden. [2]Department of Pediatrics, Institute of Clinical Sciences at Sahlgrenska Academy, Gothenburg University, Gothenburg, Sweden.

References

1. Arabin B, Kyvernitakis I. Vaginal delivery of the second nonvertex twin: avoiding a poor outcome when the presenting part is not engaged. Obstet Gynecol. 2011;118(4):950–4.
2. Barrett JF, Ritchie WK. Twin delivery. Best Pract Res Clin Obstet Gynaecol. 2002;16(1):43–56.
3. Armson BA, O'Connell C, Persad V, Joseph KS, Young DC, Baskett TF. Determinants of perinatal mortality and serious neonatal morbidity in the second twin. Obstet Gynecol. 2006;108(3 Pt 1):556–64.
4. Cruikshank DP. Intrapartum management of twin gestations. Obstet Gynecol. 2007;109(5):1167–76.
5. Kiely JL. The epidemiology of perinatal mortality in multiple births. Bull N Y Acad Med. 1990;66(6):618–37.
6. Rossi AC, Mullin PM, Chmait RH. Neonatal outcomes of twins according to birth order, presentation and mode of delivery: a systematic review and meta-analysis. BJOG. 2011;118:523–32.
7. Barrett JF, Hannah ME, Hutton EK, Willan AR, Allen AC, Armson BA, Gafni A, Joseph KS, Mason D, Ohlsson A, et al. A randomized trial of planned cesarean or vaginal delivery for twin pregnancy. N Engl J Med. 2013;369(14): 1295–305.
8. Erdemoglu E, Mungan T, Tapisiz OL, Ustunyurt E, Caglar E. Effect of inter-twin delivery time on Apgar scores of the second twin. Aust N Z J Obstet Gynaecol. 2003;43(3):203–6.
9. Stein W, Misselwitz B, Schmidt S. Twin-to-twin delivery time interval: influencing factors and effect on short-term outcome of the second twin. Acta Obstet Gynecol Scand. 2008;87(3):346–53.
10. Smith GC, Shah I, White IR, Pell JP, Dobbie R. Mode of delivery and the risk of delivery-related perinatal death among twins at term: a retrospective cohort study of 8073 births. BJOG. 2005;112(8):1139–44.
11. Leung TY, Tam WH, Leung TN, Lok IH, Lau TK. Effect of twin-to-twin delivery interval on umbilical cord blood gas in the second twins. BJOG. 2002;109(1):63–7.
12. Hjorto S, Nickelsen C, Petersen J, Secher NJ. The effect of chorionicity and twin-to-twin delivery time interval on short-term outcome of the second twin. J Matern Fetal Neonatal Med. 2014;27(1):42–7.
13. McGrail CD, Bryant DR. Intertwin time interval: how it affects the immediate neonatal outcome of the second twin. Am J Obstet Gynecol. 2005;192(5):1420–2.
14. Rayburn WF, Lavin JP Jr, Miodovnik M, Varner MW. Multiple gestation: time interval between delivery of the first and second twins. Obstet Gynecol. 1984;63(4):502–6.
15. Committee on Practice B-O, Society for Maternal-Fetal M. Practice bulletin no. 169: multifetal gestations: twin, triplet, and higher-order multifetal pregnancies. Obstet Gynecol. 2016;128(4):e131–46.
16. Marsal K, Persson PH, Larsen T, Lilja H, Selbing A, Sultan B. Intrauterine growth curves based on ultrasonically estimated foetal weights. Acta Paediatr. 1996;85(7):843–8.
17. D'Antonio F, Khalil A, Dias T, Thilaganathan B, Southwest Thames Obstetric

Research C. Weight discordance and perinatal mortality in twins: analysis of the Southwest Thames obstetric research collaborative (STORK) multiple pregnancy cohort. Ultrasound Obstet Gynecol. 2013;41(6):643–8.

18. Wolff K. Excessive use of cesarean section for the second twin? Gynecol Obstet Investig. 2000;50(1):28–32.
19. Leung TY, Lok IH, Tam WH, Leung TN, Lau TK. Deterioration in cord blood gas status during the second stage of labour is more rapid in the second twin than in the first twin. BJOG. 2004;111(6):546–9.
20. Fox NS, Silverstein M, Bender S, Klauser CK, Saltzman DH, Rebarber A. Active second-stage management in twin pregnancies undergoing planned vaginal delivery in a U.S. population. Obstet Gynecol. 2010;115(2 Pt 1):229–33.
21. Rabinovici J, Barkai G, Reichman B, Serr DM, Mashiach S. Randomized management of the second nonvertex twin: vaginal delivery or cesarean section. Am J Obstet Gynecol. 1987;156(1):52–6.
22. Schmitz T, Carnavalet Cde C, Azria E, Lopez E, Cabrol D, Goffinet F. Neonatal outcomes of twin pregnancy according to the planned mode of delivery. Obstet Gynecol. 2008;111(3):695–703.
23. Chauhan SP, Roberts WE, McLaren RA, Roach H, Morrison JC, Martin JN Jr. Delivery of the nonvertex second twin: breech extraction versus external cephalic version. Am J Obstet Gynecol. 1995;173(4):1015–20.
24. Jonsdottir F, Henriksen L, Secher NJ, Maaloe N. Does internal podalic version of the non-vertex second twin still have a place in obstetrics? A Danish national retrospective cohort study. Acta Obstet Gynecol Scand. 2015;94(1):59–64.
25. Gocke SE, Nageotte MP, Garite T, Towers CV, Dorcester W. Management of the nonvertex second twin: primary cesarean section, external version, or primary breech extraction. Am J Obstet Gynecol. 1989;161(1):111–4.
26. Murray-Davis B, McVittie J, Barrett JF, Hutton EK, Twin Birth Study Collaborative G. Exploring Women's preferences for the mode of delivery in twin gestations: results of the twin birth study. Birth. 2016;43(4):285–92.

2

Companionship during facility-based childbirth: results from a mixed-methods study with recently delivered women and providers in Kenya

Patience Afulani[1,2*], Caroline Kusi[2], Leah Kirumbi[3] and Dilys Walker[1,2]

Abstract

Background: Research suggests that birth companionship, and in particular, continuous support during labor and delivery, can improve women's childbirth experience and birth outcomes. Yet, little is known about the extent to which birth companionship is practiced, as well as women and providers' perceptions of it in low-resource settings. This study aimed to assess the prevalence and determinants of birth companionship, and women and providers' perceptions of it in health facilities in a rural County in Western Kenya.

Methods: We used quantitative and qualitative data from 3 sources: surveys with 877 women, 8 focus group discussions with 58 women, and in-depth interviews with 49 maternity providers in the County. Eligible women were 15 to 49 years old and delivered in the 9 weeks preceding the study.

Results: About 88% of women were accompanied by someone from their social network to the health facility during their childbirth, with 29% accompanied by a male partner. Sixty-seven percent were allowed continuous support during labor, but only 29% were allowed continuous support during delivery. Eighteen percent did not desire companionship during labor and 63% did not desire it during delivery. Literate, wealthy, and employed women, as well as women who delivered in health centers and did not experience birth complications, were more likely to be allowed continuous support during labor. Most women desired a companion during labor to attend to their needs. Reasons for not desiring companions included embarrassment and fear of gossip and abuse. Most providers recommended birth companionship, but stated that it is often not possible due to privacy concerns and other reasons mainly related to distrust of companions. Providers perceive companions' roles more in terms of assisting them with non-clinical tasks than providing emotional support to women.

Conclusion: Although many women desire birth companionship, their desires differ across the labor and delivery continuum, with most desiring companionship during labor but not at the time of delivery. Most, however, don't get continuous support during labor and delivery. Interventions with women, companions, and providers, as well as structural and health system interventions, are needed to promote continuous support during labor and delivery.

Keywords: Continuous support during labor and delivery, Birth companionship, Woman-centered care, Respectful maternity care, Kenya

* Correspondence: patience.afulani@ucsf.edu
[1]Obstetrics, Gynecology and Reproductive Sciences, UCSF, San Francisco, USA
[2]Institute for Global Health Sciences, UCSF, San Francisco, USA

Background

Over the past decade, the promotion of facility based delivery has been at the forefront of international efforts to reduce maternal mortality. Between 2003 and 2013, the percentage of women who delivered in health facilities increased in every region of the world [1]. However, retention, equity, dignity, and quality of care along the continuum of maternal health care remain a challenge [2–4]. Women's experiences during childbirth are a powerful determinant of use of maternal healthcare services [5]. The World Health Organization (WHO) Quality of Care Framework for maternal and newborn health outlines access to emotional and social support of women's choice as core to the experience of care and to achieving positive person-centered health outcomes [6]. Thus, WHO recommends that every woman is offered the option to experience labor and childbirth with a companion of her choice [7].

Different terms have been used for this recommendation, including companion of choice at birth, labor companion, birth companion, emotional support during birth, social support during labor and delivery, supportive companionship, and continuous support for women during childbirth [8–13]. But the evidence supporting the recommendation emphasizes continuous support during childbirth [9, 10]. The definition of continuous support during childbirth differs across studies and settings and can start at any time between conception to postpartum period. Generally, however, it involves the continuous presence of a companion during labor and delivery [9, 10]. In this paper, we use the terms birth companionship to refer to the provision of any type of support by a lay companion at any time during the intrapartum period, and continuous support during labor and delivery (CSLD) to refer to the continuous presence of the companion during labor and delivery. CSLD is thus a subset of birth companionship since not all birth companionship is continuous.

Common elements of support provided by birth companions include, emotional support (e.g. continuous presence and giving reassurance and praise), informational support (e.g. giving information about labor progress and advice regarding coping techniques), comfort measures (e.g. comforting touch, massage, warm baths/showers, encouraging mobility, and promoting adequate fluid intake and output), advocacy (e.g. helping women articulate their wishes to providers), and instrumental support (providing assistance with needs) [9, 10, 14]. Support can be provided by different types of companions, including trained support persons such as doulas (non-health care professionals trained to provide emotional and physical support to women before, during and after childbirth) or by companions chosen from a woman's social network [9, 15].

Birth companionship is associated with increased satisfaction with healthcare services [9, 16]. Some studies also suggest that women who have birth companions are less likely to experience mistreatment during childbirth [17, 18]. In addition, CSLD has been shown to impact pregnancy outcomes. A recent Cochrane review of CSLD found that women who received continuous labor support were more likely to have shorter labor and spontaneous vaginal deliveries (i.e. give birth vaginally without the use of instruments or to have a cesarean section). In addition, they were less likely to use pain medication while giving birth and their babies were less likely to have low five-minute Apgar scores [9]. The effect of CSLD differed, however, depending on the type of companion and the setting. They found that CSLD was most effective at reducing caesarean birth when the companion was present in a doula role, as well as in settings where epidural analgesia was not routinely available. The effect of CSLD on birth outcomes was also stronger in settings where women were not permitted to have companions during labor. The authors concluded that continuous support from a person who solely provides support, is not a member of the woman's own network, is experienced in providing labor support, and has a modest amount of training (such as a doula), appears to have the greatest impact on outcomes. Nonetheless, compared to having no companion, support from a chosen family member or friend appeared to increase women's satisfaction with their childbirth experience [9]. The authors noted that none of the studies included in their review were from low-income settings and, therefore, recommended that future studies explore how continuous support can be best provided in different contexts, particularly in low-income settings.

Birth companionship is increasingly being included in the maternal health guidelines of many countries, including in low- and middle-income countries in Sub-Saharan Africa (SSA). For example, the National Guidelines for Quality Obstetrics and Perinatal Care in Kenya recommends that during the first stage of labor, providers should encourage women to have their chosen companions with them and make arrangements to accommodate birth companions or male partners; and in the second stage of labor providers should "allow and encourage her birth companion/male partner to be present" [19]. Yet little is known about the extent to which this is actually practiced in Kenya, as well as in most of SSA. The research is equally limited on women's perceptions and preferences for birth companions, and on providers' perceptions of birth companions in these settings [11–13, 20, 21]. No study to our knowledge has comprehensively examined birth companionship in Kenya. Little is therefore known about the prevalence of birth companionship including CSLD, the types of companions used, women's preferences for companionship, and the factors associated with these in Kenya. In contexts where women have little autonomy and their health seeking behavior is strongly influenced by sociocultural norms; and providers have greater autonomy, but operate with very limited resources, it is important to understand women's preferences for companionship and providers perceptions about providing it, to guide efforts towards promoting birth companionship. The current study aims to fill this gap in evidence.

Furthermore, while most of the works on birth companionship have examined it as a single unit, we chose to make some distinctions based on our field experiences. The first distinction is between having a companion present and having continuous support. This is motivated by the fact that, while a woman might have a companion present, the support provided may not be continuous for various reasons. The second distinction is between labor support, delivery support, and post-delivery support. This distinction is to enable us to understand if women's preferences for support differ at these different stages of the childbirth process. In addition, these distinctions are important because, when support is not continuous and is only provided at certain time points (like during labor but not delivery), the potential benefits may differ from those stated in CSLD literature. Our objectives, therefore, were to: (1) Assess the prevalence of birth companionship and CSLD in health facilities in a rural county in western Kenya; (2) Assess women's desire for birth companionship; (3) Identify types of birth companions that women prefer; and (4) Examine factors associated with receiving CSLD, desire for companionship, and preference for male companions. In addition, we use qualitative data to examine: (1) women's perceptions of birth companionship and their preferred companions; and (2) providers' perceptions of birth companionship and barriers to ensuring CSLD for women.

Methods

We employed mixed methods for this study. Mixed methods combine elements of qualitative and quantitative approaches to provide breadth and depth in our understanding of phenomenon [22]. Quantitative methods allow objective measurement of a particular reality, with a large enough sample to increase generalizability [23]. Quantitative methods are however limited in explaining the "why" of phenomena and how personal viewpoints, context and meaning produce multiple realities [23]. Qualitative methods help to address this weakness, but have limited generalizability because of practical limitations of sample size. Mixed methods were therefore appropriate to harness the strengths and counterbalance the weaknesses of quantitative and qualitative methods to provide a holistic understanding of birth companionship [23]. The quantitative methods provide data for measuring prevalence and examining statistical associations and the qualitative data help to explain the quantitative findings and provide rich descriptions of views and beliefs about birth companionship. In addition, we collected data from recently delivered women and maternity providers to obtain the complementary perspectives of both the recipients and providers of care.

Setting

Data for this study were part of a larger study examining community perceptions of quality of maternity care in a rural county in western Kenya. The County has a population of about one million and an estimated 40,000 annual births [24]. Approximately 43% of the population live below the poverty line and only about 3% of women of reproductive age have more than a secondary education. About 24% of women of childbearing age are 15–19 years [25]. The total fertility rate of the county is 5.3 compared to the national average of 3.9. The County is one of 15 counties in Kenya that account for over 60% of maternal deaths in the country—with an estimated maternal mortality ratio of 673 deaths per 100,000 live births compared to the national average of 495 [26]. The number of nurses, clinical officers, and doctors, per 100,000 people in the county is 32, 19, and 4 respectively [27].

About 53% of births in the County occur in health facilities, compared to the national average of 61% [25]. Several factors account for low use of facility deliveries, including low perceived need of facility deliveries, poor physical and financial access to health services, and low perceived quality of care [28–30]. Additionally, sociocultural factors such as norms and values related to childbirth (e.g. beliefs about the causes of pregnancy complications) and women's autonomy (e.g. women not being final decision makers on place of birth) interact with socioeconomic factors such as wealth and education to determine whether or not women seek health care during pregnancy or delivery [5, 31–33]. Thus, the low status of most childbearing women in the County (young, uneducated, poor, and unemployed) is likely a key determinant of the low use of services in the County. These factors also affect how women are treated in the health facility, which affects future health seeking behavior. Given evidence that birth companionship improves women's birth experiences [5, 9, 17], understanding and respecting women's desires and preferences for birth companions could positively impact health seeking behavior during childbirth in the County.

Data sources

We used 3 data sources: surveys and focus group discussions with recently delivered women and in-depth interviews with providers. Eligible women were 15–49 years and delivered in the 9 weeks preceding the study. Eligible providers worked in a maternity unit in the county. Ethical approval for the study was provided by the authors' institutions. All participants provided written informed consent after receiving information about the study and received 200 KES (~$2) for their participation.

Surveys with women

Survey data were collected between August and September 2016 with eligible women. A multistage sampling approach was used to select women. First, the County was divided into eight strata based on its 8 sub-counties. Next, ten health units were randomly selected from each strata. Eligible women were then identified and recruited from the selected health units. The sampling procedures are documented elsewhere [34]. Twelve data collectors were trained to conduct the interviews—in English, Swahili, and Luo in private spaces in health facilities or in respondents' homes. Data were collected using the REDCap electronic data capture tools hosted at the University of California-San Francisco [35]. Approximately one thousand women were interviewed, with a response rate above 98%. We use data from women who delivered in a health facility (894) and had no missing data on relevant variables for this analysis ($N = 857–877$ for different outcomes).

Focus group discussions (FGDs) with women

Between October and November 2016, we conducted eight FGDs—one in each sub-county—with 58 eligible mothers. We chose a focus group design to obtain qualitative data from women because our field experience in the region suggested women were more willing to discuss their experiences in groups with their peers than with an individual interviewer not familiar to them. The FGD procedures are documented elsewhere [36]. We recruited respondents from one randomly selected health unit in each sub-county that was not included in the survey. Women who met the eligibility criteria were purposively selected from the selected health unit. Each focus group consisted of six to ten women and lasted about 90 min. Two female research assistants with college degrees were trained by the first author to moderate each group discussion; one led the discussion using a discussion guide, and the other took notes and managed audio recording. Women were asked, among other things, if they were allowed to have a companion present during labor and delivery and how they felt when they were allowed or disallowed a companion. They were also asked if they desired birth companionship and why they desired or did not desire it. The discussions were conducted in Swahili or Luo, in private spaces in the community or health facility. Discussions were audio recorded, and simultaneously translated and transcribed.

In-depth interviews with providers

We conducted 49 interviews with maternity providers from 18 facilities across all the 8 sub-counties, which were selected for an intrapartum quality improvement project based on their relatively higher volume of deliveries. With permission from the county and facility heads to conduct the study, the research assistants approached maternity providers in selected facilities, briefed them about the study, and invited them to participate in the interviews. The interviewers used an interview guide with both closed and open-ended questions. Providers were asked, among other things, if women were allowed CSLD, their perceptions of CSLD, and barriers to providing it in their facilities. Interviews were conducted in English, Swahili or Luo—in private spaces in each health facility—and lasted about an hour. The structured responses were directly entered into the REDCap application during the interview. Interviews were also audio-recorded and transcribed (with simultaneous translation where necessary).

Measures for quantitative analysis

Dependent (outcome) variables

Our dependent variables are from several survey questions on birth companionship during: (1) labor, (2) delivery, and (3) post-delivery. These include questions on whether they were accompanied by a companion to the facility, their relationship to the companion, whether they were allowed continuous support during labor and during delivery, whether they desired companionship during labor, delivery, and after delivery, and their preferred type of companion. The variables are described in Table 1 with exact wording of questions in Additional file 1.

Independent variables

These include various socio-demographic, facility, and provider related factors that might be associated with the dependent variables. These were selected based on existing literature and theoretical reasoning. They include age, marital status, parity, education, literacy, employment, household wealth, tribe, religion, prior facility delivery, antenatal attendance, pregnancy complications, labor and delivery complications, type of delivery facility, type and sex of delivery providers, and women's perceptions of crowding in the facility. In multivariate analysis, we controlled for potential reporting bias by place of interview and post-partum length.

Data analysis

Quantitative analysis

First, we conducted descriptive analysis to examine the characteristics of the sample and to assess the prevalence of birth companionship and CSLD, as well the

Table 1 Description of Birth Companionship variables

Variable	Description
Availability of a companion	Whether or not someone accompanied the woman from home to the health facility. In addition, we asked if this person stayed with them during labor, delivery, and/or after delivery.
Type of companion	Relationship to the person who accompanied them to the facility. Women were allowed to mention more than one person, and thus, the preferred companion analysis is based on whether or not a particular type of person was mentioned.
Allowed continuous support during labor	Whether or not they were allowed to have someone they wanted to stay with them during labor. A response of "yes, most of the time," or "yes, all the time" is coded as being allowed continuous labor support, and "no, never" or "yes, a few times" is coded as not being allowed continuous labor support.
Allowed continuous support during delivery	Whether they were allowed to have someone they wanted to stay with them during delivery. Recoded similarly to "allowed continuous support during labor"
Desire for companionship during labor, delivery, and after delivery	Whether or not they wanted the person who accompanied them to stay with them during labor, delivery, and/or after delivery; and if they will want a companion at each stage if they were to have another baby in the future
Preferred type of companion	The type of person they would want as a companion during labor, delivery, and/or after delivery if they were to have another baby. They could mention more than one person, so responses refer to whether or not they mentioned a particular type of person

proportion of women who desired companionship and their preferred companions. Next, we used cross tabulations and bivariate logistic regressions to examine the bivariate associations between the dependent and independent variables. We also examined whether the type of companion was associated with being allowed CSLD and women's desire for companionship. Finally, we used multivariate logistic regression to examine the factors associated with being allowed CSLD, net of other factors.

Qualitative analysis

Using the Braun & Clarke approach (2006), we analyzed the qualitative data thematically to identify patterns within data [37]. We coded data inductively, considering both the semantic (surface) and latent (underlying) meaning of the text, focusing on salience rather than frequency. We iteratively read and re-read the transcripts and coded line-by-line across the entire data set. Two coders (the first and second authors) double coded half of the transcripts and compared codes to check consistency. We then analyzed initial codes to generate categories and identify themes [37]. We again reviewed transcripts until no new themes emerged. See Additional file 2 for how open codes were used to generate categories and themes. This was however an iterative process with constant reviews and revisions. Throughout the process, we wrote analytic and reflexive memos to capture emerging ideas and examine our assumptions, preconceptions, and reactions to the data. For example, we started the study with the preconception that all women will be unhappy about being denied companions. We were thus surprised by some women's reactions to not being allowed companions and the many reasons they gave for not desiring companions. We therefore wrote a memo on this early on to ensure we adequately captured women's perceptions. We managed data using Atlas.ti. (COREQ checklist in Additional file 3).

Results

Results from interviews with women

Univariate distributions

Table 2 shows demographic characteristics of both survey and focus group respondents. Focus group participants were older and more likely to be married, had higher parity, and lower education compared to survey participants. About two-thirds of respondents in both samples belonged to the dominant tribe of the County—the Luo tribe.

The distribution of the birth companionship variables is shown in Table 3. Among survey respondents, 88% were accompanied by someone to the health facility. About a third of respondents were accompanied by a partner (29%) or mother-in-law (28%). Seventy-eight percent, 26, and 88% reported the person who accompanied them (subsequently referred to as the companion) stayed with them for some period during labor, delivery, and after delivery respectively. However, only 67 and 29% of the respondents were allowed continuous support during labor and delivery respectively. Besides, 18, 63, and 6% did not want their companion to stay with them during labor, delivery, and after delivery respectively. Also, 33, 69, and 10% reported that if they were to have another baby, they would not want a companion during labor, delivery, and after delivery respectively. For preferred companion in the future, 22% wanted their partner during labor and 43% wanted him after delivery, but only 6% wanted him during the delivery.

Bivariate results

The bivariate associations between the independent and dependent variables are shown in Tables 4, 5, and 6. We

Table 2 Demographic characteristics of Study Participants, PQCC Study 2016

	Survey respondents		FGD respondents	
	No.	%	No.	%
Total N	877	100.0	58	100
Age				
15 to 19 years	162	18.5	4	6.9
20 to 29 years	511	58.3	38	65.5
30 to 48 years	204	23.3	16	27.6
Marital status				
Single	140	16.0	5	8.6
Partnered/Cohabiting	3	0.3	1	1.7
Married	687	78.3	51	87.9
Widowed	35	4.0	1	1.7
Divorced/Separated	12	1.4		
Number of births				
1.0	290	33.1	6	10.3
2.0	185	21.1	8	13.8
3.0	163	18.6	11	19
4 or more	239	27.3	33	56.9
Education				
No school/Primary	495	56.4	46	79.3
Post-primary/Vocational/ Secondary	271	30.9	10	17.2
College or above	111	12.7	2	3.4
Literacy: writing				
No, cannot write	31	3.5	1	1.7
Yes, but with some difficulty	141	16.1	38	65.5
Yes, Very well	705	80.4	19	32.8
Literacy: reading				
No, cannot read	37	4.2	4	6.9
Yes, but with some difficulty	129	14.7	34	58.6
Yes, Very well	711	81.1	20	34.5
Employed				
No	658	75.0	39	67.2
Yes	219	25.0	19	32.8
Wealth Quintile				
Poorest	190	21.7		
Poorer	190	21.7		
Middle	135	15.4		
Richer	172	19.6		
Richest	190	21.7		
Delivery facility type				
Gov't Hospital	404	46.1	27	49.1
Gov't Health Center	362	41.3	23	41.8
Mission/Private facility	111	12.7	5	9.1
Delivery provider				
Nurse/Midwife	656	74.8		
Doctor	83	9.5		
Clinical Officer	54	6.2		
Non-skilled attendant	21	2.4		
1plus skilled providers	63	7.2		
Delivery Provider sex				
Male	329	37.5		
Female	514	58.6		
Both	34	3.9		
Labor/Delivery complications				
No	721	82.21		
Yes	156	17.79		
Past facility delivery				
No	342	39.0	11	19
Yes	535	61.0	47	81
Trimester of first ANC				
First trimester	261	29.8		
Second trimester	536	61.3		
Third Trimester	72	8.2		
No ANC	6	0.7		
Number of ANC visits				
No ANC	6	0.7		
Less than 4	281	32.2		
4 or 5	485	55.6		
6 plus	100	11.5		
Tribe				
Luo	584	66.6	38	65.5
Kuria	208	23.7	12	20.7
Other	85	9.7	8	13.8
Religion				
Catholic	242	27.6	12	20.7
Protestant/Pentecostal	191	21.8	22	37.9
Seventh Day Adventist	263	30.0	14	24.1
Other Christian	166	18.9	7	12.1
Muslim/other religion	15	1.7	3	5.2
Postpartum length				
Less than 1 week	75	8.6	1	1.7
1 week or more	802	91.4	57	98.3
Place of Interview				
Health facility	356	40.6	10	17.2
In the community/a home	521	59.4	48	82.8

Blanks were not asked of FGD respondents; PQCC is Perceived Quality of Care during Childbirth

Table 3 Distribution of Birth Companionship variables, PQCC Study 2016

Birth Companionship Variables	No.	%	No.	%	No.	%
Accompanied from home to facility						
No	106	12.4				
Yes	751	87.6				
Accompanied by						
Partner-Husband	251	29.3				
Mother-in-law	236	27.5				
Mother	100	11.7				
Sister/Sister-in-law	164	19.1				
Friend/Neighbor	112	13.1				
Other [a]	74	8.7				
Companion stayed during	Labor		Delivery		Post-delivery	
No	157	20.9	556	74	86	11.5
Yes	588	78.3	192	25.6	661	88
Don't know	6	0.8	3	0.4	4	0.5
Companion allowed during	Labor		Delivery			
No, never	162	18.9	524	61.1		
Yes, a few times	103	12	72	8.4		
Yes, most of the time	230	26.8	110	12.8		
Yes, all the time	357	41.7	138	16.1		
Wanted Companion to stay during	Labor		Delivery		Post-delivery	
No	138	18.4	476	63.4	48	6.4
Yes	608	81	267	35.6	701	93.3
Don't know	5	0.7	8	1.1	2	0.3
Will want companion in future during	Labor		Delivery		Post-delivery	
No	285	33.3	592	69.1	85	9.9
Yes	560	65.3	254	29.6	761	88.8
Don't know	12	1.4	11	1.3	11	1.3
Preferred companion type in future during	Labor		Delivery		Post-delivery	
Partner-Husband	188	21.9	49	5.7	370	43.2
Mother in Law	234	27.3	119	13.9	362	42.2
Mother	91	10.6	42	4.9	138	16.1
Sister/Sister in law	165	19.3	63	7.4	244	28.5
Friend/Neighbor	77	9	31	3.6	159	18.6
Community Health Volunteer	4	0.5	4	0.5	8	0.9
Nurse/Midwife	35	4.1	21	2.5	49	5.7
Doctor	10	1.2	10	1.2	14	1.6
Other	23	2.7	8	0.9	26	3
Acceptability of being denied a companion						
Unacceptable in all instances	722	84.2				
Acceptable in certain instances	112	13.1				
Acceptable in all instances	23	2.7				
Total	857	100	857	100	857	100

[a]Other includes co-wives, grand-mother, community health volunteers, etc.

Table 4 Bivariate distribution of selected birth companionship variables by demographic and facility characteristics, PQCC Study 2016

	Accompanied to facility		Allowed continuous support during			
			Labor		Delivery	
	No.	%	No.	%	No.	%
Age						
15 to 19 years	156	96.3**	118	72.8	58	35.8
20 to 29 years	442	86.5	352	69.2	153	29.9
30 to 48 years	172	84.3	130	63.7	56	27.5
Marital Status						
Not married	172	90.5	137	72.1	69	36.3*
Currently married	598	87	463	67.6	198	28.8
Number of births						
1.0	274	94.5***	216	74.5**	102	35.2
2.0	163	88.1	134	73.2	51	27.6
3.0	137	84	103	63.2	53	32.5
4 or more	196	82	147	61.5	61	25.5
Education						
No school/Primary	425	85.9	323	65.4*	132	26.7*
Post-primary/vocational/Secondary	246	90.8	189	70	99	36.5
College or above	99	89.2	88	79.3	36	32.4
Literacy						
No, cannot write	28	90.3	13	41.9***	7	22.6***
Yes, but with some difficulty	122	86.5	84	59.6	20	14.2
Yes, Very well	620	87.9	503	71.6	240	34
Household wealth						
Poorest/poorer	332	87.4	236	62.3**	105	27.6*
Middle	122	90.4	93	68.9	37	27.4
Richer/richest	316	87.3	271	75.1	125	34.5
Employed						
No	576	87.5	427	65.1***	198	30.1
Yes	194	88.6	173	79	69	31.5
Pregnancy complication						
No	431	87.2	349	70.8	168	34**
Yes	339	88.5	251	65.7	99	25.8
Birth Complication						
No	633	87.8	515	71.6***	242	33.6***
Yes	137	87.8	85	54.5	25	16
Past health facility delivery						
No	315	92.1**	242	70.8	117	34.2
Yes	455	85	358	67.2	150	28
ANC visits						
Less than 4	240	83.6**	200	69.7	92	32.1
4 plus	526	89.9	396	67.8	173	29.6
Tribe						
Luo	496	84.9***	426	73.1***	189	32.4

Table 4 Bivariate distribution of selected birth companionship variables by demographic and facility characteristics, PQCC Study 2016 *(Continued)*

	Accompanied to facility		Allowed continuous support during			
			Labor		Delivery	
	No.	%	No.	%	No.	%
Kuria	200	96.2	117	56.5	53	25.5
Other	74	87.1	57	67.1	25	29.4
Religion						
Catholic	215	88.8	175	72.6	68	28.1
Protestant/Pentecostal	165	86.4	122	63.9	53	27.7
Seventh Day Adventist	236	89.7	182	69.5	94	35.7
Other Christian	142	85.5	112	67.5	46	27.7
Muslim/other religion	12	80	9	60	6	40
Delivery facility type						
Gov't Hospital	369	91.3**	257	63.9**	115	28.5
Gov't Health Center	303	83.7	273	75.4	114	31.5
Mission/Private facility	98	88.3	70	63.1	38	34.2
Delivery provider						
Nurse/Midwife	578	88.1	462	70.6**	209	31.9
Doctor/Clinical Officer	119	86.9	89	65	40	29.2
Non-skilled attendant	17	81	17	81	8	38.1
1plus skilled providers	56	88.9	32	50.8	10	15.9
Delivery Provider sex						
Male	294	89.4	206	62.6*	82	24.9*
Female	445	86.6	370	72.3	173	33.7
Both	31	91.2	24	70.6	12	35.3
Accompanied by						
Partner						
No			434	69.7	208	33.3**
Yes			166	65.9	59	23.3
Mother-in-law						
No			442	70	186	29.4
Yes			158	64.8	81	33.1
Mother						
No			525	67.9	231	29.8
Yes			75	73.5	36	35.3
Sister/Sister in law						
No			465	65.7***	223	31.4
Yes			135	80.8	44	26.3
Friend/Neighbor						
No			519	68.2	238	31.2
Yes			81	71.1	29	25.4
Facility crowded						
No or a few times			425	72.2**	172	29.1
Most or all the time			173	60.9	94	33.1

Table 4 Bivariate distribution of selected birth companionship variables by demographic and facility characteristics, PQCC Study 2016 *(Continued)*

	Accompanied to facility		Allowed continuous support during			
			Labor		Delivery	
	No.	%	No.	%	No.	%
Desired labor companion						
No			68	47.9***		
Yes			459	73.9		
Don't know			3	60		
Desired delivery companion						
No					92	18.8***
Yes					135	49.6
Don't know					4	50
Total	770	87.8	600	68.6	267	30.4

* $p < 0.05$ ** $p < 0.01$ *** $p < 0.001$

find that younger and primiparous women who had no past facility delivery, as well as women from the Kuria tribe, women with four or more antenatal visits, and women who delivered in higher level facilities were more likely (than their reference groups) to be accompanied to the health facility (Table 4).

Continuous labor and delivery support Younger, wealthier, employed, college educated, and literate women were more likely to be allowed continuous labor support. On the other hand, women who were of the Kuria tribe, had birth complications, reported the facility was over crowded most of the time, delivered in hospitals, and those who did not want their companion to stay with them, were less likely to be allowed continuous labor support. Many of the factors associated with continuous delivery support in bivariate analysis are similar to those for continuous labor support (Table 4).

Desire for labor and delivery support Employed women and women accompanied by a sister or sister-in-law were more likely to desire companionship during labor. In addition, younger, unmarried, primiparous, literate, and wealthier women, as well as those accompanied by a mother or a non-relative were more likely to desire companionship at the time of delivery. Women who were accompanied by a partner were less likely to desire companionship during labor and delivery. Also, women who perceived the health facility to be over crowded most of the time were less likely to desire labor companionship. Women who were allowed CSLD at their last birth were more likely to desire it in the future (Table 5).

Preferred companion Wealthier and more educated women were more likely to be accompanied by their partners and to desire labor companionship from their partners in the future. They were also less likely to be accompanied by their mothers-in-law and to desire companionship from their mothers-in-law in the future. Kuria women were more likely to be accompanied by their mothers-in-law and to desire companionship from their mothers-in-law during labor in the future (Table 6).

Multivariate results

Table 7 shows multivariate logistic regressions of continuous labor and delivery support on various predictors. The multivariate results for desire for companionship and preference for male partners are shown in Additional file 4.

Continuous labor support Wealthier, employed, and literate women had close to two times higher odds of being allowed continuous labor support than the poorest, unemployed, and illiterate women respectively; and Kuria women had about 40% lower odds of being allowed continuous labor support than Luo women. Also, those who delivered in a health center and were accompanied by a sister or sister-in-law had close to two times higher odds of being allowed continuous labor support than those who delivered in hospitals and those not accompanied by a sister or sister-in-law respectively. Women who desired a labor companion had about 40% higher odds of being allowed continuous labor support than those who did not desire one. Additionally, women who reported the facility was over crowded most or all the time had about 35% lower odds of being allowed continuous labor support than those who said it was not crowded or crowded only a few times.

Continuous delivery support Women had lower odds of being allowed continuous delivery support if they had a birth complication and if there were two or more skilled providers present at the delivery than if they had

Table 5 Bivariate distribution of selected birth companionship variables by demographic and facility characteristics, PQCC study 2016

	Desire for labor support				Desire for delivery support			
	Last birth		Future birth		Last birth		Future birth	
	No.	%	No.	%	No.	%	No.	%
Age								
15 to 19 years	128	82.1	108	66.7*	73	46.8*	58	35.8
20 to 29 years	352	79.6	327	64	144	32.6	137	26.9
30 to 48 years	142	82.6	139	68.1	55	32	62	30.4
Marital Status								
Not married	149	86.6	125	65.8**	81	47.1**	65	34.2*
Currently married	473	79.1	449	65.4	191	31.9	192	28
Number of births								
1.0	233	85	190	65.5	122	44.5**	108	37.2*
2.0	134	82.2	132	71.4	55	33.7	51	27.7
3.0	105	76.6	103	63.2	38	27.7	37	22.7
4 or more	150	76.5	149	62.3	57	29.1	61	25.5
Education								
No school/Primary	336	79.1	321	64.8	137	32.2	141	28.5
Post-primary/Vocational/Secondary	202	82.1	182	67.2	99	40.2	78	28.8
College or above	84	84.8	71	64	36	36.4	38	34.2
Literacy								
No, cannot write	22	78.6	22	71	9	32.1*	6	19.4
Yes, but with some difficulty	94	77	98	69.5	28	23	38	27
Yes, Very well	506	81.6	454	64.4	235	37.9	213	30.3
Household wealth								
Poorest/poorer	260	78.3	251	66.1	103	31**	104	27.4
Middle	98	80.3	86	63.7	39	32	33	24.4
Richer/richest	264	83.5	237	65.5	130	41.1	120	33.1
Employed								
No	452	78.5*	402	61.1***	200	34.7	184	28
Yes	170	87.6	172	78.5	72	37.1	73	33.3
Pregnancy complication								
No	346	80.3	309	62.6*	149	34.6	144	29.1
Yes	276	81.4	265	69.2	123	36.3	113	29.6
Birth Complication								
No	517	81.7	468	64.9	224	35.4	210	29.2
Yes	105	76.6	106	67.9	48	35	47	30.1
Past health facility delivery								
No	265	84.1	225	65.8	140	44.4***	122	35.7**
Yes	357	78.5	349	65.2	132	29	135	25.3
ANC visits								
Less than 4	196	81.7	190	66.2	86	35.8	91	31.8
4 plus	423	80.4	380	65	183	34.8	163	27.9
Tribe								
Luo	407	82.1	370	63.4	167	33.7	143	24.5***

Table 5 Bivariate distribution of selected birth companionship variables by demographic and facility characteristics, PQCC study 2016 *(Continued)*

	Desire for labor support				Desire for delivery support			
	Last birth		Future birth		Last birth		Future birth	
	No.	%	No.	%	No.	%	No.	%
Kuria	160	80	146	70.2	71	35.5	79	38
Other	55	74.3	58	68.2	34	45.9	35	41.2
Religion								
Catholic	180	83.7	155	64	73	34	72	29.8**
Protestant/Pentecostal	129	78.2	125	65.4	72	43.6	77	40.5
Seventh Day Adventist	196	83.1	184	70	79	33.5	73	27.8
Other Christian	108	76.1	102	61.4	44	31	33	19.9
Muslim/other religion	9	75	8	53.3	4	33.3	2	13.3
Delivery facility type								
Gov't Hospital	294	79.7	256	63.4	133	36	130	32.3
Gov't Health Center	251	82.8	248	68.5	100	33	89	24.6
Mission/Private facility	77	78.6	70	63.1	39	39.8	38	34.2
Delivery provider								
Nurse/Midwife	472	81.7	438	66.8	211	36.5	203	31
Doctor/Clinical Officer	94	79	84	61.3	35	29.4	29	21.2
Non-skilled attendant	13	76.5	14	66.7	6	35.3	6	28.6
1plus skilled providers	43	76.8	38	60.3	20	35.7	19	30.2
Delivery Provider sex								
Male	235	79.9	215	65.3	108	36.7	104	31.6
Female	363	81.6	337	65.6	152	34.2	141	27.5
Both	24	77.4	22	64.7	12	38.7	12	35.3
Accompanied by								
Partner								
No	443	85.7***	412	66	209	40.4***	195	31.3*
Yes	179	70.8	162	64	63	24.9	62	24.5
Mother-in-law								
No	419	79.8	401	63.4	180	34.3	168	26.6*
Yes	203	82.9	173	70.6	92	37.6	89	36.5
Mother								
No	534	79.9	504	65*	224	33.5*	221	28.6
Yes	88	86.3	70	68.6	48	47.1	36	35.3
Sister/Sister in law								
No	476	78.9*	456	64.2	212	35.2	206	29.1
Yes	146	87.4	118	70.7	60	35.9	51	30.5
Friend/Neighbor								
No	532	81.1	504	66.1	222	33.8*	222	29.1
Yes	90	78.9	70	61.4	50	43.9	35	30.7
Facility crowded								
No or a few times	428	83.4*	400	67.7	185	36.1	174	29.4
Most or all the time	192	75.3	172	60.6	86	33.7	82	28.9

Table 5 Bivariate distribution of selected birth companionship variables by demographic and facility characteristics, PQCC study 2016 *(Continued)*

	Desire for labor support				Desire for delivery support			
	Last birth		Future birth		Last birth		Future birth	
	No.	%	No.	%	No.	%	No.	%
Allowed continuous labor support								
No or a few times	162	68.1***	146	53.1***				
Most or all the time	459	86.6	428	71.3				
Allowed continuous delivery support								
No or a few times					137	25.4***	139	22.8***
Most or all the time					135	58.4	118	44.2
Total	622	80.8	574	65.5	272	35.3	257	29.3

* $p < 0.05$ ** $p < 0.01$ *** $p < 0.001$

no complication and were assisted by only a nurse or midwife respectively. In spite of the fact that there was no significant association between being allowed continuous delivery support and perception of overcrowding in the bivariate analysis, this association became significant in the multivariate model, but in an unexpected direction—women who reported that the health facility was overcrowded most or all the time had about 69% higher odds of being allowed continuous delivery support than those who perceived that the facility was not overcrowded. Also, women accompanied by a partner had about 40% lower odds of being allowed continuous delivery support than those not accompanied by a partner; and those who desired a companion at delivery had close to two times higher odds of being allowed continuous delivery support.

Women's perspectives on labor and delivery support: Qualitative data from FGDs with women

The overarching themes from the analysis of the data from FGD with women are on their feelings about being allowed or denied a companion during labor and delivery, reasons why they do or do not want a companion, and their preferences for different types of companions.

Feelings about being allowed or denied a companion during labor and delivery

Most women were happy when their companions were allowed to stay with them during labor, and unhappy when they were not allowed to stay with them.

> *"They allowed the relatives to be with us ....I felt good because there are times you can be going to bath, and so they will remain and take care of the baby for you." (KP5)*

> *"No they didn't [allow relative to stay] and I did not like it because they are busy with their own things and it is this relative of yours who can help you with your problem..." (WP1)*

Companions were however only allowed at certain times, like during labor but not at the time of delivery, or only after the baby was born; or during certain times of the day like at night, but not in the morning. Many felt it was inappropriate to not be allowed a companion during labor and after delivery.

> *"I wanted her to be with me so that I can explain to her how am feeling so that in case I need help then I send her to go and call the doctor or nurse to come and help me quickly and they kept on telling them that "get out care takers your time is not now, wait until they give birth is when you can come in", and yet after giving birth am not as serious as when I still have my labor pains when am not supposed to be alone and so I felt bad." (WP2)*

However, many did not mind not being allowed a companion at the time of delivery for various reasons described in later sections.

> *"I felt it was good if they were allowed to be with me after having my baby. But before, it was good that they were not allowed to be with me." (CP10)*

It appeared some providers did not take time to explain to women about why they were not allowed a birth companion, and were sometimes abusive when disallowing the companion.

> *"They refused and even chased the person who accompanied me and told her 'leave her alone .... you did not give her the pregnancy she will deliver it herself'.... that was not good." (MP2)*

Women therefore inferred various reasons why their companions were not allowed to stay with them. Some felt that it was a facility requirement that applied to

Table 6 Bivariate distribution of selected birth companionship variables by demographic and facility characteristics, PQCC Study 2016

	Accompanied by Partner			Accompanied by mother-in-law		
	No.	%	*p*-value	No.	%	*p*-value
Age						
15 to 19 years	26	16	***	43	26.5	
20 to 29 years	154	30.1		150	29.4	
30 to 48 years	73	35.8		52	25.5	
Marital Status						
Not married	12	6.3	***	21	11.1	***
Currently married	241	35.1		224	32.6	
Number of births						
1.0	57	19.7	***	67	23.1	*
2.0	70	37.8		62	33.5	
3.0	50	30.7		53	32.5	
4 or more	76	31.8		63	26.4	
Education						
No school/Primary	117	23.6	***	150	30.3	*
Post-primary/vocational/Secondary	86	31.7		76	28	
College or above	50	45		19	17.1	
Literacy						
No, cannot write	11	35.5		11	35.5	
Yes, but with some difficulty	39	27.7		40	28.4	
Yes, Very well	203	28.8		194	27.5	
Household wealth						
Poorest/poorer	93	24.5	*	135	35.5	***
Middle	40	29.6		33	24.4	
Richer/richest	120	33.1		77	21.3	
Employed						
No	176	26.7	*	177	26.9	
Yes	77	35.2		68	31.1	
Has Health Insurance						
No	175	24.2	***	207	28.7	
Yes	78	50.3		38	24.5	
Pregnancy complication						
No	149	30.2		131	26.5	
Yes	104	27.2		114	29.8	
Birth Complication						
No	204	28.3		202	28	
Yes	49	31.4		43	27.6	
Past health facility delivery						
No	68	19.9	***	83	24.3	
Yes	185	34.6		162	30.3	
ANC visits						
Less than 4	58	20.2	***	85	29.6	

Table 6 Bivariate distribution of selected birth companionship variables by demographic and facility characteristics, PQCC Study 2016 *(Continued)*

	Accompanied by Partner			Accompanied by mother-in-law		
	No.	%	*p*-value	No.	%	*p*-value
4 plus	192	32.8		158	27	
Tribe						
Luo	176	30.1		114	19.5	***
Kuria	53	25.5		114	54.8	
Other	24	28.2		17	20	
Religion						
Catholic	72	29.8		68	28.1	
Protestant/Pentecostal	46	24.1		59	30.9	
Seventh Day Adventist	84	31.9		75	28.5	
Other Christian	48	28.9		39	23.5	
Muslim/other religion	3	20		4	26.7	
Delivery facility type						
Gov't Hospital	120	29.7		122	30.2	
Gov't HC/Disp	94	26		96	26.5	
Mission/Private facility	39	35.1		27	24.3	
Delivery provider						
Nurse/Midwife	190	29		188	28.7	
Doctor/Clinical Officer	40	29.2		35	25.5	
Non-skilled attendant	6	28.6		5	23.8	
1plus skilled providers	17	27		17	27	
Delivery Provider sex						
Male	100	30.4		97	29.5	
Female	142	27.6		138	26.8	
Both	11	32.4		10	29.4	
Total	253	28.8		245	27.9	

* $p < 0.05$ ** $p < 0.01$ *** $p < 0.001$

everyone. However, others felt that it was the providers who did not want them to have someone close to them.

> *"They refused so I just stayed alone in the hospital until I stayed two days in the hospital... It is required that I just stay alone.... I felt bad" (MP4)*

> *"They do not always allow somebody to be with you, it is the doctor and you alone. Whoever has brought you is to wait outside" (OP5)*

> *"They do not want someone to be close to you, even after giving birth, they tell them that time for visiting patients is over and they send them away." (CP10)*

Some women also thought companions were less likely to be allowed during delivery if they were male compared to if they were female companions.

> *"I was allowed to be with a woman relative but not a man... The woman relative was allowed for when there is a problem she can assist the nurse, but a male relative they do not allow them to stay." (P10)*

Reasons for desiring a companion

Instrumental support The most common reason for desiring a labor companion was to have someone readily available to attend to their needs. This was important because they often felt helpless in labor, and providers were not with them all the time. Also, because providers were usually busy with other things, the presence of their companion ensured that there was someone readily available to help them if they needed help for things such as going to the bathroom room and to call the provider if they developed a problem or went into the second stage of labor.

Table 7 Multivariate logistic regression of continuous support during labor and delivery on potential predictors, PQCC study 2016

	Allowed Continuous support during					
	Labor			Delivery		
	OR	95% CI		OR	95% CI	
Age						
15 to 19 years	1	[1	1]	1	[1	1]
20 to 29 years	0.79	[0.46	1.35]	0.86	[0.50	1.47]
30 to 48 years	0.74	[0.36	1.54]	0.92	[0.43	1.95]
Currently married	1.35	[0.79	2.29]	0.98	[0.57	1.69]
Number of births						
1	1	[1	1]	1	[1	1]
2	0.61	[0.26	1.43]	1.24	[0.51	3.04]
3	0.37*	[0.15	0.95]	2.06	[0.77	5.50]
4 or more	0.39	[0.15	1.01]	1.45	[0.53	3.93]
Education						
No school/Primary	1	[1	1]	1	[1	1]
Post-primary/vocational/Secondary	0.73	[0.47	1.14]	1.27	[0.83	1.96]
College or above	0.75	[0.36	1.56]	1.21	[0.61	2.39]
Literacy						
No, cannot write	1	[1	1]	1	[1	1]
Yes, but with some difficulty	1.9	[0.72	5.05]	0.73	[0.22	2.42]
Yes, very well	2.89*	[1.13	7.37]	1.92	[0.63	5.90]
Household wealth						
Poorest/poorer	1	[1	1]	1	[1	1]
Middle	1.73*	[1.04	2.90]	0.81	[0.47	1.40]
Richer/richest	1.91**	[1.20	3.03]	1.16	[0.74	1.84]
Employed	1.97**	[1.24	3.12]	0.91	[0.58	1.42]
Past health facility delivery	2.19*	[1.05	4.57]	0.71	[0.32	1.58]
4plus ANC visits	0.68	[0.46	1.01]	0.82	[0.56	1.20]
Birth Complication	0.67	[0.43	1.04]	0.34***	[0.19	0.60]
Tribe						
Luo	1	[1	1]	1	[1	1]
Kuria	0.57*	[0.37	0.90]	0.79	[0.48	1.29]
Other	0.79	[0.44	1.43]	0.79	[0.43	1.45]
Religion						
Catholic	1	[1	1]	1	[1	1]
Protestant/Pentecostal	0.68	[0.41	1.12]	1.06	[0.62	1.79]
Seventh Day Adventist	0.7	[0.44	1.12]	1.55	[0.99	2.44]
Other Christian	0.79	[0.46	1.35]	0.93	[0.54	1.59]
Muslim/other religion	0.86	[0.21	3.44]	1.8	[0.43	7.52]
Delivery facility type						
Gov't Hospital	1	[1	1]	1	[1	1]
Gov't Health Center	1.98***	[1.32	2.97]	1.46	[0.98	2.17]
Mission/Private facility	0.86	[0.49	1.51]	1.67	[0.95	2.95]

Table 7 Multivariate logistic regression of continuous support during labor and delivery on potential predictors, PQCC study 2016 *(Continued)*

	Allowed Continuous support during					
	Labor			Delivery		
	OR	95% CI		OR	95% CI	
Delivery provider						
Nurse/Midwife	1	[1	1]	1	[1	1]
Doctor/Clinical Officer	0.8	[0.46	1.39]	1.13	[0.63	2.00]
Non-skilled attendant	1	[0.28	3.60]	0.88	[0.28	2.79]
1plus skilled providers	0.27**	[0.12	0.63]	0.19**	[0.060	0.59]
Delivery Provider sex						
Male	1	[1	1]	1	[1	1]
Female	1.24	[0.82	1.89]	1.42	[0.92	2.19]
Both	4.68**	[1.54	14.2]	5.40**	[1.67	17.5]
Accompanied by						
Partner	0.81	[0.53	1.24]	0.61*	[0.39	0.97]
Mother-in-law	0.92	[0.59	1.44]	1.19	[0.74	1.91]
Mother	1.3	[0.70	2.42]	1.01	[0.54	1.90]
Sister/Sister in law	1.85*	[1.13	3.01]	0.73	[0.45	1.18]
Friend- Neighbor	0.87	[0.51	1.46]	0.61	[0.35	1.06]
Facility crowded	0.65*	[0.45	0.93]	1.69**	[1.15	2.50]
Desired labor companion	1.42*	[1.01	2.00]			
Desired delivery companion				1.97***	[1.48	2.62]
Interviews in community (ref = HF)	1.02	[0.70	1.49]	0.79	[0.54	1.14]
Postpartum length= > 1 week (ref < 1	0.99	[0.53	1.83]	1.24	[0.64	2.38]
Constant	0.87	[0.22	3.42]	0.15*	[0.033	0.64]
N	763			764		

* $p < 0.05$ ** $p < 0.01$ *** $p < 0.001$

> *"They did not allow them just as the other person has said, you want to be with your relative and they are sent out. You know sometimes they the doctors are out and have gone wherever places. For you your labor is bad and you are bleeding, so the energy that you will have to walk and go to call the doctor you do not have and so it is your relative whom you can send to go and get you the doctor and so that is why I was not happy with this." (WP6)*

> *"I feel it is good to have someone with you because sister [the nurse] can show you the bed to go and sleep, then she goes to sit somewhere else. So if you are about to give birth then you can send her to go and call for you the nurse so that she can come and help you." (CP4)*

Companions were also needed to help run errands: like going to buy drugs and supplies that might not be available on the ward or arranging additional help if they were referred.

> *" I feel that they should be next to you because, the doctor can tell you that there is some drug that you should be treated with, and so he can be sent to go to the chemist to go and buy." (CP1)*

> *"They should be around because sometimes you can develop complications and you are being referred and so if you are alone then you may not be able to get help." (OP6)*

In addition, companions were needed after delivery to help care for the baby, including holding the baby when they needed to go to the bathroom.

> *"They should be allowed. Because they can help you with carrying the baby." (CP10)*

> *"I felt good because there are times you can be going to bath, and so they will remain and take care of the baby for you." (KP5)*

Informational support and advocacy For others, the companion helped meet their informational needs by telling them what to do, helping them make decisions, and advocating for their care—as they felt they were not in a state to make decisions on their own during labor. Others wanted the companion around in order to have someone who could remind them later of what happened during labor.

> *"They should allow your relatives to be with you at that particular time in case that anything happens then they can share with the nurses to know what next is to be done to you, because at that time, you are in so much pain that you cannot make any wise decision." (KP3)*

> *"For me I like it because at that time I do not know anything that am doing so when she is there then she will be able to tell me that at that time you did this and that until the doctor either did this to you is when you were able to put to birth." (OP3)*

Emotional support Emotional support was barely mentioned as a reason for desiring a companion. Only one woman's response to why she was unhappy about being denied a companion related to a desire for emotional support during labor.

> *"That was not good because when you have someone near, she will try to make your heart relax, yes, but when they refuse you are just alone you will surely have some problems." (MP2)*

Reasons for not desiring for a companion

Some women did not desire companionship during labor, and in particular at the time of delivery, and so did not mind that their companions were not allowed to stay. Reasons for not desiring companionship included the following.

They cannot help you A common reason women gave for not desiring a companion was that "they can't help you." Some mentioned that the reason why they come to deliver in the facility was because their relatives could not help them at home, and so there was no need for them to be around once they had brought them to the facility.

> *"I do not want because when you left home...they could not help you and so that is why you came to get help from the hospital." (CP4)*

Others felt it was only the provider who could help them, and that they felt safe with the providers. Thus, there was no need for their companion to be around.

> *"I feel that it is the right thing [that companion was asked to wait outside] because whoever has brought you is not the doctor, and he has brought you in safe hands of the doctor and so he should just stay out and wait .... because there is nothing he will do apart from just looking at you and so it is only when the doctor is not able then he will refer you." (OP4)*

In particular at the time of delivery, many felt it was the provider who knew everything and so should be the only one with them.

> *"It is the doctor who knows everything and so he is the one who should be with you alone in the delivery room but the other person I would not like him to be next to me when I am giving birth." (OP3)*

Some also felt lay companions, in addition to not being able to help them, might laugh at them if they saw their condition at the time of delivery.

> *" I should be with the doctor alone because she is the one with all the know-how but this relative of mine, all he will do is just look and laugh at you." (WP2)*

Others felt at the time of delivery it was only "between you and your God" and so there was no need for a relative to be there to see their nakedness

> *"We did not say that it is bad to have someone with you...let them just come. But when time comes that you are in a state of between you and your God, then let them stay outside and wait for you....At that time, he should not see my nakedness." (OP3)*

Embarrassment Some women felt embarrassed to have someone other than a provider see them during labor, and particularly during delivery. They also felt that providers had seen a lot to not be surprised at their condition or nakedness, but did not feel the same way about lay companions.

> *"No, I feel embarrassed and [will] rather be with the doctor alone in that hospital." (CP5)*

> *"I refused because when you are giving birth, maybe you do not have clothes and you are with your mother-in-law so you feel embarrassed." (CP8)*

"It is better if you are with the nurse alone because for her she has seen a lot but the other person can exclaim that 'ei and this person." (CP10)

Certain roles companions were asked to play made women particularly vulnerable, as well as decrease their desire for companionship. For example, one woman reported she felt very embarrassed because the provider asked the relative to hold the flashlight for him to conduct the delivery (because there was no electricity) and she felt completely exposed to this relative.

"I did not like it because whoever escorted me is the one that the doctor made to carry for him the sport light and was pointing it at me and I did not like it at all....but it is only that I was in a problem and I was praying to God to help me, but my inner heart did not like the fact that this person was seeing my nakedness." (OP3)

Fear that support persons may go outside the facility and discuss private matters Some feared that the support person may discuss what they saw about them with others outside the facility. They were confident that providers could not discuss what they saw about them outside the facility, but did not feel the same about lay companions.

"At that time they should not allow someone to be in, the doctor is the only person who should see my nakedness...people are so mouthy. Some people when they leave the hospital they go and say so many strange things about you, how they saw you, but the doctor is not allowed to go out and talk about what has happened in the facility." (KP4)

"For me I don't want because they can look at you then go and tell other women that ei.. so and so is like this." (CP2)

"For me I liked it and felt good [that the person was not allowed inside] because whoever is taking care of you can go out and talk about your secret but the doctor cannot." (CP5)

Fear of abuse Some did not want the companion to stay with them because they feared that they might unknowingly abuse the support person when they are in pain.

"After reaching with her at the door, then he should stay aside because you are very angry at that time and so you can find yourself insulting her." (CP10)

Others feared that the support person may abuse them—like shouting at them at them during labor pains. The fear of being abused was mentioned in relation to the type of support person. Some women felt that their mothers-in-law were more likely to be abusive, hence they preferred to have their mother as a support person.

"it's good to be with a parent when giving birth, like me I was with my mother when I was giving birth and I was attended to well but when you are with your mother in law, when taking care of you, she will shout at you that stop disturbing me but when you are with your mother then she will take good care of you, it's good to be with your mother than any other person." (CP9)

Reasons for not desiring birth companionship from their partner

Women spontaneously talked about preferring a female relative, and not their partners, as birth companions. Reasons for this included that their partners could not help them and so did not need to be there.

" He will not help you with anything...so it is better for him to be away." (KP2)

Others did not want to see their partners during the time of delivery because they hated him at that time.

" While I was giving birth, I went with my husband as my mum lives in [another town]. But my husband was waiting for me far away.... I really did hate him at that time (...Laughs...) when that time came I felt hatred for him and I told him you sit that side" (CP6)

Another reason was fear that their partners might lose sexual desire for them if they saw them at the time of delivery. It appeared that providers reinforced this belief by using it as a reason to discourage the women from having male partners present at the time of delivery.

"When I am inside, I would want him just to stay outside there...The time the baby is coming out, is not a good sight for a man to be there...They always say that when a woman is delivering and the time the baby is coming out, your body is not looking good so when the husband sees that, after delivery, he will not have a desire (sexual desire) for you. That is what is said and most of us mothers know about this {laughter...}. They prevent the husbands from seeing this so that later he may have a desire for you. That is why the nurse will enter inside with you only unless there is something she cannot handle is when he will

be allowed in (WP4). M: This is what nurses are saying or who?{All in chorus, nurses...}"

There were also some cultural beliefs around allowing men in the delivery room. Some mentioned their tribes required a mother-in-law to accompany the women at the time of delivery, because the presence of a man can prolong the delivery. Thus, partners were not allowed even during deliveries conducted by traditional birth attendants [TBA].

> *My third child I delivered at the TBA place. I was accompanied by my husband and other mother-in-laws. When we arrived there the baby was almost coming out, he was told to stay outside [and] not to go in. This was because the Luo culture says that when your husband goes inside with you where you are going to deliver, he will tie you and the baby might delay in coming out, so it is not good that we go with our husbands to where we are delivering (WP7).*

Others did not want their partners present because they wanted them to go home and take care of other children.

> *"For me in most occasions when am going to deliver, I usually go with my husband, and when we go when we reach, after I have been admitted, Like this one, they asked me whoever he was to me and I told them that he is my husband and they asked me if I wanted him to stay behind and be with me. But I told them that no the children are home alone and so he must go back home as I was in safe hands and he was to go back and only call him in case there is anything that needs his attention then they could call him come back...I did not see the point of having [him] around because when giving birth, even if he is my own husband I do not want him to be with me at that time, I want only a doctor." (KP2)*

Providers' perspectives: quantitative and qualitative data from in-depth-interviews with providers

We conducted in-depth-interviews with seven clinical officers, 25 nurses and midwives, and 17 non-clinical staff including cleaners and cooks. Thirty of them worked in public hospitals, 13 in health centers, and 6 in mission hospitals (Table 8). Most of the providers reported that women were usually allowed a companion during labor: 84% reported that during labor, companions were allowed all or most of the time. Fewer, however, reported that women were usually allowed a companion during delivery: only 39% reported that during delivery, companions were allowed all or most of the time. Clinical staff were also more likely to report that women were allowed continuous delivery support compared to non-clinical staff. Additionally, compared to female providers, male providers were more likely to report that women were allowed continuous labor and delivery support (Table 8).

Role birth companions play in the facility

The reasons given by providers for allowing birth companions were generally consistent with those given by women. Providers however also implied that the companions were useful not just to the mother but to them the providers. Providers reported companions sometimes helped them with various chores, such as going to purchase supplies and drugs, calling on them to attend to the women, helping women to and from the delivery bed, holding items like a flashlight during delivery, helping them pick up delivery supplies, and cleaning up. The role of the companion was particularly useful in the face of staff shortages, where only one provider may be on duty.

> *"You know after that like now we have staff shortage, so maybe after examining a mother maybe I am alone in the facility, I may run to come and see clients here but when they are almost ready, she will come and call me. Even after delivery helping them to do one, two, three, like cleaning the clothes something like that."*

> *"Most of the time we need one caretaker to be around. In case of any eventuality they can be asked to go may be to organize for example in a case of complicated delivery and you want things like gloves somebody at least you can send to get for you the things you want, so most of the times we allow one caretaker to be around the mother who is giving birth."*

Some providers insisted that they almost always allow birth companions, because they can't do without them when they are alone assisting with the delivery.

> *"Rarely do we not allow birth companions, rarely, not unless the mother came alone. There are some who come without Birth companions though during ANC they are encouraged to have with Birth partners, but when they come without they are equally just served as others. But when they come with a birth partner, especially X facility, if they do not assist us I don't know how we would do it, because they do assist us even wheeling the patient to the bedside post delivery they do a lot to us especially to me when I am on duty, they do a lot."*

"We have no problem, if the mother has allowed someone who escorted her to labor to get in then we have no problem with the person as there was a time when a mother was delivering and it is the husband who was holding for us the touch."

Some support staff mentioned that some clinical providers only allowed birth companions who could be helpful to them.

"The delivery room is small so the nurse will only need the person who will assist her get things like cotton wool, bucket for the placenta and water."

"The relative may only come in when it is at night and the lights are off so the care taker gets in to hold for the nurse the torch only."

In addition, although companions were usually not allowed at the time of delivery, they were sometimes called on to help with non-compliant women. This was mostly noted by the non-clinical staff.

"This time is more private, he does not allow anyone to be with the mother unless he is alone and the mother is not cooperative...[that] is when he will call a relative to come and talk to the mother to push the baby."

"No, it is only the nurses who are in there. The person is to wait outside. Only if the woman is difficult to deal with is when they call the caretaker to come in and help them."

Reasons why companions may not be allowed in the ward

The reasons why birth companions were sometimes not allowed in the ward are related to privacy and ward set up, distrust of companions, lack of confidence in companions in the event of complications, and respecting the woman's wishes.

Privacy and ward set up Most providers reported that companions were sometimes not allowed in the ward because of limited space and overcrowding, hence privacy concerns for other women in the labor and delivery wards. Some also mentioned that the set-up of the labor wards is not conducive for companions, including limited seating, which may cause companions to use beds meant for the laboring woman.

If they are two in labor then now you see the privacy will [be a problem] ...but if that woman is all alone there, then we will just allow, so it is more of the setup which is preventing us but we know...that if they want even their spouses to come to the delivery room they should be allowed but because of the setup and the environment now it is not really conducive.

Privacy was the main reason given for not allowing companions at the time of delivery.

"Yes, we allow them but it is not a normal practice here and at second stage we do not allow them. Here you find maybe they came with them, they stay with them but when we are going to second stage we tell them to wait until the time they have delivered. But that one is done because of space as I was saying. Maybe...the relative of this mother A is there and another mother B is delivering so when I bring these relatives here they will also be watching this mother B, so we say let me counsel them when we need them we can always call them after delivery"

Distrust of companions Another set of reasons for sometimes not allowing companions were related to distrust of the companions. Providers had several fears of inappropriate things companions did (or which they thought companions might do), which made them reluctant to allow companions. These included the following:

Fear companions will practice things usually done in home deliveries like giving the laboring woman herbs: Several providers mentioned they sometimes refuse to let the companions into the ward because some of them bring traditional herbs that are thought to hasten labor to the health facility to give to the laboring woman. They also mentioned that some companions attempt to apply fundal pressure and touch women with unclean hands.

"like here they like coming with the herbs, since the nurse is one, you leave the mother with the care taker and by the time you are back, you find that they have place for the mother the herb, so it depends on who has brought the client."

"Sometimes you find the mother in second stage, a mother comes in, there are certain things they usually practice home deliveries, so you can find that they start practicing that so we don't allow that in health care so this is why. Mothers at home give fundal [pressure] and they can touch anywhere with bare hands, yeah so in a normal delivery procedure they remain outside the delivery room."

They were particularly distrustful of older birth companions, particularly mothers-in-law, whom they said

Table 8 Univariate and Bivariate distribution of Provider data, PQCC study 2016

	Characteristics of Providers		Percent reporting women are allowed continuous support during			
			Labor		Delivery	
	No.	%	No.	%	No.	%
Facility type						
Govt. Hospital	30	61.2	22	73.3	10	33.3
Govt. Health Center	13	26.5	13	100	6	46.2
Mission Hospital	6	12	6	100	3	50
Position in facility						
Clinical officer	7	14.3	7	100	4	57.1*
Nurse/Midwife	25	51	19	76	12	48
Support staff	17	34.7	15	88.2	3	17.6
Gender						
Male	14	28.6	14	100	9	64.3*
Female	35	71.4	27	77.1	10	28.6
Age						
24 to 39 years	30	61.2	26	86.7	12	40
40 to 58 years	19	38.8	15	78.9	7	36.8
Marital status						
Single/Widowed	8	17	7	87.5	3	37.5
Married	39	83	32	82	15	38.5
Parity						
0 to 3	34	72.34	28	82.4	13	38.2
4 to 7	13	27.66	11	84.6	5	38.5
Feels Facility is crowded						
No, never	14	28.6	12	85.7	5	35.7
Yes, a few times	6	12.2	5	83.3	3	50
Yes, most of the time	23	46.9	21	91.3	9	39.1
Yes, all the time	6	12.2	3	50	2	33.3
Women allowed labor support						
No, never	1	2				
Yes, a few times	6	12.2				
Yes, most of the time	12	24.5				
Yes, all the time	29	59.2				
Women allowed delivery support						
No, never	18	36.7				
Yes, a few times	12	24.5				
Yes, most of the time	9	18.4				
Yes, all the time	10	20.4				
Total	49	100	41	83.7	19	38.8

* $p < 0.05$ ** $p < 0.01$ *** $p < 0.001$

were more likely to give women concoctions to try to hasten labor.

> *"Mostly those old mothers, the grannies, the mother in laws who are old. They believe that once a mother comes to the labor ward to deliver, maybe to get a baby as fast as possible, so once they are around, they can discuss and give the mother some medicine to fasten delivery so [because of] that most of us who are midwives are very keen and we don't want those mothers to come so many of them, they can give herbal medicine or they boil tea concentrated without sugar*

as they believe that this one will hasten the delivery. That act most of us are not ready to entertain."

Fear companions will force mothers to do things against their will: Some providers did not trust companions because they feared they may force women to do things against their will such as forcing the women to take the herbs.

"some mothers come with the herbs and force the laboring woman to drink or chew and so that is why we don't usually allow them to come in where the woman is"

Fear companions may misinform mothers: There was also the suspicion that companions may misinform the laboring women when they are with them in the labor ward, such as asking them to push before they are fully dilated.

"Mmm sometimes you get, okay personally, the mothers who come with a companion, give misinformation to the mothers, they force the mothers to push before they are fully dilated, and that is why many a times I do not allow them because they give a lot of misinformation to the mothers while they are in labor. [It causes] those things like cervical tear which are not supposed to be there."

Fear that companions may misinterpret what they see in the facility and discuss it outside: Providers also sometimes prevented companions from staying in the ward because of fears that when they observe certain procedures and something goes wrong (like the baby dies), the companions will go out and spread rumors that the baby died because of the procedure the provider performed.

"When you have invasive procedure... the companion is not supposed to be around to see, for they can feel that you did that thing wrongly and yet we were helping the mother or the baby. I: Like what procedures? R1: Like vacuum extraction you cannot allow the companion to be there. There is fear they can take the information at home that they did this that killed our baby by using the instruments."

A support staff mentioned that clinical providers also sometimes disallowed companions because of fears that companions will go out and gossip about the woman's condition to others, including adding their own interpretations to what they saw.

Some women after seeing the woman delivering, they go and talk about how the woman's private part is. Some women also give birth to babies who are white with a lot of whitish things in them, so they go and start gossiping how the woman was having sex until the last minute is why the baby is born dirty. So that is why the nurses want to do everything and clean the baby. [That] is when she is taken to the other room for the relatives and friends to see the baby.

Fear of companions being disrespectful to providers and not taking instructions: Another reason some providers gave for sometimes disallowing companions was that some of them were disrespectful: they talk rudely to them, do not take instructions, want to order the providers around, and are naughty and noisy.

"...some care takers are so stubborn they talk to the nurses as if they know everything that the nurse should be doing."

"Sometimes, some people want to be the nurse and so they give the nurse orders in there. So such people are told to wait in the labor room."

"...also it depends on the understanding as some of them will come and don't want to listen to the instructions of the provider."

Disallowing companions for women with complications

Women with chronic medical conditions or pregnancy complications were sometimes not allowed companions because of the following:

Need to keep the woman's health information confidential: Some providers mentioned not allowing companions to maintain the woman's confidentiality, especially if she had a condition like HIV.

"Like when the patient is positive (HIV) the doctor will first talk to her and find out from the patient whom to inform and not everybody because at times is a neighbor who brought her. Also find out from her who will collect the drugs for her. In such a case is only the doctor who will be with the patient until she says whom she would want to be closer to her."

Need to monitor woman frequently: Some also mentioned not allowing companions if the woman had a condition that they needed to monitor frequently.

"Okay, sometimes if a woman has a chronic condition that you need to monitor, so we may not like a lot of relatives to be there but we have to inform the relative

that we are doing this and this. So you will find at that time [only] the health worker will be so near to the patient to monitor."

Inappropriate companion behavior: Providers were also concerned that in the event of a complication, the companion's behaviors may discourage the woman.

"Sometimes just in case of any complication as those people, the family people, they will tend to change to discourage the patient by the way they behave. Like they are so anxious about the patient and they try to discourage."

"Some relatives are so scared and so they are not allowed to get in because they will make the woman to also be scared."

A provider mentioned fear of companions collapsing because of what they saw, giving them additional work of caring for the companion as well as the woman.

"There are a few cases the condition of a mother does not warrant the relatives to be near the mother because of big number like sometimes we had seen somebody who has escorted the patient after seeing the thing fainted, now you will have double work, you are struggling with the mother and somebody has just fainted. So in such scenarios in some cases we do tell some not to. Or you are seriously resuscitating a child and the person who has escorted the mother is crying, you tell her to be out as we do the resuscitation process."

Respecting the woman and companions wishes

Sometimes companions were asked to stay outside the labor or delivery ward to respect the woman's wishes.

" If the mother who is in labor says, me I do not want anyone around until I deliver. [1] *just preserve that as her right, but most of the times we just allow the relatives to be around."*

Other times, it was the companion who did not want to stay with the woman, because some women, in their pain, were cruel to their companions.

R: During labor pains, most of the women become very cruel or very rude. So some of the family members may be afraid to go and be with them in there. [Laughs]We tell her to choose the best person so if she does not want you then we tell you to leave.

Perceptions about partners as birth companions

Providers spontaneously mentioned that they were more likely to allow continuous labor and delivery support if the companion was a partner. They mentioned that partners are the first selected to support women when there is limited space, because they did not trust other companions.

" Mostly we allow the husband, we allow them to be with the wife but if another care taker, sometimes we don't allow. I: Why, what is the reason? R1: Because you never know who is the caretaker"

"we do not know the caretaker and you know family issues we don't interfere, only the husband we allow in the delivery room if the patient is willing, some patients are not willing; they tell the husband go away"

They, however, acknowledged that many women did not want their partners in the delivery room because they wanted their privacy.

"Maybe the mother will just say let him [partner] or her go outside for sometime. They do not like when they are pushing especially their husbands [to be around]."

"Sometimes it is the husband who has come, and the woman is the one who sends him away so we also tell them to keep off and wait outside as she is putting to birth"

Other times, it was the partners who did not want to be in the delivery room: because they did not want to see the nakedness of women, didn't find it appropriate to enter the room, or because of cultural reasons.

"They are allowed, but men mostly don't come...One said that he didn't want to see the lady naked, he doesn't want to see her being handled during delivery. But us we do allow them"

"I may say its culture, let me say if it's a husband who has brought the wife, some of them do not want to go where the woman is laboring."

Some providers also discouraged partners from being birth companions, due to the perception that the presence of a partner may cause women to desire more attention.

"when the husband is around this might affect her psychologically as when she sees the husband she

might want the sympathy from him. When the husband is away she will be with the nurses who should take care of her."

Discussion

This study is the first study, to our knowledge, to comprehensively examine the prevalence and nature of labor and delivery support from the perspective of both mothers and providers in Kenya, and among the first of such studies in SSA. We found that most women are accompanied to the facility for childbirth and most of them want to have a companion stay with them during labor and after delivery, but fewer want that person around at the time of delivery. Women's reasons for desiring a companion were mostly related to having someone around to help them meet their physical needs; more so than for emotional support. Those who expressed that they did not want a companion felt that companions could not help them, were embarrassed to have the companion see their nakedness, feared that companions may gossip about what they saw, or were afraid the companion might abuse them or vice-versa. Most providers acknowledged the importance of having a birth companion but stated that it is often not possible due to privacy concerns and other reasons related to distrust and lack of confidence in companions. Some providers, however, thought of companions' roles as assisting them with non-clinical tasks rather than providing emotional support to women.

The findings from this study support the few other studies in SSA that challenge the assumption that all women want a birth companion [13]. In addition, continuous support is often examined as a single unit, but our findings suggest that combining labor and delivery together may not align with women's preferences. By examining labor and delivery separately we show that women have different desires for companionship at different stages of labor and delivery. Furthermore, we show that having a companion present doesn't guarantee that the woman will be supported or feel supported. Where providers think of companions as providing support to them, women's needs might be overlooked. Nonetheless, women who were allowed CSLD in their last pregnancy were more likely to desire it in the future, suggesting that they valued the experience.

We also extend the discussion on women's preferences for companionship at labor and delivery. Less than a quarter of women mentioned a partner as their preferred companion during labor, and even fewer (only 6%) wanted a partner as a companion during delivery. Most women preferred a female companion, such as their mother, mother-in-law, sister, sister-in-law, or friend. A few mentioned co-wives, but notably no one mentioned a traditional birth attendant (TBA) as their preferred companion. The reasons for the low preference male partners included fear that their partners might lose sexual desire for them if they saw the baby coming out, as well as cultural beliefs about how the presence of a partner could affect the delivery. The preferred type of companion is also influenced by tribal norms, with a mother-in-law being preferred over the partner among the Kuria tribe. Our findings are consistent with that of a study in Ghana, where 24% of respondents preferred a male labor companion [13], but much lower than that from a study in Nigeria where most women (86%) preferred their husband as their labor companion [21]. A reason for this might be that the study in Nigeria involved women with higher socio-economic status than our respondents. We found that wealthier and more educated women were more likely to desire their partners as both labor and delivery companions than poorer and less educated women.

The national guideline for Obstetrics and Perinatal Care in Kenya specifically mentions partners as birth companions, and, currently, there are initiatives to promote male involvement in maternal and child health in Kenya. These may be reasons why providers spontaneously discussed a preference for partners as companions during interviews. The survey results, however, suggest that women are less likely to be allowed continuous support at delivery if the companion was a male partner. In addition, women perceive that providers are less likely to allow them to have continuous labor and delivery support if their companions are male partners. This inconsistency between providers' and women's report might be due to providers responding in a socially desirable manner in spite of the fact that both groups are not particularly supportive of having male partners as birth companions. Moreover, the spontaneous discussion among women about male companions may suggest that they are not entirely supportive of the emphasis on having their partners as companions. These findings suggest that we need to find better ways of changing social norms around the role of men during labor and delivery and promoting the involvement of male partners in maternal and child healthcare, while prioritizing women's preferences.

Morhason-Bello et al., found that emotional support was the most cited reason for women's desire for birth companionship (80%). This finding is not consistent with that of our study, and the demographics of our sample may explain the difference. The limited reference to emotional support should, however, not be misconstrued as a lack of desire for emotional support. We did not specifically ask our participants about emotional support or other types of support. The reasons women give for desiring labor companions are therefore likely the top reasons based on the realities of their situation—which in this case is a need for instrumental support to meet their practical needs at the facility. In addition, Alexander et al., in their study in Ghana, found that male companions were expected to provide emotional support, while female companions were expected to provide other types of support [13]. The limited reference to emotional support in our study may therefore be due to the low preference for male companions.

Beyond women's desires and preferences are health system barriers to providing continuous labor and delivery support. Providers cite overcrowding and privacy issues are the main reasons for disallowing birth companions. This is consistent with our survey results, where women who perceived the facility as crowded were less likely to be allowed a labor companion. It is also consistent with findings related to barriers to promoting CLSD in other low resource settings [8]. Our findings suggest that providers sometimes have to prioritize different aspects of respectful maternity care—and they tend to choose privacy over CSLD. Overcrowding, however, did not predict continuous delivery support in the way we expected—women who felt that the facility was overcrowded were more likely to have continuous delivery support. It is unclear why this is so, but this finding highlights the importance of other factors besides crowding that may affect CSLD.

Providers gave other reasons for disallowing companions, such as mistrust and lack of confidence in companions. In contrast, women frequently expressed confidence and trust in providers, obviating the need for a companion. Providers seemed particularly distrustful of older women, and especially mothers-in-law, who are the most common companions among Kuria women. Kuria women were therefore less likely to be allowed continuous labor support, compared to Luo women, even though they were more likely to have a companion present at the facility. Providers' preference for younger female companions is reflected in women being more likely to be allowed continuous labor support if they had a sister or sister-in-law as their companion. Furthermore, being allowed labor support is predicted by socioeconomic status (SES), with wealthier, employed, and literate women being more likely to be allowed continuous labor support than poorer, unemployed, and illiterate women. This finding is consistent with the literature on differential care in health facilities based SES [38, 39]. Additionally, women with complications were less likely to be allowed continuous labor and delivery support than those without complications. The reasons for this include, a perceived need by providers to keep women's health information confidential, avoid interruptions during the care process, and protect women from companions who might not be helpful in supporting them to deal with complications. Again, it appears that providers feel the need to prioritize, and companionship is often not considered as a top priority.

Health system weaknesses also dictate the role of companions. The shortage of clinical and support staff and the burden placed on families to purchase medicines and supplies outside of the facility, have caused providers to redefine the role of companions. This is inferred when providers mostly mention instrumental support from companions as a reason for permitting women to have companions. The instrumental role of companions was mentioned as very useful in the face of staff shortages. This perspective may account for companions being more likely to be allowed in health centers, as there are usually fewer providers on duty in lower-level facilities. In addition, providers, just like the women, hardly mentioned emotional support as a reason for companionship. There is likely limited understanding among providers, as well as women, about what emotional support or woman-centered care should look like. These findings imply a complex interaction between women's needs and preferences, as well as providers needs and preferences, within facilities and systems that might not be set up to provide CSLD.

Our findings have some implications for research. First, despite WHO recommendations on birth companionship, there have been very few studies on it in SSA and other low resource settings. We need rigorous studies to better understand the effectiveness of different forms of birth companionship in these settings. For example, when women have a companion present only during labor and not at delivery, does it reduce the positive effects of CSLD and by how much? Also, given most companions in this setting are relatives and not professional support persons like doulas, how can we improve the effectiveness of CSLD? Can we learn from doula programs in developed settings and develop a cadre of providers for CSLD with whom patients can feel comfortable? Can TBAs be trained as doulas and will that be acceptable to women? (noting that none of the women in our sample was accompanied by a TBA and none mentioned a TBA as their preferred companion). Given reasons for not desiring companionship at delivery, should family members be companions during labor and post-partum and another cadre like a doula be companions for delivery? Will doula programs be feasible, acceptable, and sustainable in low resource settings? What level of training for companions is sufficient to have an impact and be cost-effective for low resource settings? Given privacy concerns and larger health systems barriers, what changes can be made to promote labor and delivery support? And how can we address the concerns of both women and providers to ensure that labor and delivery support is effective and reflects their needs and concerns.

The study has some limitations. First, the data are based on self-report. Social desirability and recall bias are thus potential limitations. Second, the findings may not be generalizable to all women and providers. in Kenya, given the peculiarities of the study County. In addition, the qualitative data may not reflect the perceptions of all women in the study County. Nonetheless, the consistency of these findings with other data from the study suggests some transferability. Despite these limitations, this study makes valuable contributions to the existing literature on social support in low resource settings. It is one of the largest and most comprehensive studies on labor and delivery support in SSA.

Conclusions

This study provides important insights that can be used to improve practice and policies on birth companionship in low-resource settings. The findings suggest that there are differences in women's desire for companionship at different phases of labor and delivery, as well as their preference for different types of companions—and these are associated with factors such as age, SES, and tribe. Therefore, it is essential for providers to understand and respect women's preferences and desires. For example, women may desire support during labor, delivery, and post-delivery; only during labor or post-delivery; or not at all; these preferences should be respected. It is also essential that providers identify women's preferred companions, and that the person who takes the woman to the facility may not be her preferred companion. Antenatal care is an opportunity to help women understand the importance of emotional support and the need to have their preferred companions with them when they go to the facility to deliver. Training providers, as well as companions, could help address the distrust and lack of confidence in companions as a barrier to allowing CSLD. It will also provide more role clarity and help highlight the value of emotional support during childbirth. In general, we need better definitions of appropriate support and interventions to sensitize women, family, and providers about the role of birth companions. Finally, many health systems in low resource settings do not have the capacity to provide CSLD. Thus, we need structural interventions within health systems to ensure that labor and delivery wards are organized in ways that facilitate CSLD. These include redesigning labor and delivery wards to have adequate space to accommodate companions and partitioning them to ensure patient privacy. Addressing the shortage of health care providers and the lack of needed drugs and supplies within maternity units (which requires family members to acquire them outside the unit) will help reduce the perceived role of the companion as an aide to providers (and one needed to run errands) and increase emphasis on their emotional support role. Without system strengthening it will be difficult to provide truly woman-centered care.

Additional files

Additional file 1: Interview guides.

Additional file 2: Coding example.

Additional file 3: COREQ checklist.

Additional file 4: Multivariate regression of desire for labor companionship and male companions on potential predictors.

Abbreviations

CSLD: Continuous support during labor and delivery; FGD: Focus group discussions; PQCC: Perceived Quality of Care during Childbirth; SSA: Sub-Saharan Africa; WHO: World Health Organization

Acknowledgments

We will like to thank Linet Ouma and Beryl Akinyi Ogola, who organized and moderated the focus group discussions and conducted the provider interviews; and all our survey data collectors. We are grateful to the PTBI-East Africa and PTBI-Kenya teams, PTBI fellowship leaders and PA's other mentors—Craig Cohen, Dominic Montagu, and Audrey Lyndon—for supporting the study. We thank the leadership of Migori County, sub-counties, and health facilities, and the community health extension workers and community health volunteers, who facilitated our entry into the County, facilities, and communities. Finally, we will like to express our gratitude to all our study participants for their willingness to share their birth stories with us.

Funding

This work was supported by the University of California, San Francisco, Preterm Birth Initiative (PTBi) transdisciplinary post-doctoral fellowship, which is funded by the Bill and Melinda Gates Foundation [OPP1107312]; and Marc and Lynne Benioff. The funders had no role in the study design, data collection and analysis, decision to publish, or preparation of the manuscript.

Authors' contributions

PA led the design and implementation of the study, conceived the manuscript, conducted the analysis, and led the writing. CK supported the analysis and writing of the manuscript. LK and DW served as mentors to PA and supported in the design and implementation of the study and writing of the manuscript. All authors read and approved the final manuscript.

Competing interests

The authors declare that they have no competing interests.

Author details

[1]Obstetrics, Gynecology and Reproductive Sciences, UCSF, San Francisco, USA. [2]Institute for Global Health Sciences, UCSF, San Francisco, USA. [3]Kenya Medical Research Institute, Nairobi, Kenya.

References

1. Montagu D, Sudhinaraset M, Diamond-Smith N, Campbell O, Gabrysch S, Freedman L, et al. Where women go to deliver: understanding the changing landscape of childbirth in Africa and Asia. Health Policy Plan. 2017;32:1146–52.
2. Graham WJ, Varghese B. Quality, quality, quality: gaps in the continuum of care. Lancet. 2012;379:e5–6.
3. Souza JP, Gülmezoglu AM, Vogel J, Carroli G, Lumbiganon P, Qureshi Z, et al. Moving beyond essential interventions for reduction of maternal mortality (the WHO multicountry survey on maternal and newborn health): a cross-sectional study. Lancet. 2013;381:1747–55.
4. Kinney MV, Boldosser-Boesch A, McCallon B. Quality, equity, and dignity for women and babies. Lancet. 2016; Available from: http://linkinghub.elsevier.com/retrieve/pii/S0140673616315252. Cited 24 Sep 2016.

5. Bohren MA, Hunter EC, Munthe-Kaas HM, Souza JP, Vogel JP, Gülmezoglu AM. Facilitators and barriers to facility-based delivery in low- and middle-income countries: a qualitative evidence synthesis. Reprod Health. 2014;11:71.
6. Tunçalp Ö, Were W, MacLennan C, Oladapo O, Gülmezoglu A, Bahl R, et al. Quality of care for pregnant women and newborns—the WHO vision. BJOG. 2015;122:1045–9.
7. WHO | Standards for improving quality of maternal and newborn care in health facilities. WHO. Available from: http://www.who.int/maternal_child_adolescent/documents/improving-maternal-newborn-care-quality/en/. Cited 4 Apr 2017.
8. Kabakian-Khasholian T, Portela A. Companion of choice at birth: factors affecting implementation. BMC Pregnancy Childbirth. 2017;17 Available from: http://bmcpregnancychildbirth.biomedcentral.com/articles/10.1186/s12884-017-1447-9
9. Bohren MA, Hofmeyr GJ, Sakala C, Fukuzawa RK, Cuthbert A. Continuous support for women during childbirth. Cochrane Database Syst Rev. John Wiley & Sons, Ltd; 2017. Available from: http://onlinelibrary.wiley.com/doi/10.1002/14651858.CD003766.pub6/abstract. Cited 29 Jul 2017.
10. Hodnett ED, Gates S, Hofmeyr GJ, Sakala C. Continuous support for women during childbirth. In: The Cochrane Collaboration, Hodnett ED, editors. Cochrane Database Syst. Rev. Chichester, UK: John Wiley & Sons, Ltd; 2013. Available from: http://doi.wiley.com/10.1002/14651858.CD003766.pub5. Cited 6 Aug 2013.
11. Maimbolwa MC, Sikazwe N, Yamba B, Diwan V, Ransjö-Arvidson A-B. Views on involving a social support person during labor in zambian maternities. J Midwifery Womens Health. 2001;46:226–34.
12. Banda G, Kafulafula G, Nyirenda E, Taulo F, Kalilani L. Acceptability and experience of supportive companionship during childbirth in Malawi. BJOG. 2010;117:937–45.
13. Alexander A, Mustafa A, Emil SAV, Amekah E, Engmann C, Adanu R, et al. Social Support During Delivery in Rural Central Ghana: A Mixed Methods Study of Women's Preferences for and Against Inclusion of a Lay Companion in the Delivery Room. J Biosoc Sci. 2014;46:669–85.
14. Berkman LF, Glass T, Brissette I, Seeman TE. From social integration to health: Durkheim in the new millennium. Soc Sci Med. 2000;51:843–57.
15. Rosen P. Supporting women in labor: analysis of different types of caregivers. J Midwifery Women's Health. 2004;49:24–31.
16. Srivastava A, Avan BI, Rajbangshi P, Bhattacharyya S. Determinants of women's satisfaction with maternal health care: a review of literature from developing countries. BMC Pregnancy Childbirth. 2015;15:97.
17. Diamond-Smith N, Sudhinaraset M, Melo J, Murthy N. The relationship between women's experiences of mistreatment at facilities during childbirth, types of support received and person providing the support in Lucknow, India. Midwifery. 2016;40:114–23.
18. Abuya T, Warren CE, Miller N, Njuki R, Ndwiga C, Maranga A, et al. Exploring the prevalence of disrespect and abuse during childbirth in Kenya. PLoS One. 2015;10. Available from: http://www.ncbi.nlm.nih.gov/pmc/articles/PMC4401776/. Cited 31 Aug 2015.
19. Ministry of Public Health and Sanitation and Ministry of Medical Services. National Guidelines for quality obstetrics and perinatal care, Kenya. 2012. Available from: https://www.k4health.org/toolkits/kenya-health/national-guidelines-quality-obstetrics-and-perinatal-care. Cited 26 Aug 2017.
20. Kabakian-Khasholian T, El-Nemer A, Bashour H. Perceptions about labor companionship at public teaching hospitals in three Arab countries. Int J Gynaecol Obstet. 2015;129:223–6.
21. Morhason-Bello IO, Olayemi O, Ojengbede OA, Adedokun BO, Okuyemi OO, Orji B. Attitude and preferences of Nigerian antenatal women to social support during labour. J Biosoc Sci. 2008;40:553–62.
22. Burke Johnson R, Onwuegbuzie AJ, Turner LA. Toward a definition of mixed methods research. J Mix Methods Res. 2007;1:112–33.
23. Tariq S, Woodman J. Using mixed methods in health research. JRSM Short Rep. 2013;4. Available from: https://www.ncbi.nlm.nih.gov/pmc/articles/PMC3697857/. Cited 5 Jan 2018
24. Migori County Health at a Glance. Available from: https://www.healthpolicyproject.com/pubs/291/Migori%20County-FINAL.pdf. Cited 2 Jun 2017.
25. Kenya National Bureau of Statistics, Ministry of Health, National AIDS Control Council, Kenya Medical Research Institute, National Council for Population and Development, Nairobi, Kenya, and The DHS Program, ICF International, Rockville, Maryland, USA. The DHS Program - Kenya: DHS, 2014 - Final Report (English). 2015. Available from: http://dhsprogram.com/publications/publication-FR308-DHS-Final-Reports.cfm. Cited 18 Feb 2016.
26. Migori County fact sheet, 2017. Available from: https://www.afidep.org/download/fact-sheets/Migori-County-fact-sheetF.pdf. Cited 12 Sep 2017.
27. Health Policy Project. Kenya County Health Fact Sheets. 2015. Available from: https://www.healthpolicyproject.com/index.cfm?id=kenyaCHFS. Cited 2 Jun 2017.
28. Thaddeus S, Maine D. Too far to walk: maternal mortality in context. Soc Sci Med. 1994;38:1091–110.
29. Gabrysch S, Campbell OM. Still too far to walk: literature review of the determinants of delivery service use. BMC Pregnancy Childbirth. 2009;9:34.
30. Afulani PA, Moyer C. Explaining disparities in use of skilled birth attendants in developing countries: a conceptual framework. PLoS One. 2016;11:e0154110.
31. Bohren MA, Vogel JP, Hunter EC, Lutsiv O, Makh SK, Souza JP, et al. The mistreatment of women during childbirth in health facilities globally: a mixed-methods systematic review. PLoS Med. 2015;12:e1001847.
32. Karanja S, Gichuki R, Igunza P, Muhula S, Ofware P, Lesiamon J, et al. Factors influencing deliveries at health facilities in a rural Maasai Community in Magadi sub-county, Kenya. BMC Pregnancy Childbirth. 2018;18:5.
33. Wanjira C, Mwangi M, Mathenge E, Mbugua G, Ng'ang'a Z. Delivery practices and associated factors among mothers seeking child welfare services in selected health facilities in Nyandarua south district, Kenya. BMC Public Health. 2011;11:360.
34. Afulani PA, Diamond-Smith N, Golub G, Sudhinaraset M. Development of a tool to measure person-centered maternity care in developing settings: validation in a rural and urban Kenyan population. Reprod Health. 2017;14:118.
35. Harris PA, Taylor R, Thielke R, Payne J, Gonzalez N, Conde JG. Research electronic data capture (REDCap) - a metadata-driven methodology and workflow process for providing translational research informatics support. J Biomed Inform. 2009;42:377–81.
36. Afulani PA, Kirumbi L, Lyndon A. What makes or mars the facility-based childbirth experience: thematic analysis of women's childbirth experiences in western Kenya. Reprod Health. 2017;14. Available from: https://www.ncbi.nlm.nih.gov/pmc/articles/PMC5747138/. Cited 7 Jan 2018.
37. Braun V, Clarke V. Using thematic analysis in psychology. Qual Res Psychol. 2006;3:77–101.
38. Andersen HM. "Villagers": differential treatment in a Ghanaian hospital. Soc Sci Med. 2004;59:2003–12.
39. Afulani PA. Rural/Urban and socioeconomic differentials in quality of antenatal care in Ghana. PLoS One. 2015;10:e0117996.

3

Midwives' experience of their education, knowledge and practice around immersion in water for labour or birth

Lucy Lewis[1,2*], Yvonne L. Hauck[1,2], Janice Butt[2], Chloe Western[2], Helen Overing[2], Corrinne Poletti[2], Jessica Priest[2], Dawn Hudd[3] and Brooke Thomson[1]

Abstract

Background: There is limited research examining midwives' education, knowledge and practice around immersion in water for labour or birth. Our aim was to address this gap in evidence and build knowledge around this important topic.

Methods: This mixed method study was performed in two phases, between August and December 2016, in the birth centre of a tertiary public maternity hospital in Western Australia. Phase one utilised a cross sectional design to examine perceptions of education, knowledge and practice around immersion in water for labour or birth through a questionnaire. Phase two employed a qualitative descriptive design and focus groups to explore what midwives enjoyed about caring for women who labour or birth in water and the challenges midwives experienced with waterbirth. Frequency distributions were employed for quantitative data. Thematic analysis was undertaken to extract common themes from focus group transcripts.

Results: The majority (85%; 29 of 34) of midwives surveyed returned a questionnaire. Results from phase one confirmed that following training, 93% (27 of 29) of midwives felt equipped to facilitate waterbirth and the mean waterbirths required to facilitate confidence was seven. Midwives were confident caring for women in water during the first, second and third stage of labour and enjoyed facilitating water immersion for labour and birth. Finally, responses to labour and birth scenarios indicated midwives were practicing according to state-wide clinical guidance.

Phase two included two focus groups of seven and five midwives. Exploration of what midwives enjoyed about caring for women who used water immersion revealed three themes: instinctive birthing; woman-centred atmosphere; and undisturbed space. Exploration of the challenges experienced with waterbirth revealed two themes: learning through reflection and facilities required to support waterbirth.

Conclusions: This research contributes to the growing knowledge base examining midwives' education, knowledge and practice around immersion in water for labour or birth. It also highlights the importance of exploring what immersion in water for labour and birth offers midwives, as this research suggests they are integral to sustaining waterbirth as an option for low risk women.

Keywords: Waterbirth, Mixed methods, Clinical confidence, Practice guideline, Learning, Education

* Correspondence: Lucy.lewis@curtin.edu.au; Lucy.Lewis@health.wa.gov.au
[1]School of Nursing, Midwifery and Paramedicine, Curtin University, Bentley, Perth, Western Australia 6102, Australia
[2]Department of Nursing and Midwifery Education and Research, King Edward Memorial Hospital, Subiaco, Western Australia 6008, Australia

Background

The provision of water immersion for labour and birth is facilitated by midwives working within low risk midwifery-led models of care who are deemed competent to provide this method of birth [1, 2]. The concept of competence is often aligned with confidence [3], but distinguishing between these two concepts is important as they are not always synonymous. A midwife may be a competent waterbirth practitioner having met all the professional competency requirements, but becoming confident is an individual journey that is dependent upon trust in clinical guidelines, presence of peer support and the challenge of achieving consistent exposure to waterbirth [4]. Additionally, midwives with extensive experience of conventional birth on land may be challenged to unlearn old skills and develop new practices required for water immersion in labour and birth. Whilst midwives working within low risk continuity of care models where physiological birth was the norm, researchers concluded that a supportive culture assisted in the development of their confidence, irrespective of clinical experience [4].

Individual midwives can act as gate keepers to water immersion which is more likely to be accepted into an organisation's culture when it is supported by midwifery managers and championed by experienced waterbirth practitioners [5]. These champions can mentor midwives who wish to achieve waterbirth competency [5]. In this situation, mentors may not always be the most senior midwives who have extensive experience with conventional birth on land. Caution is recommended to recognise and consider ways to minimise the possible hierarchical tensions that may occur when experienced midwives are mentored by junior midwives who have achieved waterbirth competency [4]. Indeed, promoting and sustaining change in midwives' waterbirth practice can be challenging. A study, undertaken in the United Kingdom (UK), utilised problem solving workshops to identify interventions that could develop and sustain a waterbirth culture. These interventions included: publishing monthly waterbirth statistics; setting a target of 100 waterbirths per annum; keeping portable birthing pools partially inflated; and appointing a waterbirth champion. Co-ordinators were able to positively influence midwifery practice through social support which was found to be pivotal in relation to developing and sustaining a waterbirth culture [6].

Access to immersion in water for labour and birth is reliant on both the care provider and the policies and procedures that guide clinical practice. Policies and guidelines in relation to water immersion for birth in Australia usually reflect the organisation's interpretation of the current literature [7]. Additionally, more evidence is required around the effect of immersion in water on neonatal morbidity [1, 8, 9] and management of the third stage of labour [7]. A literature review exploring midwives concerns around waterbirth [10] identified three clinical issues (neonatal water aspiration and neonatal and maternal infection and thermo-regulation) and two practice issues (midwives skills and education and emergency procedures around maternal collapse). The clinical issues were not evidence based and the practice issues could 'be addressed by appropriate policy, guidelines and practice' [10]. Other work exploring how a convenience sample of 249 Australian midwives utilised normal birth guidelines, found that although the majority (90%) were aware that specific guidelines existed, only 71% reported routinely using them to guide their clinical practice [11].

It has been suggested that the waterbirth environment nurtures woman-centred care by facilitating shared decision making and perceptions of control around their care [8]. However, recent Australian research found some midwives perceive waterbirth policies and guidelines can limit their scope to facilitate water immersion and did not always support women's informed choice [12].

There is limited research examining midwives' education, knowledge and practice around immersion in water for labour or birth. To address this gap in evidence and build our knowledge around this topic, our intention was to obtain a contemporary overview of midwives' experience of their education, knowledge and practice around immersion in water for labour or birth in Western Australia (WA).

Methods

The specific aim of this WA study was to assess Midwifery Group Practice (MGP) and Community Midwifery Program (CMP) midwives' experience of their education, knowledge and practice around immersion in water for labour or birth. This mixed method study was performed in two sequential phases. Phase one incorporated a cross sectional design and examined midwives' perceptions of education, knowledge and practice around immersion in water for labour or birth through a questionnaire; 34 midwives were invited to participate. Phase two employed a qualitative descriptive design to explore what midwives enjoyed about caring for women who labour or birth in water and the challenges midwives experienced with waterbirth; two focus groups were held.

Design

Mixed methods were utilised to provide in-depth knowledge [13, 14] relating to the education, knowledge and practice around immersion in water for labour or birth. This methodology offers researchers using quantitative methods the opportunity to utilise qualitative research to gain deeper understanding of the investigated phenomenon [15]. Utilising this two phase mixed methodology provided a more informative, constructive and thorough integration of the research results, building on the links between methods rather than within methods [15]. We envisaged being able to utilise both numbers and words would give greater insight into the bigger picture around midwives' experience of their education, knowledge and practice around immersion in water for labour or birth.

Participants and setting

The study was performed at the sole tertiary public maternity hospital in WA, which has approximately 5200 births annually. Women can labour and birth in the tertiary maternity hospital's Labour Ward and Birth Suite or the Family Birth Centre (an adjacent building within the hospital grounds).

Perinatal data collected in 2016, by King Edward Memorial Hospital (KEMH) in WA confirmed that 5% (228 of 4402) of infants ≥37 weeks gestation were born immersed in water. Currently WA and South Australia are the only Australian states with state-wide policies and guidance supporting immersion in water for labour and birth, although waterbirth is available in every state and territory [16, 17]. In WA midwives are guided by state-wide clinical waterbirth guidelines [16]. Between August and November 2016 we invited the 34 midwives who provided care for women who opted to use water for labour and/or birth to participate. Throughout the study, women choosing to labour and/or birth in water were cared for by midwives working within two publically funded services: the MGP and CMP. These low risk continuity of care models [18] are ideally suited to provide care for women who labour and/or birth in water, as this model facilitates a shift from high risk obstetric-led care to low risk midwifery-led care [18, 19]. Both the MGP and CMP operate their services (antenatal, intrapartum and postnatal care) from the Family Birth Centre (FBC) with the CMP also providing antenatal, intrapartum and postnatal care to women in their homes and local community clinics. In these midwifery care models, a primary midwife is supported by a small team of midwives who provide continuity of care 24 h a day throughout pregnancy, birth and up to two weeks post birth. Perinatal data collected in 2016 at KEMH confirmed MGP and CMP midwives birthed 16% (813 of 5189) of all women at KEMH. Although, no women received immersion in water for labour and birth in the tertiary maternity hospital's Labour Ward and Birth Suite throughout the duration of the study, in the last two weeks of the study the tertiary maternity hospital agreed that immersion in water for labour and birth could be facilitated in their main Labour and Birth Suite.

Recruitment and data collection

Phase one

Midwives were invited to participate in the study through an information letter and in-house designed questionnaire (Additional file 1), both of which were sent to their workplace mobile phone. Midwives who did not want to complete the online questionnaire were given the option to complete a hard copy and return it to the research team by placing it in a locked box situated in the FBC. Returning a completed questionnaire was deemed implied consent. Ethics approval was gained from the Women and Newborn Health Service Ethics Committee (Approval Number 2016103QK) at the study centre.

The questionnaire was validated through a review process with an expert panel involving a midwifery educator and three midwives who had experience caring for women who had birthed in water. Feedback from the panel resulted in changes to questions around being competent to facilitate water immersion for labour or birth and actively promoting this birth choice for labour and birth. This question was divided into two questions, one focused upon labour and another concerning birth.

The aim of the questionnaire was to examine midwives' perceptions of education, knowledge and practice around immersion in water for labour. Midwives were asked about: their employment status (if they worked in the MGP or CMP and how long they had been working as a midwife and facilitating water immersion for labour or birth); their education (training undertaken to facilitate immersion in water for labour or birth and number of births required to develop waterbirth confidence); their practice (two factors they would discuss with women in relation to water immersion for labour or birth); their confidence caring for women immersed in water for labour and birth (in the first, second and third stages of labour); their enjoyment facilitating immersion in water for labour and birth; whether they actively promote water immersion for labour and birth; and their interpretation of four scenarios around antenatal, early labour, birth and third stage clinical care. The scenarios required a written response, were scored and were based on information relating to the state-wide clinical waterbirth guidelines [16]. It was decided to give midwives completing the questionnaire a website link to the state-wide guidelines [16], in the information letter accompanying the questionnaire. By providing a website link to this guidance, we were examining how midwives interpreted and applied the guidance in their clinical practice. In relation to confidence and enjoyment, midwives were asked to place a cross on a 10 cm line (where zero was 'not confident' or 'does not enjoy' and 10 was 'very confident' or 'enjoys'), to quantify their perceptions on the continuum from zero to ten.

Phase two

An item was included at the end of the questionnaire (phase one) inviting midwives to participate in a focus group to discuss their experiences around immersion in water for labour or birth. The first author conducted the two focus groups. Observations were documented by the fourth author in the form of field notes. Each focus group lasted approximately 45 min. The focus groups were held at the study centre in an interview room that was convenient to all interested midwives. Prior to commencing the focus group, midwives were reminded that their privacy would be maintained by issuing each of them a unique identifier; the discussions linked to an individual's identity should 'remain in the room'; and that the focus group would be audio recorded. All midwives verbally consented to these conditions.

The final questions for the focus groups (Additional file 2) were based around the results from phase one, with two questions being developed: question one asked 'What contributes to your enjoyment of waterbirth?' Two prompts were utilised for this question. The first one addressed the promotion of natural birth and the second was around supporting women's choice. Question two asked 'Are there any issues with waterbirth?' One prompt was utilised around the issue of exploring which stage of labour midwives found most challenging.

Data analysis

Phase one: Quantitative data

Each of the four clinical scenarios was allocated a maximum score according to whether a midwife correctly identified key aspects of clinical practice based on the state-wide clinical waterbirth guidelines [16]. Four members of the research team independently scored each scenario. The team then met to compare scores. Any disagreement in relation to the scores was discussed and a consensus reached by referring back to the data.

Means, and interquartile ranges were used to summarise continuous data (such as the scores for each scenario). Frequency distributions were used to summarise categorical data (such as feeling equipped to facilitate waterbirth following training). Statistical software (SPSS version 22) was used for analysis.

Phase two: Qualitative data

Transcribed focus groups were subjected to thematic analysis [20] by five members of the research team, who analysed a cross-section of transcripts and field notes ensuring each data source was reviewed by at least two members [21]. Analysis required the research team to become submerged in the data. Transcripts and field notes were deconstructed enabling the research team to identify patterns, similarities and themes from the midwives' words or sentences [13, 20, 21]. The team met weekly over three months to negotiate, clarify and refine the themes. Any disagreements on interpretation were negotiated by referring back to the data. All the researchers were clinical or academic midwives, with varying experiences of facilitating immersion in water for labour or birth. As a process of member checking, preliminary themes were presented to five midwife participants who confirmed agreement with the themes.

Results

Phase one

Table 1 summarises the midwives' perception of their education, knowledge and practice around immersion in water for labour and birth. A total of 29 (85%) out of a potential 34 midwives returned a questionnaire. The mean time midwives were qualified was 162 months (13 years and 5 months), with the mean time midwives had been facilitating waterbirth being 83 months (eight years and 9 months). Most (59%; $n = 17$) midwives worked in the MGP. The majority (93%; $n = 27$) of midwives used the WA state-wide clinical guidelines for waterbirth [16] for their education and training, with 90% ($n = 26$) accessing the E-learning package developed by the study hospital's education department. Following waterbirth training, 93% ($n = 27$) felt equipped to facilitate waterbirth with the mean number of waterbirths required to facilitate confidence being seven.

On a scale of 0 to 10 (where zero was 'not confident' and 10 was 'very confident'), midwives were very confident caring for women in water during the first stage of labour (mean score of 10). They were also confident caring for women in the second stage (mean score of 9) and third stage of labour (mean score of 8). The mean score in relation to confidence using the emergency evacuation to get the woman out of the bath was eight. On a scale of 0 to 10 (where zero was 'does not enjoy' and 10 was 'enjoys'), midwives enjoyed facilitating immersion in water and birth, obtaining a mean score of 10. Finally, mean scores for the antenatal, early labour, birth and third stage of labour scenarios indicated midwives were practicing according to the WA state-wide clinical guidelines for waterbirth [16].

Phase two

Two focus groups comprising of seven and five midwives were performed. Findings are presented with supportive quotes in italics from the midwives. For confidentiality a pseudo-name was allocated to each midwife.

Caring for women who labour or birth in water

Exploration of what midwives enjoyed about caring for women who labour or birth in water revealed three distinctive themes: instinctive birthing; woman-centred atmosphere; and undisturbed space (Table 2).

Table 1 Midwives' perception of their education, knowledge and practice around immersion in water for labour and birth

Outcomes	n=29 (n%)
Months qualified as midwife[a]	162(64-247)[10-454]
Months been facilitating water immersion for labour or birth[a]	83(36-120)[4-286]
Where do you work?	
Community Midwifery Program	12(41)
Midwifery Group Practice	17 (59)
Waterbirth training	
West Australian guidelines	27(93)
Hospital based E-learning	26(90)
Observed waterbirth by midwife competent in waterbirth	26(90)
Waterbirth supervised by midwife competent in waterbirth	25(86)
Hospital study day	15(52)
Following training felt well equipped to facilitate waterbirth	27(93)
Number of waterbirths required to facilitate confidence[a]	7(4-10)[0-30]
Primary factor discussed with women	
Safety	9(31)
Eligibility	8(28)
Benefits of waterbirth	7(24)
Waterbirth process	5(17)
Confidence caring for women in water during 1st stage labour[a,b]	10(10-10)[8-10]
Confidence caring for women in water during 2nd stage labour[a,b]	9(9-10)[6-10]
Confidence caring for women in water during 3rd stage labour[a,b]	8(6-10)[2-10]
Confidence using emergency evacuation system[a,b]	8(8-10)[3-10]
Enjoy facilitating immersion in water for labour[a,c]	10(10-10)[8-10]
Enjoy facilitating immersion in water for birth[a,c]	10(10-10)[8-10]
Actively promote use of water for labour for all eligible women	28(97)
Actively promote use of water for birth for all eligible women	26(90)
Scenario 1 (Antenatal); Maximum 2 points[a]	2(1-2)[0-2]
Scenario 2 (Early labour); Maximum 3 points[a]	2(2-3)[0-3]
Scenario 3 (Birth); Maximum 2 points[a]	2(1-2)[0-2]
Scenario 4 (Third stage); Maximum 3 points[a]	2(2-3)[0-3]

[a]Mean (interquartile range)[range]
[b]Scale of 0-10. Where 0 'Not confident' and 10 'Very confident'
[c]Scale of 0-10. Where 0 'Do not enjoy' and 10 'Enjoy'

Instinctive birthing

The theme 'instinctive birthing' described how midwives perceived labouring or birthing in water nurtured an instinctive birthing behaviour led by the woman. Anna reflected '*You absolutely see the hormones that promote labour take over. You know labour progresses better and the woman relaxes into labour*'. Noreen agreed; they '*Really feel what the body is able to do and how birth feels*', whilst Kate described how she perceived water enabled her to trust a woman's ability to instinctively birth:

> *I think they progress really well. I don't do many vaginal exams, but they are getting in* [the water] *and they are well established, they are fully before you know it and they don't push early. Like sometimes with their first grunt the heads on view...They're not asking for epidurals, they're not asking for gas.*

Jasmine agreed with Kate's sentiments: '*Because you can't see as the vagina is submerged, the first sign she needs to push is she's pushing*' whilst Anna summarised her experience was that '*They're more likely to reach down and lift the baby up themselves*'.

Table 2 What midwives enjoy about caring for women who labour or birth in water

Theme	Definition of Theme
Instinctive birthing	Nurtures instinctive birthing behaviour led by the woman
Woman-centred atmosphere	Provides an environment which is woman centred, calm and peaceful and relaxed.
Undisturbed space	Creates an undisturbed space where access is mediated by the water.

Woman-centred atmosphere

The theme 'woman-centred atmosphere' described a labour and birth environment which was woman centred, calm, peaceful and relaxed. Initially midwives discussed how labouring and birthing in water empowered women. Jacquie noted '*I feel women have more control*'. Anna agreed suggesting she thought it was to do with power stating '*The woman holds more of the power in labour*'. Noreen continued the discussion '*the thing is society brings up pictures of women with somebody doing it* [the birth] *for them, there is a cultural thing of having somebody delivering the baby whilst* [with water] *there is themselves and their body*'. Bonnie reflected on Noreen's comments suggesting water promoted a change in the woman's demeanour '*You can see the change in the woman's face and in her body when she gets in the water, it's nice and relaxed*'. Beth agreed water '*Promotes the environment to be quiet and peaceful*'. Jacquie thought this may be because '*The space between contractions is very different from a land birth, they are very much more focused on their breathing and calmer*'. Whilst Noreen shared how a woman's relaxed state affected the care she gave '*You know it's all relaxed and you can concentrate more on the signs, the natural signs of a woman giving birth*'. Sophie agreed '*It's so calming for the women. I think it relaxes them which then relaxes us*'.

Undisturbed space

The theme 'undisturbed space', described how water creates an undisturbed space where access to the woman is mediated by the water. Jasmine noted that '*If you're in the bath people knock and they stay out, they leave you alone. As far as society is concerned, it's not acceptable to walk into the room when someone's in the bath. If someone's in lithotomy, fine*'. Kerry reflected it also had an impact on how safe the woman felt. '*Especially for the women who have a sexual abuse history, they feel safer in the water, they feel like you can't get at them*'. The topic of safety led to a discussion around privacy with Olivia commenting that '*It's* ['water] *their 'own space and you have to really reach into their space, rather than them being poked and prodded* [with a land birth]'. Dorothy agreed stating '*It's more undisturbed*'. Kerry continued '*Even though you can see beneath the water and everything, I think for them it just feels, more private under the water*'. Kate reflected on her experiences by recounting a scenario '*A woman that came back to the waterbirth study day and spoke about when she got in* [the pool] *there was a real sense of privacy, even though she had nothing on, the water was like a veil*'. Baily also remarked on how the 'dynamics' of a labour in water effects the partner '*I get a sense they quite like it too, because they are able to just sit and observe and hold that silent still place...my experience is that even men feel quite comfortable in that space*'.

The challenges midwives experienced with waterbirth

Analysis of the focus group transcripts exploring the question 'are there any issues with waterbirth' revealed that issues highlighted by the midwives were perceived as challenges. Two themes were identified: learning through reflection and facilities required to support waterbirth.

Learning through reflection

The theme 'learning through reflection' illustrates how midwives learnt by documenting and then reflecting on the clinical challenges encountered during their day to day clinical practice around water immersion for labour and birth. Kerry shared '*I didn't used to but since we've been doing group practice... when you look at your records you can see most of them are waterbirths*'. Olivia continued '*I don't remember all of the waterbirths...I've got a little book that I just pop them in*'. Kate reflected on her colleagues comments sharing she did not keep records of each waterbirth and that her confidence caring for women in water '*took a long time. I've probably done, I don't know over 150 now*'. Kate went on to explain why '*You had to flex the head and then move the hand and then sweep the perineum, it was really hands on. But that's how we were taught. So to move to totally hands off* [waterbirth] *where you're not even poised is challenging*'. Olivia agreed with Kate's sentiments describing a waterbirth scenario where '*I remember taking over from somebody else and it was a hypno-birth and so there was no talking...it was a good learning experience*'.

To illustrate, the topic of learning through clinical experience led to a discussion around placental cord snapping. Bonnie shared '*I've had a few cord snaps now. Like quite a few issues, but it hasn't changed my feeling of how to perform waterbirth because I know it's going to be fine and we just deal with it as it comes*'. Kerry empathised, supporting Bonnie by acknowledging '*I think a lot of midwives get anxious even though they may pretend they don't get anxious about waterbirths. They want to get the baby out as fast as possible. But I think if you make them* [the women] *aware you don't just yank it* [the baby up]*...you need to check how long it* [the cord] *is before you can go yanking*'.

Facilities required to support waterbirth

The theme 'facilities required to support waterbirth' related to ensuring waterbirth facilities were suitable, available and accessible for women and identified challenges relating to the provision of infrastructure around waterbirth. Jasmine stated:

> *If we want this option* [waterbirth] *open for all women then we need to provide the facilities for that to happen. I have an issue with it being inequitable at the moment. The Birth Centre has the birth pool and blow up pools that are free of charge whilst clients* [women] *in the main hospital and CMP have to pay and hire their own...how come one group of clients under the same public system get it for nothing and the other group have to pay?*

Sophie was also concerned by the rollout of waterbirths to the main hospital but her frustration was around the referral process. '*When waterbith was approved in the main hospital...I had a patient come over and say 'I want a waterbirth but they* [the main hospital] *won't facilitate one for me over there and they've told me to come to the Birth Centre and I was quite surprised*'. Whilst Kate's sentiments concerned the content of the waterbirth guidelines. '*When it* [the waterbirth guideline] *was first developed we didn't have telemetry and now we do. So I think waterbirth telemetry needs to be incorporated into the guideline*'. Other midwives did not appear sure of how often in-service needed to be provided in relation to emergency management, pool evacuation and assessment of blood loss. There was debate between midwives in relation to how often these drills should be performed. Dorothy confirmed *'In the CMP we have to do like a quiz, you know we put the blood in the water every six months and estimate it'*. Whilst Jacquie confirmed *'We do up a calendar* [of available professional development sessions]' and it was up to individuals to ensure their development was up to date.

Discussion

This mixed methods study enabled us to explore midwives' experience of their education, knowledge and practice around immersion in water for labour or birth in WA. Quantitative analysis found the majority of midwives felt equipped following waterbirth training to facilitate labour and birth in water, with scenario responses indicating midwives were practicing according to the WA state-wide guidance. Additionally, midwives were confident and enjoyed caring for women who used water immersion. Qualitative exploration of what midwives enjoyed about caring for women who used water immersion for labour and/or birth revealed three distinctive themes: instinctive birthing; woman-centred atmosphere; and undisturbed space. Whilst exploration of the challenges experienced with waterbirth revealed two themes: learning through reflection and facilities required to support waterbirth. Our discussion will focus on what waterbirth offers midwives.

Labouring and birthing in water is centred around the philosophy that pregnancy and birth are normal life events [19]. The importance of sustaining a waterbirth culture highlighted by these WA midwives aligns with the belief that maintaining low risk birth cultures is essential to meet the needs of healthy, low risk women through recognition and respect of midwives' contribution [22]. Midwives in this study were experts in their field, who had been qualified for a mean of 13 years and five months and facilitating waterbirth for a mean of eight years and nine months; similar to other research [6]. During the study it was agreed that immersion in water for labour and birth could be facilitated in the tertiary Labour and Birth Suite. We suggest this expertise will be integral in relation to supporting midwives in the tertiary Labour and Birth Suite to become skilled waterbirth practitioners. Indeed, an action research study introducing a problem solving waterbirth workshop with UK midwives and their co-ordinators positively affected change in waterbirth practice and was recognised for its potential shift toward normalising low risk midwifery care [6].

Midwives are guided by the International Confederation of Midwives (ICM) Position Statement on 'keeping birth normal' [23] which asserts that midwives are advocates and experts in low risk childbirth. The ICM acknowledges that 'women should have access to midwifery-led care, one-to-one support, including the choice of a home birth and immersion in water' [23] which aligns with the international recommended pathway towards evidence based respectful maternity care [24]. Utilising immersion for labour and/or birth provides midwives with an opportunity to facilitate this experience for women.

The theme of 'learning through reflection' articulated by the midwives supports the ICM Philosophy of Midwifery Care [25] ensuring competent midwifery care is informed and guided by continuous education. The association between workplace learning and competence was confirmed in a Japanese study with nurse/midwives who related learning through reflection to their self-reported competence [26]. Differences were noted based upon level of experience whereby learning from feedback and training were associated with competence for more experienced clinicians compared to learning through practice and from others for self-reported competence for those with less experience [26]. Fittingly, the Australian national competency standards for the midwife [27] present domains around the provision of woman-centred care, with one domain suitably entitled 'reflective and ethical practice'. Midwives in this study reinforce the relevance of this domain in their practice as both the clinical scenarios and focus group findings illustrated they valued having the ability and skills to analyse and reflect in, on and about practice to ultimately maintain clinical competence and confidence. In short, when care is provided by midwives who are educated [28, 29], regulated [21, 30] and provide respectful evidence based care [24], the outcomes are improved for women and their infants [1, 24, 28, 29]. The midwives in this study adhered to these principles empowering women to realise their potential to birth, though the medium of water.

Strengths and limitations

Although the quantitative methods employed provided limited scope to explore the wide range of experiences midwives in our study encountered caring for women who laboured and/or birthed in water, they did provide the research team with an objective starting point for further exploration of specific aspects of the questionnaire [21, 30]. For example, utilising a question for the focus groups gleaned from a phase one question asking midwives to score their enjoyment facilitating immersion in water for labour and birth, gave us the opportunity to contextualise what they enjoyed; providing a connection between the quantitative and qualitative components that could not be answered by mono-methods alone. By utilising both numbers and words to explore this topic [14, 15], the qualitative and quantitative components became cohesively integrated, producing research findings around midwives enjoyment which were greater than the sum of individual parts of the research [31]. This approach exposed the importance of instinctive birthing; woman-centred atmosphere; and undisturbed space.

Midwives in this study were self-selected from the MGP and CMP midwives based within the sole tertiary public maternity hospital in WA. Providing midwives with a website link to the WA state-wide waterbirth guidelines may have influenced their responses. This was a self-assessment of competence which is a subjective aptitude. The research would have been strengthened by comparing the midwives responses to their actions. Participating midwives may have been motivated and confident in their waterbirth practice. The sample of midwives included in phase one was small and may not be representative of all midwives who provide care for women who labour and/or birth in water. We acknowledge these factors could have had an impact in relation to the findings and should be considered when interpreting transferability of the findings to other settings.

Conclusion

This research contributes to the growing knowledge base examining midwives' education, knowledge and practice around immersion in water for labour or birth. It also highlights the importance of exploring what immersion in water for labour and birth offers midwives, as this research suggests they are an integral component in relation to supporting and sustaining a waterbirth culture. Midwives in this WA study were both competent and confident and enjoyed caring for women who used water immersion. Perhaps this was because the medium of water not only empowered women to realise their potential, but also themselves.

Abbreviations

CMP: Community Midwifery Program; FBC: Family Birth Centre; ICM: International Confederation of Midwives; KEMH: King Edward Memorial Hospital; MGP: Midwifery Group Practice; UK: United Kindgom; WA: Western Australia

Acknowledgements

We would like to thank King Edward Memorial Hospital for providing funding for the research staff and the midwives for graciously sharing their experiences.

Funding

The research was not supported by a research grant. King Edward Memorial Hospital provided funding for the research staff to undertake and complete the project with no role in study design, data collection, analysis, interpretation and writing the manuscript.

Authors' contributions

All authors read and approved the final version of the manuscript. LL was responsible for the proposal, ethics approval development of the data collection tool/questions and coordination of the study. For the quantitative data she assisted data entry into SPSS. She also performed the quantitative data analysis. For the qualitative data she ran the focus groups and participated in thematic analysis. She drafted the article and was responsible for the final editing which incorporated the team member's comments. YH assisted LL with the proposal and ethics approval and development of the data collection tool. For the qualitative data she participated in the thematic analysis. She assisted LL with the drafting of the article. JB assisted with development of the data collection tool/questions and made comments on the final article. CW assisted with the coordination of the study. For the qualitative data she assisted with the focus groups. She made comment on the final article. HO participated in thematic analysis. She made comment on the final article. CP participated in thematic analysis. She made comment on the final article. JP participated in thematic analysis. She made comment on the final article. DH assisted with coordination of the study. She made comment on the final article. BT contributed and approved the final article.

Competing interests

The authors declare that they have no competing interests.

Author details

[1]School of Nursing, Midwifery and Paramedicine, Curtin University, Bentley, Perth, Western Australia 6102, Australia. [2]Department of Nursing and Midwifery Education and Research, King Edward Memorial Hospital, Subiaco, Western Australia 6008, Australia. [3]Family Birth Centre, Midwifery Group Practice and Community Midwifery Program, King Edward Memorial Hospital, Subiaco 6008, Western Australia, Australia.

References

1. Lewis L, Hauck Y, Butt J, Hornbuckle J. Obstetric and neonatal outcomes for women intending to use immersion in water for labour and birth in Western Australia (2015-2016): a retrospective audit of clinical outcomes. Aust N Z J Obstet Gynaecol. 2018:1–9. https://doi.org/10.1111/ajo.12758.
2. Lewis L, Hauck Y, Crichton C, Barnes C, Poletti C, Overing H, Keyes L, Thomon B. The perceptions and experiences of women who achieved and did not achieve a waterbirth. BMC Pregnancy Childbirth. 2018;18:23. https://doi.org/10.1186/s12884-017-1637-5.
3. Ulrich B, Krozek C, Early S, Ashlock CH, Africa LM, Carman ML. Improving retention, confidence, and competence of new graduate nurses: results from a 10-year longitudinal database. Nurs Econ. 2010;28:363–76.
4. Nicholls S, Hauck YL, Bayes S, Butt J. Exploring midwives' perception of confidence around facilitating water birth in Western Australia: a qualitative descriptive study. Midwifery. 2016;33:73–81.
5. Russell K. Struggling to get into the pool room. A critical discourse analysis of midwives water birth practices. Int J Childbirth. 2011;1:52–60.
6. Russell K, Walsh D, Scott I, McIntosh T. Effecting change in midwives' waterbirth practice behaviours on labour ward: an action research study. Midwifery. 2014;30:e96–e101. https://doi.org/10.1016/j.midw.2013.11.001.
7. Cooper M, McCutcheon H, Warland J. A critical analysis of Australian policies and guidelines for water immersion during labour and birth. Women Birth. 2017;30(5):431–41.
8. Cluett ER, Burns E. Immersion in water in labour and birth. Cochrane Database Syst Rev. 2009;2:CD000111.
9. Nutter E, Meyer S, Shaw-Battista J, et al. Waterbirth: an integrative analysis of peer-reviewed literature. J Midwifery Womens Health. 2014;59(3):286–319.
10. Young K, Kruske S. How valid are the common concerns raised against water birth? A focused review of the literature. Women Birth. 2013; 26(2):105–9.
11. Toohill J, Sidebotham M, Gamble J, Fenwick J, Creedy DK. Factors influencing midwives' use of an evidenced based normal birth guideline. Women Birth. 2017;30(5):415–23.
12. Cooper M, Warland J, McCutcheon H. Australian midwives views and experiences of practice and politics related to water immersion for labour and birth: a web based survey. Women Birth. 2017; https://doi.org/10.1016/j.wombi.2017.09.001.
13. Creswell J, Plano Clark V. The foundations of mixed methods research. In: Creswell J, Plano Clark V, editors. Designing and conducting mixed methods research. London: Sage; 2011. p. 19–52.

14. Polit D, Beck C. Designing and conducting mixed methods studies to generate evidence for nursing. In: Polit D, Beck C, editors. Generating and assessing evidence for nursing practice. Sydney: Lippincott, Williams & Wilkins; 2012. p. 149–62.
15. Johnson B, Onwuegbuzie A, Turner L. Toward a definition of mixed methods research. J Mix Methods Res. 2007;1:112–33.
16. Department of Health, Western Australia (WA). WA water birth clinical guidelines. Perth: Health Networks Branch, Department of Health, Western Australia; 2009. Updated February 2017. [Cited 2017 November 22]. Available from: http://www.health.wa.gov.au/circularsnew/attachments/1195.pdf
17. Department of Health, South Australia. South Australia (SA). SA policy for first stage labour and birth in water. Government of South Australia, Department of Health. 2010. [Cited 2017 November 22]. Available from: https://www.sahealth.sa.gov.au/wps/wcm/connect/ae527200465ec14d8572ff2e504170d4/Policy-FirstStageBirthInWater-SAHealth-20101221.pdf?MOD=AJPERES&CACHEID=ae527200465ec14d8572ff2e504170d
18. Homer CS. Models of maternity care: evidence for midwifery continuity of care. Med J Aust. 2016;205(8):370–4.
19. Sandall J, Soltani H, Gates S, Shennan A, Devane D. Midwife-led continuity models versus other models of care for childbearing women. Cochrane Database Syst Rev. 2016;28:4. CD004667
20. Braun V, Clarke V. Using thematic analysis in psychology. Qual Res Psychol. 2006;3(2):77–101.
21. Lewis L, Hauck Y, Ronchi F, Crichton C, Waller L. Gaining insight into how women conceptualize satisfaction: western Australian women's perception of their maternity care experiences. BMC Pregnancy Childbirth. 2016;16:29. https://doi.org/10.1186/s12884-015-0759-x.
22. Akileswaran CP, Hutchison MS. Making room at the table for obstetrics, midwifery, and a culture of normalcy within maternity care. Obstet Gynecol. 2016;128(1):176–80.
23. International Confederation of Midwives (ICM). Position statement: keeping birth normal. 2014 [Cited 2017 November 22]. Available from: https://internationalmidwives.org/assets/uploads/documents/Position%20Statements%20-%20English/Reviewed%20PS%20in%202014/PS2008_007%20V2014%20Keeping%20Birth%20Normal%20ENG.pdf.
24. Miller S, Abalos E, Chamillard M, Ciapponi A, Colaci D, Comandé D. Beyond too little, too late and too much, too soon: a pathway towards evidence-based, respectful maternity care worldwide. Lancet. 2016;388(10056):2176–92.
25. International Confederation of Midwives (ICM). Philosophy and model of midwifery care: core document. 2014[Cited 2017 November 22]. Available from: https://internationalmidwives.org/assets/uploads/documents/CoreDocuments/CD2005_001%20V2014%20ENG%20Philosophy%20and%20model%20of%20midwifery%20care.pdf.
26. Takase M, Yamamoto M, Sato Y, Niitani M, Uemura C. The relationship between workplace learning and midwives' and nurses' self-reported competence: a cross –sectional survey. Int J Nurs Stud. 2015;52(12):1804–15.
27. Nursing and Midwifery Board of Australia (NMBA). National competency standards for the midwife. 2006: Melbourne. [Cited 2017 November 22]. Available from: http://www.nursingmidwiferyboard.gov.au/Codes-Guidelines-Statements/Professional-standards.aspx
28. Renfrew MJ, McFadden A, Bastos MH, et al. Midwifery and quality care: findings from a new evidence-informed framework for maternal and newborn care. Lancet. 2014;384(9948):1129–45.
29. Hoope-Bender P, de Bernis L, Campbell J, et al. Improvement of maternal and newborn health through midwifery. Lancet. 2014;384(994):1226–35.
30. Newton MS, McLachlan HL, Forster DA, Willis KF. Understanding the 'work' of caseload midwives: a mixed-methods exploration of two caseload midwifery models in Victoria, Australia. Women Birth. 2016;29(3):223–33.
31. Woolly CM. Meeting the mixed methods challenge of integration in a sociological study of structure and agency. J Mix Methods Res. 2009; 3(1):7–25.

4

Support provided by midwives to women during labour in a public hospital, Limpopo Province, South Africa

Maria S. Maputle

Abstract

Background: Physical presence during labour offer women opportunity of having positive childbirth experiences as well as childbirth outcomes. The study aimed to determine what support provided by midwives during intrapartum care at a public hospital in Limpopo Province. The study was conducted at a tertiary hospital in Limpopo Province.

Methods: A participant observation approach was used to achieve the objectives of the study. The population comprised of all women who were admitted with labour and for delivery and midwives who were providing midwifery care in the obstetric unit of a tertiary public hospital in Limpopo Province. Non-probability, purposive and convenience sampling were used to sample 24 women and 12 midwives. Data were collected through participant observations which included unstructured conversations with the use of observational guide, field notes of all events and conversations that occurred when women interact with midwives were recorded verbatim and a Visual Analog Scale to complement the observations. Data were analysed qualitatively but were presented in the tables and bar graphs.

Results: Five themes emerged as support provided by midwives during labour, namely; communication between women and midwives, informational support, emotional support activities, interpretation of the experienced labour pain and supportive care activities during labour.

Conclusion: The communication between woman and midwife was occurring as part of midwifery care and very limited for empowering. The information sharing focused on the assistive actions rather than on the activities that would promote mothers' participation. The emotional support activities indicated lack of respect and disregard cultural preferences and this contributed to inability to exercise choices in decision-making. The study recommended the implementation of Batho Pele principles in order to provide woman-centred care during labour.

Keywords: Support offered, Labour pains, Communication between women and midwives, Informational support, Emotional support, Physical comforting measures

Correspondence: sonto.maputle@univen.ac.za
Department of Advanced Nursing, University of Venda, Private Bag X5050, Thohoyandou 0950, South Africa

Background

The Batho-Pele Principles in the White Paper introduced a customer-focused approach with the aim of transforming systems, procedures, attitudes and behaviour within the childbirth units and re-orient midwives in the customers' favour, an approach which put people first [1]. In this study, the observations were focused on consultation, standard, courtesy and information. These would be evident when women were treated with courtesy and consideration; it was observed whether mothers were allowed to practice their preferences during childbirth (courtesy). The practice in public hospitals, mothers were provided with full and accurate information regarding childbirth process and midwifery and intrapartum care which they were entitled to receive (information). Hence, the researcher conducted the study to determine the support provided by midwives to women during labour at a public hospital in Limpopo Province. Support provision during labour was viewed to be having impact on the childbirth experience as well as on childbirth outcomes [2]. Midwives are there to provide support to women to offer them strength of facing challenge of giving birth without losing control [3, 4].

Provision of support during labour is important and is continuous, so as reduce the risk of medical interventions, like emergency caesarean section or regional analgesia maybe less prevalent and labour maybe shorter [5]. The labour supporter could play a major role in increasing women's chances to have a positive initial breastfeeding experience. Rosen [6] describes support as an interactive process which may be affected by persons' age, experience, and personality as well as by the environment [6]. Whereas Simkin [7] views labour support as continuous presence, emotional support that includes encouragement, guidance, and reassurance; physical comforting which was assistance in carrying out coping techniques, use of touch, massage, positioning, and movement) [7]. Simkin further indicate that labour support includes provision of information and guidance to the woman and her partner; and to further assist the woman to express her needs and wishes; and provision of advice, anticipatory guidance, and explanations of procedures [7]. Labour support was viewed as an affordable intervention that responds to the basic emotional and physical needs of a woman during a painful and vulnerable moment of her reproductive carrier – child birth.

The pain during labour is a physiological phenomenon [8]. Ralph et al. [8] further pointed that, sources of pain during the first stage was associated with reduced blood supply to the uterine muscles during contractions. In the second stage, the source of pain was associated with the stretching of vaginal wall and perineum and compression of pelvic structures during the passage of descending head. The pain that women experienced during labour was affected by multiple physiological and psychological factors and its intensity varied greatly.

In studies "*Experiences of mothers of care provided by midwives during childbirth* by Maputle and Nolte [9] and *Experiences of midwives of providing care to women during childbirth*" by Maputle and Hiss [10] it was noted that the labour ward of a tertiary hospital was experiencing shortage of staff and open plan labour ward with no privacy and this had negative impact on the allowing the male partner to support to women during labour. There was shortage of midwives wherein, one midwife would care for more than one woman at the same time. The remarks cited by mother transcripts' were: *"I couldn't communicate freely with the midwife because she was very busy, but she examined me when I reported/ requested help. The midwife was busy with other mothers; she was not in my cubicle throughout the childbirth".* This was supported by the study of Schafheutle et al. [11]., who indicated that inadequate nursing staff in a shift may contribute to lack of time in providing adequate care and this is cited as barrier to effective pain management, by interfering with applying non-pharmacological pain relief methods.

In the same study by Maputle and Nolte [9], authors found that one participant preferred the male partner to be available during childbirth; however, her wish was not honoured because of the physical structure of the ward. Tournaire and Theau-Yonneau [12] pointed out that the availability of doula to provide support was considered an important part of natural pain relief methods. Leeman et al., [13] advocated for the effective use of conventional approaches to emphasize the interaction between mind, body and environment [13]. Lack of social and emotional support from partner/ doula or excessive medical intervention to women during labour is factors that may be related to increased intensity of pain [14]. Labour support could be perceived as the presence of an empathic person who offers information, comforting measures and other forms of tangible assistance to enable a woman cope with the stress of labour and birth. At this public hospital, women were always alone during labour. In South Africa, the provision of midwifery care during labour should be aligned to Batho-Pele Principles, namely; consultation, service standard, courtesy, access, information, openness and transparency, redress and value for money [1]. It was against this background that the study was conducted.

Methods

Study design

A qualitative participatory research approach was used to determine the support provided by midwives to women during labour at a public hospital in Limpopo Province.

Study setting

The study was conducted in the labour ward of a public hospital in Limpopo province, South Africa. The hospital is a 509 bed hospital, out of these beds only 45 were allocated to labouring women. The total number of normal deliveries would be ±10 per day. The total number of midwives who were allocated in the units during the day was twenty (but on duty there would be eight midwives, because some would be on leave or off duty).

Population and sample

Population comprised of all women, admitted in labour to deliver their babies and the midwives who were providing midwifery care and who consented to participate in the study. Non-probability, convenience and purposive sampling in De Vos et al., [15] were used. Only women who were found to be in labour during the day of data collection were included in the study. The selection of midwife was guided by whether the midwife who is on duty had been already observed when providing care. The inclusion criteria for women were: full term pregnancy (38–42 weeks) and should be in early active phase of labour (cervical dilatation of 3–10 cm, regular uterine contractions), with the presence of the foetal heart beat. All the midwives who had at least two years' experience in the labour unit who agreed to participate in the study. The researcher sampled women and midwives [16]. The sample comprised of 24 women and 12 midwives.

Data collection

Data were collected by researcher who is a holder of PhD in Midwifery and Neonatal nursing, during the day shift in August – December 2015. The researcher was also shared the same culture and language with participants. The researcher collected data through participant observations which included semi-structured observational guide, observing the activities, interactions and conversations between the women and the midwives during intrapartum care (Additional file 1). The use of participant observation gave additional and more accurate information on behaviour of people [17]. This semi-structured observation method enabled the researcher to describe events and behaviour as they occurred during labour [17]. Observations were limited to the interaction between a woman and a midwife during labour and the midwifery care rendered that is; communication, informational support, emotional support activities, physical comforting measures rendered and supportive care activities when the woman is experiencing labour pains. Observations were carried when a woman was in the active phase of labour, when the cervical dilatation was 3 cm to the delivery of the placenta. The unstructured conversations were held informally with women and midwives throughout labour, because these conversations were spontaneous and emerged out of natural social interaction and contributed to the depth and richness of information that otherwise would have been difficult to capture through more structured interviews. Field notes of events were recorded in a notebook and conversations that occurred when women interact with midwives were recorded verbatim by the use of a voice recorder. To complement the informal conversations, Visual Analog Scale (VAS) which is an instrument and a simple scale was completed by the women and midwives independently during the following dilatations of the cervix 0–3, 4–7 and > 8 cm. Recording of field notes form a core of record [17]. It entailed both the empirical observations and their interpretation.

Data analysis

Biographical data of both women and midwives and the data obtained through the unstructured observation guide, the VAS were analysed through frequency distribution and the data were presented as percentages in tables and bar graphs and clustered into 5 themes [18]. The field notes and informal voice conversations were analyzed qualitatively through open coding and were mergered with the 5 themes.

Ethical considerations

Ethical clearance was obtained from the Ethics Committee of the University of Venda (SHS/11/PDC/001) and permission to access the health facility and conduct the study from the Provincial Department of Health. The principles of informed consent, beneficence and right to privacy were observed. Participation in the study was voluntary and no remuneration was given. The consent of participants was obtained before data collection.

Results

Theme 1: Communication between women and midwives during labour

Communication between women and midwives during labour was determined by observing the interactions and activities as presented in Fig. 1:

- Ability of midwife to empower the woman
- Enabling the woman to feel special and relaxed (by explaining the physiological changes and encouraging relaxation exercises)
- Advocacy skill
- Determining the woman's cultural and personal preferences
- Continuous updating on foetal and maternal progress

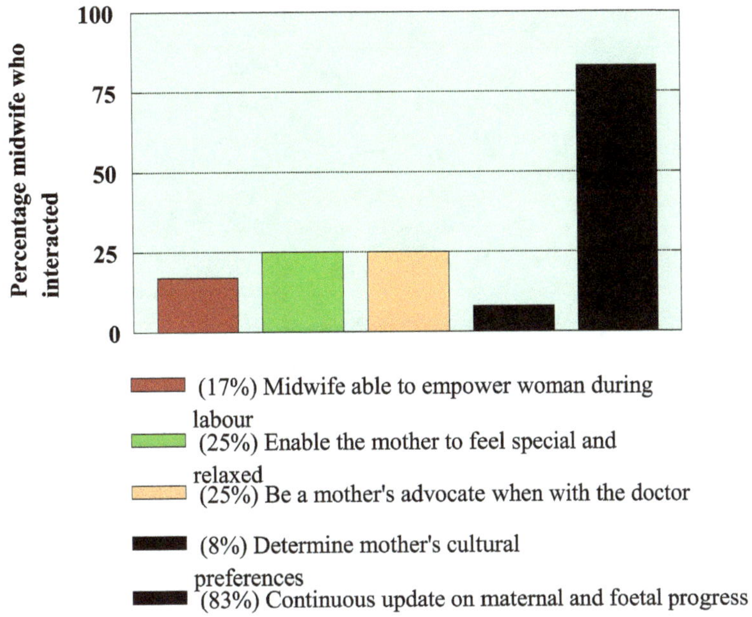

Fig. 1 Interaction/ communication between women and midwives

The observation showed that (10) 83% of midwives where continuously updated the mother on maternal labour progress and on foetal well-being. Limited affective communication was displayed which was thought to facilitate mutual participation as evidenced by (3) 25% of midwives advocating mothers when with the doctor, (2) 17% of the midwives were able to empower mothers, (3) 25% of the midwives were enabling the mother to feel special and relaxed and (1) 8% of the midwives determined the mother's cultural/personal preferences. Some of the direct quotes from participants that indicate limited empowering during labour were *"my midwife was not telling me what is happening and I think she must be patient and at least listen to what I want to say"*. With regard to determining the mother's cultural preferences, one participant said *"Hmm ... I didn't clearly understand the language of the midwife"*, so this indicated that cultural preferences were not determined. Another participant said *"if I indicate the cultural preference she didn't allow or even listen to why I was making such a preference."*

Theme 2: Informational support during childbirth

From the profile of mothers recruited for the study (Table 1), 23 (96%) did not participate in childbirth preparation classes. Only 1 (4%) mother participated in childbirth classes, hence it can be inferred that mothers probably had limited information support from the attending midwives during childbirth. To determine whether informational support was given by the attending midwives to mothers during childbirth, the observed informational support as presented in Fig. 2, namely;

- Answering of mother's questions
- Allowing/encouraging mothers to ask questions
- Advising mothers on the physiological changes of labour
- Offering mothers opportunities to come up with suggestions
- Extending advice and encouragement
- Guiding and assisting mothers throughout delivery

It was noted that (9) 75% of the midwives advised mothers on changes taking place during childbirth and guided and assisted them throughout childbirth. Actions that were promoting mothers' participation were limited as only (4) 33% of the midwives extended encouragements, (1) 8% offered opportunities for mother to give suggestions whilst (1) 8% of attending midwives allowed mothers to ask questions which were answered during childbirth.

The observation was supported by the direct quotes from a labouring woman who said *"my midwife was telling me to breathe in and out but I didn't know why."* This showed that midwives are giving advice and encouragement but not advising on the labour changes. However, the other participant said *"Midwives should give me information, and then I would be able to make choices. So as I'm updated with the progress of labour I'm able to make informed choices like relaxation techniques."*

Table 1 Demographic profile of mothers and midwives recruited for the study

Mothers	N = 24	%	Midwives	N = 12	%
1. Age in years on your last birthday			1. Gender		
16–20	7	29	Male	0	0
21–30	12	50	Female	12	100
31+	05	21			
2. Parity:			2. Qualifications		
Primigravida	13	54	Registered midwife	10	83
Para 2–3	07	29	Advanced midwife	02	17
Para 4+	04	17			
3. Delivery outcome (exclude fetal deaths			3. Duration of allocation in labour ward - years		
Normal vaginal delivery	19	79	2–4	06	50
Forceps or vacuum extraction delivery	0	0	5–6	04	33
Caesarian section (not elective)	05	21	> 7	02	17
4. Duration of labour (hours)			4. Cultural/ Ethnic group		
2–4	2	8	Northern Sotho	9	75
5–8	4	17	Tsonga	2	17
> 9	18	75	Venda	1	8
			Others	0	0
5. Pain relief during labour			5. Religious affiliation		
Pharmacological	03	13	Protestants	4	33
Non-pharmacological	21	87	Apostolic church	2	17
			Zion Christian church	2	17
			Others	4	33
6. Cultural/ Ethnic group					
Northern Sotho	15	63			
Tsonga	4	17			
Venda	3	12			
Others	2	08			
7. Family status					
Married	10	42			
Single	14	58			
Divorced	0	0			
Widow	0	0			
8. Religious affiliation					
Protestants	14	58			
Apostolic church	3	13			
Zion Christian church	7	29			
Others	0	0			
9. Educational status					
Never literate	2	8			
Primary school literate	5	21			
Secondary school literate	9	38			
Tertiary institution	8	33			
10. Companion present?					
Yes	0	0			

Table 1 Demographic profile of mothers and midwives recruited for the study *(Continued)*

Mothers	*N* = 24	%	Midwives	*N* = 12	%
No	24	100			
11. Participation in childbirth preparation classes					
Yes	1	4			
No	23	96			
12. Transfer from another hospital					
Yes	5	21			
No	19	79			

Theme 3: Emotional support during childbirth

To determine the emotional support given by the attending midwives to mothers during childbirth, the following were observed:

- Instilling of confidence (with information provided) and encouragement of companion to be present during labour
- Be understanding, friendly and reassuring
- Encouraging free choice and full participation
- Fostering the integration of cultural/personal preferences
- Show of respect

It was observed that midwives offered limited emotional support during childbirth as evidenced by the observation that (0) none of the midwives encouraged the presence of a companion and integration of cultural/personal preferences during childbirth. Only (4) 33% of attending midwives showed respect for mothers during labour whereas (3) 25% were encouraging free choice and full participation of the mothers. A significant number of attending midwives (8) 67% displayed an understanding, friendly and reassuring attitude to mothers during childbirth. Figure 3 illustrates that only (4) 33% of the midwives showed respect for mothers. Some midwives were encouraging participation and this was

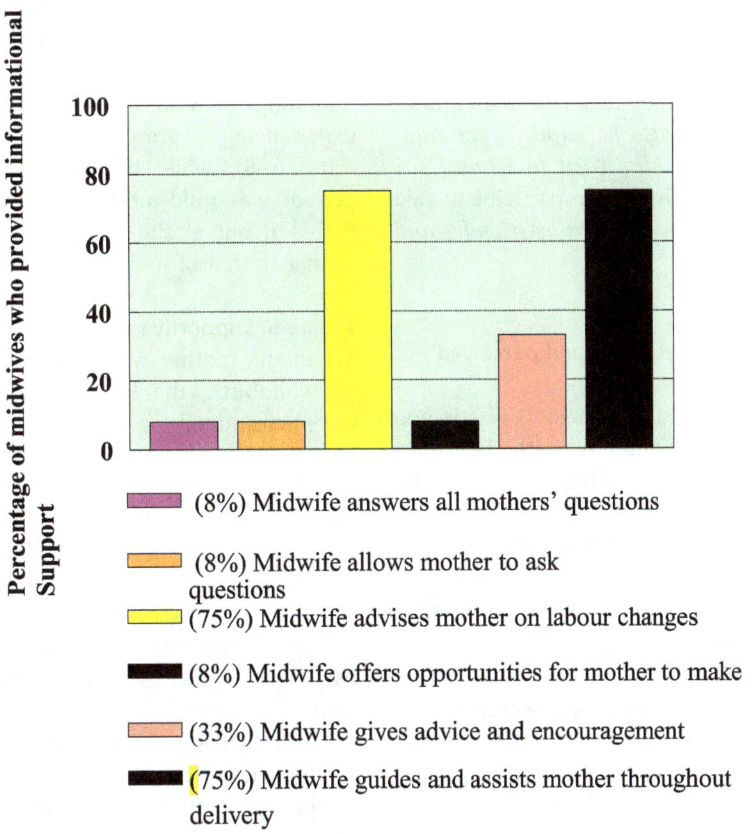

Fig. 2 Informational support and exchange between mothers and attending midwives

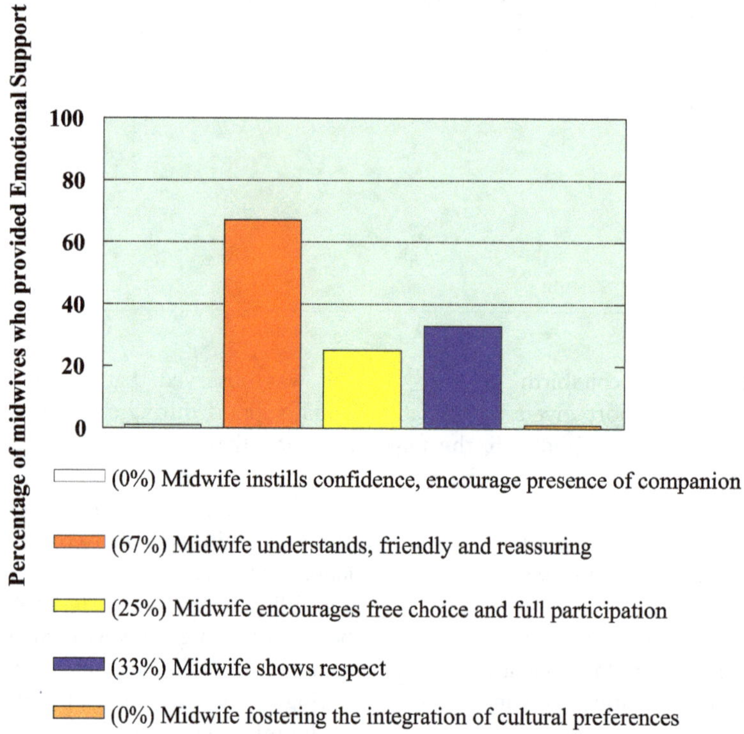

Fig. 3 Emotional support activities by attending midwives during labour

confirmed by one participant who said "*When I was experiencing severe pain, she told me to lie on the side, sit or adopt any position that I feel comfortable.*" However, contrary to the observed friendliness and reassurance the participant said "*I would also be happy if the midwives can be more approachable, listen to what I say and not to be too harsh.*" The other participant said "*During childbirth I expect midwives to be friendly and to respect me as an adult.*"

Theme 4: Interpretation of experienced and perceived pain during labour

The visual analog scale (VAS, 100 mm tool) was issued to mothers and their attending midwives with the aim of comparing the pain experienced among mothers during childbirth and to observe the awareness and responses of the attending midwives to the pain exhibited by mothers. Mothers and their attending midwives had to complete the scale independently during the following phases of cervical dilatation:

- 0–3 cm, mothers were experiencing moderate pain while attending midwives perceived as mild pain
- 4–7 cm, mothers experienced severe pain while midwives still perceived this as mild pain
- 8–10 cm, both groups experienced and perceived pain as severe.

All assessments were completed independently and without reference to the previous rating. Findings as presented in Fig. 4.

Findings on VAS on Fig. 4 indicated that mothers were experiencing severe pain throughout labour (with a pain score 6–8), while the pain midwives exhibited (perceived) was mild-moderate at the beginning of labour (2.5–4.5) but at the end of labour, the pain score was similar to that of mothers (9.5).

Theme 5: Supportive care activities during labour

When the mother was responding to contractions during childbirth, the following supportive care activities were determined:

- Provision of physical care
- Attendance to the elimination needs
- Midwife caring for more than one mother at the same time

Figure 5 presents the findings of supportive care activities by midwives when mothers were experiencing pain.

All midwives provided care for mothers' elimination needs. Midwives could not give individual care to mothers, as they were caring for more than one mother at the same time. There was a shortage of staff as (2) 17% of the midwives were caring for more

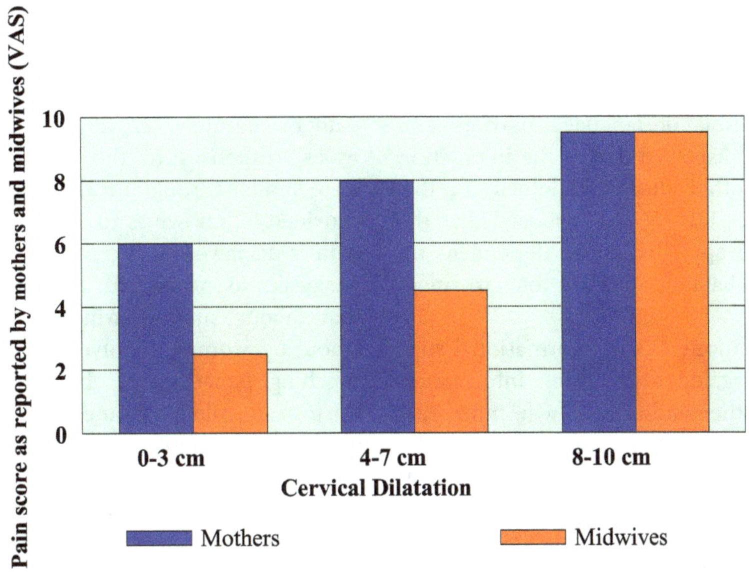

Fig. 4 Pain scores by visual analogue scale

than one mother. Only (3) 25% of midwives provided physical care during childbirth (physical care include touching, rubbing/ massaging).

The quotes from participants that supported the observation as cited by one participant was *"the midwife was good to me, because she was assisting me with my elimination needs, hence I was able to deal with my pain."* However, another woman said *"I am waiting for that other midwife, as the one who was helping me has left".* For this woman, the midwife was caring for more women.

Discussion

Five themes emerged as support provided by midwives during labour, namely; communication between women and midwives, informational support, emotional support activities, interpretation of the experienced labour pain and supportive care activities during labour. It was noted that communication between the woman and the midwife occurred more when the midwife was rendering midwifery care and very limited during affective communication. Watkins [19] pointed out that determining women's preferences for their care in labour is a

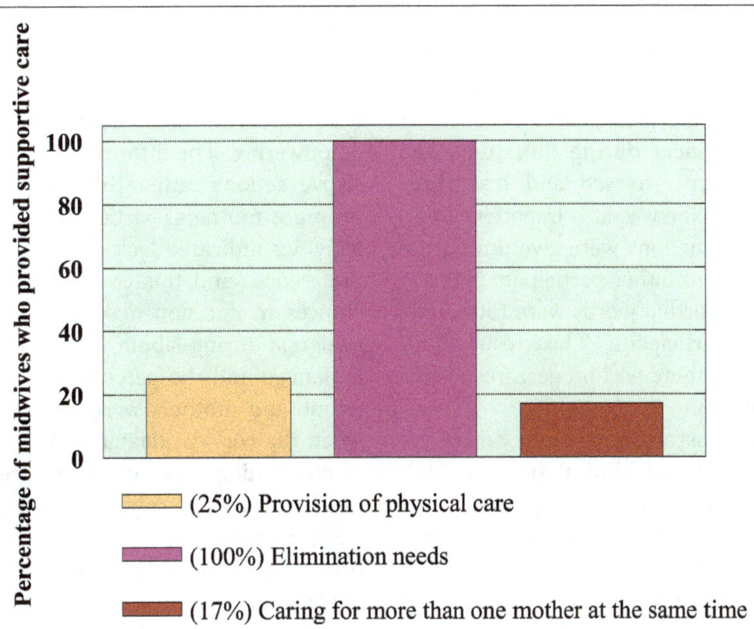

Fig. 5 Supportive care activities by attending midwives during labour

reasonable basis for caregiving activities. Table 1 indicates that from the total population of mothers ($n = 24$) recruited in the study, 9 (37%) did not share the same language with the attending midwives. Hindered verbal communication as a result of language barriers and non-listening skills were displayed during the interaction of a midwife and a mother during childbirth in this study. Persson and Dykes [20] firmly supposed that the experience of good care appeared to be dependent on communication and behaviour to be able to meet mothers just as they are.

Analysis of the observations in the informational support theme, (Fig. 2) revealed that during information sharing between the mother and the midwife more emphasis was placed on the assistive actions than on the activities that would promote mothers' participation. Bergstrom et al., [21] indicated that women want information about pain and fear and how to mitigate both, explanations about the instruments and processes involved in birth, and positive communication. The amount and type of information sharing, to include explanations about the process of birth, reports about descent of the foetus's head, and soliciting information about the woman's well-being. Bryanton et al., [22] supported that when women have more information about what is happening to and around them and are given options about position changes and timing of pushing, they can take control of the birth.

Rice [23] indicated that lack of respect and disregard of the choices for mothers, in the mothers' narratives, contribute to apathy towards respect in their treatment and inability to exercise choices in decision-making. Respect empowers women [24]. Results also indicated that none of the midwives encouraged the presence of a companion during childbirth. Brown [25] wrote that the reasons for this restriction may include negative attitude of labour ward staff toward the presence of outsiders in the labour ward. In an incident during the study, one midwife participant was very stressed and insensitive with an instructive attitude. She was also impatient to an extent that little or no explanations were give during the provision of care. Hence, the mother participant was absolutely terrified as no comforting words were forthcoming from the midwife participant. This resulted in mother not co-operating as there was no gestures of understanding between the two.

The VAS is one of the most used pain assessment instruments, both in research and clinical practice [26]. With the VAS, mothers were experiencing severe pain throughout labour while the pain perceived by midwives was mild-moderate. This was supported by Baker et al. [27] who found that midwives were less able to assess pain accurately when women described their pain as severe. The patient's verbal report is considered to be the single most reliable indicator of how much pain she is experiencing [28]. However, at the end of labour pain score for both mothers and midwives was similar. Pain research indicated that midwives often assess patients' pain inaccurately [27, 29]. On observation of the midwives' responses to the mothers' pain, the responses were similar throughout the childbirth process. The care provided by midwives to the mothers when experiencing pain is displayed in Fig. 5. Very few mothers were given analgesics as prescribed. Hodnett, et al., [30] reinforced that labour support which is non-medical care of a labouring woman, involves physical comforting such as touching, massaging, bathing, grooming, applying warmth or cold Teshome et al., [31] emotional support such as continuous companion, reassurance, encouragement, anticipatory guidance, information provision, and non-medical advice. Whereas Mackey [32]; Lundgren [33] considered praise, flexibility, acceptance, information giving, encouragement, friendliness, presence, confidence, and assisting with breathing and relaxing to be aspects of helpful nursing qualities during labour.

Limitations

Data was only collected during the day shift from 07 h00 to 18 h00 the support provided by night shift staff could have given different results. The use of participatory observations by semi-structured observational guide may have been influence observer preconceived ideas, which may affect the results of the study.

Conclusions

The tertiary hospital was challenged with the shortage of staff and this contributed to one midwife to caring for more than one woman at a time. Hence, midwives were mainly providing care for mothers' elimination needs. The communication was occurring when the midwife was rendering midwifery care and very limited for empowering. The information sharing focused on the assistive actions rather than on the activities that would promote mothers' participation. The emotional support activities indicated lack of respect and disregard cultural preferences and this contributed to inability to exercise choices in decision-making. Mothers were never given analgesic during labour because the interpretation of experienced and the perceived pain by midwives were different, and mothers were perceived to be in severe pain when the cervical dilatation was 9–10 cm. The presence of companion was not encouraged, hence physical care include touching, rubbing/ massaging were limited. The study recommended the implementation of Batho Pele principles in order to provide woman-centred care during labour.

The recommendations were aimed at improving the standard of the public service and effective service delivery to support women during labour. Services should be based on a customer-orientated framework. These principles were integrated within the framework to provide woman-centered care as follows:

- Midwives are to consult mothers about the level of midwifery care to be received and, where possible, should give (allow) involvement and support choices about the services that are offered (consultation).
- Mothers should be told what level and quality of midwifery care (intervention are to be provided so that they would be aware of what to expect (service standard).
- Mothers are to be treated with courtesy and consideration; they should be allowed to practice their preferences during childbirth (courtesy).
- Midwives should allow all mothers equal access to personal control and decision-making (access).
- Mothers should be given full and accurate information about the childbirth process and midwifery care which they are entitled to receive (information). The Department of Public Service and Administration [1] indicates that the importance of the public service delivery lies in the need to build confidence and trust between the provider (midwife) and the user (mother) through openness and transparency.

Sandall [34] and Midmer [35] were in support of customer-oriented service delivery when they pointed out that the philosophy and focus should shift from technologization to personalization, and to building of the paradigm of woman-centered practice that will be based on equal partnership between mothers and attending midwives.

Abbreviation

VAS: Visual Analog Scale

Acknowledgements

Acknowledgements are extended to the midwives and mothers for agreeing to participate in this study. Limpopo Department of Health for providing permission to access the facilities.

Author's contribution

MS (University of Venda) used the framework from the Doctoral thesis to conceptualise data collection, analysis, literature search and article writing. The author read and approved the final manuscript.

Competing interest

The author declares that she has no financial or personal relationship(s) which may have inappropriately influenced her in writing this article.

References

1. Department of Public Services and Administration. White paper on transforming public service delivery, Government Gazette 388 (18340), Government Printer, Pretoria. 1997.
2. Raphael-Leff J. Psychological processes of childbearing. 4th ed. Guildford, UK: Anna Freud Centre; 2005.
3. Lundgren I. Releasing and relieving encounters. Experiences of Pregnancy and Childbirth: Faculty of medicine, Uppsala University, Uppsala, Sweden; 2002.
4. Kennedy HP. The midwife as an "instrument" of care. Am J Public Health. 2002;92(11):1759–60.
5. Hodnett ED, Gates S, Hofmeyr GJ, Sakala C, Weston J. Continuous support for women during childbirth. Cochrane Database Syst Rev. 2013;2: CD003766.
6. Rosen P. Supporting women in labor: analysis of different types of caregivers. Journal of Midwifery and Women's Health. 2004;49(1):24–31.
7. Simkin P. Reducing pain and enhancing progress in labour: a guide to non-pharmacologic methods for maternity caregivers. Birth. 1995;22(3):161–71.
8. Almushait M, Ghani RA. Perceptiontoward non-pharmacological strategies in relieving labour pain: An analytical descriptive study. J Nat Sci Res.4(2):2014.
9. Maputle MS, Nolte AWG. Mothers' experience of labour in a tertiary care hospital. Health SA Gesondheid. 2008;13(1):55–62.
10. Maputle MS, Hiss DC. Experiences of midwives managing women during labour at a tertiary care hospital in the Limpopo Province. Curationis. 2010; 33(3):5–14.
11. Schafheutle EI, Cantrill JA, Noyce PR. Why is pain management suboptimal on surgical wards? J Adv Nurs. 2001;33(6):728–37.
12. Tournaire M, Theau-Yonneau A. Complementary and alternative approaches to pain relief during labor. Evidence Based and Complementary Alternative Medicine. 2007;4(4):409–17.
13. Leeman L, Fontaine P, King V, Klein MC, Ratcliffe S. The nature and management of labour pain: part 1. Non-pharmacological pain relief. Am Fam Physician. 2003;68(6):1109–13.
14. Zwelling E, Johnson K, Allen J. How to implement complementary therapies for laboring women. American Journal of Maternal and Child Nursing. 2006; 31(6):364–70.
15. De Vos A, Strydom H, Fouche C, Delport C. Research at grassroots for the social sciences and human professions. 3rd ed. Pretoria: JL Van Schaick; 2011.
16. Strauss A, Corbin J. Basics of qualitative research: grounded theory procedures and techniques. 3rd ed. Newbury Park, CA: Sage; 2008.
17. Hardon AP, Boonmongkon P, Streefland P, et al. Qualitative data collection techniques. In: Applied Health Research Manual: Anthropology of Health and Health Care, Module 17; 1994.
18. Brink H. Fundamentals of research methodology for health care professionals. Juta: Cape Town; 2012.
19. Iliadou M. Supporting women in labour. Health science. Journal. 2012;6(3): 385–91.
20. Persson EK, Dykes AK. Parents experience of early discharge from hospital after birth in Sweden. Midwifery. 2002;18:53–60.
21. Bergstrom L, Richards L, Proctor A, Bohrer-Avila L, Morse JM, Roberts JE. Birth talk in second stage labor. Qual Health Res. 2009;19:954–64.
22. Bryanton J, Gagon AJ, Johnston C, Hatem M. Predictors of women's perceptions of childbirth experience. J Obstet Gynecol Neonatal Nurs. 2008; 37:24–34.
23. Rice PL. What women say about their childbirth experiences: the case of Hmong women in Australia. Journal of Reproductive and Infant Psychology. 1999;17(3):237–53.
24. Gibbins J, Thomson AM. Women's expectations and experiences of childbirth. Midwifery. 2001;17(4):302–13.
25. Brown H, Hofmeyr GJ, Nikodem VC, Smith H, Garner P. Promoting childbirth companions in South Africa: a randomised pilot study. BioMedCentral Medicine. 2007:5–7.
26. Myles PS, Urquhart N. The linearity of the visual analogue scale in patients with severe acute pain. Anaesth Intensive Care. 2005;33:54–8.
27. Baker A, Ferguson SA, Roach GD, Dawson D. Perceptions of labour pain by mothers and attitudes of their midwives. J Adv Nurs. 2001;35:171–9.

28. Jensen MP, Karoly P. Self-report scales and procedures for assessing pain in adults. In: Turk DC, Meltzack R, editors. Handbook of pain assessment. New York: The Guilford press; 2001.
29. Solomon P. Congruence between health professionals 'and patients 'pain ratings: a review of the literature. Scandinavian Journal Caring science. 2001; 15:174–80.
30. Hodnett ED, Gates S, Hofmeyr GJ, Sakala C. Continuous support for women during childbirth. Cochrane Database Systematic Review. 2007;18(3): CD003766.
31. Teshome M, Abdella A, Kumbi S. Parturients' need of continuous labor support in labor wards. Ethiop J Health Dev. 2007;21(1):35–9.
32. Mackey MC, Stepans ME. Women's evaluations of their labor and delivery nurses. J Obstet Gynecol Neonatal Nurs. 2006;23(5):413–20.
33. Lundgren I. Releasing and relieving encounters: experiences of pregnancy and childbirth. Scand J Caring Sci. 2004;18(4):368–75.
34. Sandall JSH, Gates S, Shennan A, Devane D. Midwife-led continuity models versus other models of care for childbearing women. Cochrane Database Syst Rev. 2013;8:CD004667.
35. Midmer DK. Does family-centered maternity care empower women? The development of the woman-centered childbirth model. Fam Med. 1992; 24(3):216–21.

5

Male adolescents' role in pregnancy prevention and unintended pregnancy in rural Victoria: health care Professional's and educators' perspectives

S. Connor[1*], K. Edvardsson[2,3] and E. Spelten[4]

Abstract

Background: While there has been a steady decline in adolescent pregnancies worldwide and in Australia over the last three decades, Australian rates still rank third highest among developed countries. Adolescent pregnancies are defined as those that occur to girls between the ages of 15 and 19. The current pregnancy rate of 15 to 19 year old females rural Victoria is 21.19%, this is more than double the Victorian state rate of 8.2% and almost double the national Australian rate at 13.1% The aim of this study was to explore Health Care Professionals and Educator perspectives on these high adolescent pregnancy rates, with particular focus on the role of adolescent males, in a rural region in Victoria, Australia.

Methods: A qualitative descriptive study using focus group discussion was undertaken with Health Care Providers and Educators ($N = 8$) in 2016. Data was analysed using thematic analysis.

Results: Four themes emerged from analysis. The first, 'Gender Stereotyping' focused on the acceptance of traditional masculinities; the second 'Adolescent males as health consumers' was based on the consensus that adolescent males are poor consumers of health and 'invisible'; the third 'Complexity of Issues' identified that, particularly in a rural region, contributing issues are varied and complex; and the fourth 'Focus on Fatherhood', saw the participants diverge from the discussion about pregnancy prevention and the adolescent males' role in unintended pregnancy, and focus on the role adolescent males may have as unintended fathers.

Conclusions: Participants did not consider young males to be of importance in the prevention of adolescent pregnancy. There is a need to further explore the role of young males in pregnancy prevention, including what role traditional gender stereotyping, from health professionals' and young males' perspectives, plays in provision of adolescent sexual health services.

Keywords: Rural adolescent males, Health care providers, Educators, Teenage pregnancy, Qualitative study

Background

Despite the worldwide decline in adolescent pregnancies, rural adolescent teen pregnancy rates continue to rise in Australia. Adolescent pregnancies are defined as those that occur to girls between the ages of 15 and 19 and while there has been a steady decline in adolescent pregnancies and births worldwide since 1990, currently 11% of all births are to girls aged 15–19, and 95% of these births occur in low and middle-income countries [1]. In Australia adolescent pregnancy, rates have also declined but in rural Victoria, the current pregnancy rate for 15 to 19 year old females is 21.19%. This is more than double the Victorian state rate of 8.2% and almost double the national Australian rate at 13.1% [2].

While not all adolescent pregnancies and births are unplanned, the often negative consequences of being an adolescent single parent and the effects for the children and society, are well documented. Among the most

* Correspondence: s.connor@latrobe.edu.au
[1]Department of Rural Nursing & Midwifery, La Trobe Rural Health School, Vic, Mildura 3500, Australia

significant consequences for adolescent single mothers and their children, are an increase in welfare dependency and poverty. Young mothers are also at high risk of poor emotional health including depression and anxiety, which may be linked to social isolation due to disengaging from high school and becoming isolated from peers [3, 4]. Non-completion of secondary schooling reduces employment opportunities [3, 4]. Children of adolescent mothers are also at higher risk of developing behavioural problems, being injured in an accident, and having lower levels of literacy and numeracy skills [1, 3–5].

The focus of this study is adolescent males in a rural Victoria region. The particular region was identified for several reasons. The region has a population of approximately 59,000 and includes an indigenous population of 2516 people, a further 30.7% of total population were born overseas [6]. The region has been identified as the third most disadvantaged region in Victoria, with only 22.9% of residents completing Year 12 level schooling and an unemployment rate at 6.6% compared with the Victorian state average of 5.4% [7].

With a rate of adolescent pregnancy at over half the national average, this region has a significant number of adolescent females and males who experience unintentional pregnancy. The purpose of this study was to explore Health Care Professionals' and Educators' perspectives on prevention of adolescent pregnancy and the male adolescents' role in unintended pregnancy and pregnancy prevention, as a growing body of evidence suggests that Health Care Professionals are failing to provide adolescent males with support services, equivalent to those, that are made available to young adolescent women [8–12].

Methods

Research design

This study utilised qualitative descriptive methodology. Qualitative description is a paradigm of qualitative research that requires the researcher to provide a detailed interpretation of the data that is explained in every day terms rather than through a theoretical lens. Qualitative descriptive studies draw on naturalistic inquiry to enable the researcher to establish solid and meaningful findings [13–16].

Purposive sampling was used to recruit participants, and inclusion criteria for participants included being a Health Care Provider or Educator currently working in the identified rural Victorian region. There was no pre-requisite regarding experience with either adolescent pregnancy or male adolescent sexual health.

Twenty-three potential participants were contacted via email and provided with written information about the study, aim and procedures, eight of whom took part in the focus group. Three potential participants responded but declined for various reasons including work and family commitments. Eight potential participants did not respond to the invitation or the two email reminders. Twelve potential participants in total accepted the invitation; however, four did not attend on the day. An overview of the participants is presented in Table 1.

A focus group discussion was chosen as the best method for data collection as this forum allows homogenous groups to come together to explore views, feelings and experiences regarding a specific topic for the purpose of collecting research data [17–20].

Five questions were developed that were intended to provoke in-depth discussion amongst the group members. The participants were asked to consider and share their experiences with adolescent males that they may have had in regard to pregnancy prevention and unintended pregnancy, in their role as professional caregivers and educators. To aid in the generation of meaningful data, further question were then posed regarding the participants knowledge of current health services for adolescent males, and any challenges they were aware of in this area. Finally the participants were offered the opportunity to add a final comment to the discussion.

The discussion was moderated by the first author (SC) and was recorded for verbatim transcription. Field notes were taken during the discussion to add richness to the data set by both co-authors (KE & ES). All participants were provided with a pseudonym, de-identified transcripts were returned to the participants for comment and member checking, prior to commencing analysis.

Thematic analysis was determined as a suitable approach to use with qualitative descriptive research. It is a rigorous systematic framework used to identify themes within the collected data, that lead to an understanding of the participants' experience [14–16, 21]. Analysis commenced with the familiarisation of the transcribed Focus Group discussion and field notes, by first author, SC. All data was read repeatedly and patterns and meanings, both manifest and latent, were actively looked for during this phase [22]. Once familiarity with the data was achieved, a list of initial codes was produced. Each code included relevant content from the data [16]. The codes where then clustered into potential categories

Table 1 Participant overview

Midwives	2
Social worker	3
Sexual health nurse	1
Mental health nurse	1
GP	1
Females	6
Males	2
Education sector	1
Health care sector	7

using colour codes to identify the category with the code and data. These categories were reviewed and collated into larger themes, ensuring that the data included within each was both distinct and meaningful. A thematic map was developed at this stage to help describe the relationship between the codes, categories and the themes [16, 22]. The thematic map and coded data sets were then shared with the co-authors, ES and KE, for further review. A detailed analysis of each theme was conducted ensuring that each theme was authentic and congruent with the overall narrative [16, 22].

The consolidated criteria for reporting qualitative research (COREQ) checklist, was utilised to determine rigor of research design and transparency of reporting of results [23].

Results

Analysis of the focus group transcripts provided four clear themes, emerging from the categories and codes. The following discussion will provide a description of the themes using quotations from the focus group to illustrate.

Gender stereotyping

The first focus group question 'what is your experience of adolescent males in relation to pregnancy and pregnancy prevention' was posed as a way of initiating conversation around adolescent males within the participant group. The participants responses clearly indicated themes relating to gender stereotyping (Table 2).

The initial response from all participants was a strong feeling that 'boys will be boys'

> *"They're quite proud of spreading their seed around and making lots of babies and not sticking around with the mums, where I am from"*
>
> Participant B, Sexual-Health Nurse.

However, this initial response quickly faded away to be replaced with a real sense that adolescent males are rarely seen by Health Professionals or Educators in relation to sexual health and adolescent pregnancies. Several participants expressed this opinion quite strongly,

> *"I would say where I work, with the community that I work with, they are almost invisible."*
> Participant C, Community Midwife

> *"I have very few health encounters where an adolescent male will come in to talk about pregnancy or pregnancy prevention."*
>
> Participant E, General Practitioner.

The discussion regarding the male adolescent role was very limited. Moreover, perhaps can be best summed up by one participant, who stated,

> *"This [adolescent pregnancy] wasn't something that I had ever considered from the male perspective."*
>
> Participant H, Primary Mental Health.

The participants however did express more detailed views regarding how they saw the female in this situation. The two main schools of thought regarding the young females, related to what they considered 'feminist' issues and their own professional standards. The participants felt that young women had to some degree taken on board a feminist stance and in doing so perhaps prevented the male's right to contribute to a decision.

> *"You know where it's [continuing with the pregnancy] considered a female decision."*

Table 2 Gender stereotyping

	Codes	Categories	Theme
• Adolescent boys are not seen in Health care services • They don't often seek help/support at school • We don't consider the needs of boys in our service • I've never thought about teenage pregnancy from the male perspective	Invisibility	Masculinity	Gender stereotyping
• Young boys sow their wild oats • They refuse to wear condoms • They wouldn't take a male pill if it was available • Boys have no responsibility	Boys will be boys		
• Young girls want to become pregnant • Once she is pregnant it is her choice -not his • The female has the right to choose	Her body -Her choice	Femininity	
• I only see the female once she is pregnant • The female is my patient/client not her boyfriend • The focus of care is on the mother to be	She is the client		

Participant F, Social worker [Education]

"[the girls say] this is my body my rights."

Participant A, Social worker.

One of the strongest views to arise at this time however was around professionalism. The health professionals in particular were quite adamant that the female, whether seeking pregnancy prevention advise or care during pregnancy, was their client and the male partner was not. Therefore, the focus for them was on the female.

"When we had a young person that was pregnant all the focus would be about getting the female to appointments and putting all the supports around her."

Participant F, Social worker

"...and, well they're [the male] not your client per se."

Participant C, Community Midwife

Well I can only speak from a medical professional, I've no right to see their [the males] medical history. I'm her carer so unless there is a reason to know or he chooses to tell me I don't have any real need.

Participant E, General Practitioner.

Adolescent males as health consumers

Overwhelmingly all participants agreed that adolescent males were difficult to engage in any form of health initiatives let alone sexual health and pregnancy prevention (Table 3). Unlike adolescent females who need to present to a sexual health service or GP clinic for contraception or health checks, there is limited need for an adolescent male to seek health advice.

"You don't need a script for condom you know, so, that's taken out of the face to face contact, but, so you miss that opportunity to have that discussion."

Participant E, General Practitioner

"Occasionally I'll see a boy, a male, in that age group if he actually has some weird something coming out of his penis. Otherwise we rarely see them..."

Participant B, Sexual-Health Nurse.

All the participants were able to discuss a wide range of services that they knew of that were available to young adolescent males in the region. These services however were in the whole, related more to Mental Health and Wellbeing than sexual health. There was only one dedicated sexual health service represented and they admitted to not seeing many young males.

"We rarely get boys in unless they are either dragged in by their partner or they have actually got symptoms that worry them."

Participant B, Sexual-Health Nurse.

This prompted discussion around adolescent males and Sexually Transmitted Infections (STIs), most participants felt that targeting the young male's health from this perspective might be more successful than trying to engage

Table 3 Adolescent males as health consumers

	Codes	Categories	Theme
• Services at High Schools with Mental Health Focus • Sexuality Education focused on females	Mental Health & Wellbeing	High School Services	Adolescent Males as health Consumers
• Boys are lost after primary school • No incentive for boys to seek health care	Disengagement	Sex Education	
• Religion has an influence on sex education in private schools	Religion		
• Focus on STIs not pregnancy • Males respond more to STIs as they are affected • STIs are treatable so they (boys) don't care	Boys & STIs		
• Males only seek health care in emergencies • Males rarely engage with our sexual health service • We only see them if they are dragged in by their partner • It's difficult enough to engage adult males let alone adolescents	Getting males to see a HP	Accessing Health	
• There is a need for male sexual health workers	Male health Workers		

them in pregnancy prevention. STI's present and actual immediate impact to their lifestyle.

> *I guess talking about the use of condoms and things, and not just saying that it prevents pregnancy but also sexual disease. You know we keep saying um, you need condoms to prevent pregnancy but what about the sexual health.*
>
> Participant D, Community Midwife

> *"It may actually be generally a better approach. Men may actually respond to that because there is an outcome that they don't want."*
>
> Participant A, Social worker.

Once the participants had identified this lack of need for adolescent males to seek health care, they linked this back to Sex Education in schools. The participants felt that this was the last chance they had to interact with young boys before they left primary school and entered adolescence. Those services that provided Sex Education did so to either the grade five or six class, making the children around 10–12 years of age. There were several different programs depending on state and school. One service had begun an 'Advanced Sex Ed' class, which included the parents and contained some explicit information regarding consent, pornography and body image.

> *Just going that one step further about consent and um, a little bit more a bit about, bit about pornography and um, body image and that sort of stuff and stepped it up just that little bit further into talking about sex really.*
>
> Participant B, Sexual-Health Nurse.

School based sex education however appears to be ad-hoc at best. One health care professional expressed her frustration at needing to be 'slotted' in amongst the school's other curriculum requirements.

> *It's very difficult these days to actually get into the schools, they plan their curriculum the year before if not two years before um and unless you factor that in.*
>
> Participant B, Sexual Health Nurse.

There is also the issue of the type and quality of sex education that is being provided through school-based programs. In particular, the parochial schools in the region do not participate in nurse led sex education programs. There was concern amongst the focus group participants that this may lead to the students being taught sex education based on the tenants of their religion rather than evidenced based best practice.

> *I did talk to the, one of the Vice Principal's there [Parochial School] about what they do in terms of contraception education, he said they talk about everything except termination and the morning after pill because they are abortion.*
>
> Participant B, Sexual Health Nurse.

However, the group consensus was that school based sex education programs often felt futile, as this was often the last contact that that any health service has with the males and they become disengaged from this point until well into adulthood.

> *"We have identified that they get lost once they go to high school."*
>
> Participant B, Sexual-Health Nurse

> *"Men's health in general is difficult, it's hard to get men engaged generally so young men who just don't care about anything apart from themselves really is even more difficult."*
>
> Participant B, Sexual-Health Nurse.

All participants of the focus group bar two were female and this was an accurate representation of the regions workforce. The participants all felt that one area that may go a long way to improve adolescent male health interactions was in developing a more gender balanced health work force within the health care and education sectors.

> *I think it's a disadvantage being a female, when we had a young male health worker we seemed to get more young men in but they don't want to see, someone the age of their mother*
>
> Participant B, Sexual-Health Nurse

> *"I just think if there were more perhaps male nurses doing sexual health, we would have better access to young males".*
>
> Participant C, Community Midwife.

Complexity of issues

All participants agreed that the issue of adolescent males and their sexual health needs was a complex issue involving, but not confined to, risk taking behaviors such as alcohol and illicit substance abuse. The issue is complicated further by the rural location and the implication of low socio-economic status, limited access to sexual health services and a real or perceived lack of confidentiality within a small community. These themes came up repeatedly throughout the focus group discussion (Table 4).

A noteworthy consideration at this point, is that, while the participants all acknowledged adolescent males as the more likely risk takers, the focus of their discussion continually returned to their experiences with adolescent females.

Risk taking was seen by the participants to be a generally accepted adolescent behavior, which led to poor decision-making followed by ambivalence of the consequences. In particular they had concerns regarding use of drugs and alcohol in the community for both genders, but were only able to relate instances regarding adolescent females.

> *"Yeah I think systemically we have got significant issues with risk taking behaviours like drugs and alcohol".*
>
> Participant F, Social worker [Education]

> *Somebody who comes in and says. 'oh, I would never do that, or I would never consider myself to be someone who is promiscuous but, it was the drugs and the alcohol*
>
> Participant E, General Practitioner

> *One of the things that we haven't really talked about in this particular question is around drugs, in particular, and the impact on choices that they {females] make with regard to their sexual behaviour and I think it's really disturbing, frankly, you start being substance affected and you don't care.*
>
> Participant A, Social worker.

The participants also felt that adolescents of both gender where ambivalent regarding the outcomes of unprotected sex.

> *I think there's ambivalence on both parts though, like from what I see they're pregnant, they're not actually wrapt about it, but they're not too bothered that's just what happened, go on with it, and he kind of just, is the same um probably there is less expectation that he will be involved but, everybody seems reasonably okay with that scenario, is what I kind of see, yeah*
>
> Participant C, Community Midwife

All participants agreed that the regions geography played an important part in the high statistics for unintended adolescent pregnancy as does, a lack of access to family planning services and a perceived lack of confidentiality amid the services that are available in a small community However they were unable to discuss this from the adolescent male perspective and focused instead on the adolescent female who was unintentionally pregnant.

Table 4 Complexity of issues

	Codes	Categories	Theme
• Perceived & real lack of confidentiality • Family or friends work in health services • Local issues with confidentiality	Confidentiality	Rurality	Complexity of Issues
• Not enough services for adolescents in general • Limited access to choices such as termination • There is a need to travel to many services	Access		
• Parents of adolescents often uneducated • Adolescent motherhood is a generational issue • There are low expectations for adolescents in this region • Many don't finish school	Socio-Economic Status		
• Alcohol and drugs are often involved • Alcohol and drugs lead to poor choices	Drugs/Alcohol	Risk Taking Behaviours	
• The boys just don't care • It can be seen as 'cool' to be a young parent	Ambivalence		
• Its normal for indigenous community • There are cultural issues involved • Our indigenous boys' health checks are not focused on sexuality	Cultural	Indigenous	

To get a termination in [this region] you've got to go see your GP by 13 weeks you can't just get on the train and go to Melbourne whereas if your somewhere in a town closer to Melbourne it's not as difficult to get a termination

Participant C, Community Midwife.

This was the same for the discussion around socio – economic status. It was generally agreed that one of the major reasons for the high adolescent pregnancy rates was directly related to the low socio-economic status of the region. However the focus for this discussion was limited to the population in general rather than the adolescent males.

"I also do think that the population that we have and the demographics that we have has a big bearing on the outcomes so, the high teenage pregnancy rates".

Participant D, Community Midwife

The socio-demographics really need to be looked at, and education, possibilities, options, opportunities that are in [the region], and how its [education] valued here or not valued here, and the percentage of parents who are not employed.

Participant A, Social Worker.

One smaller sub-theme, adolescent Indigenous health, emerged in this category; it is limited to a sub-theme, as it did not generate a significant amount of data. However, considering the rural location of the region and the large indigenous population, as previously outlined, it warrants inclusion. Only one participant, differentiated between indigenous and non-indigenous adolescents.

We also have the highest aboriginal population and it its normal for aboriginal girls to start their families younger. We have the highest per capita aboriginal population in the state so.

Participant C, community Midwife

The research team did not separate indigenous adolescent males from the research question cohort as, at this stage, the study is exploring Health Care providers and educators' perspectives on adolescent males in general, not specific groups of the population.

There was considerable knowledge amongst the focus group participants regarding various Health Education Programs aimed at Adolescent Indigenous Males, though none of these has a focus on Sexual Health or Pregnancy prevention.

Focus on fatherhood

One of the strongest themes to emerge from the data was Focus on Fatherhood (Table 5). It was evident from previous themes that consideration of adolescent males in relation to pregnancy prevention and unintended pregnancy was a new perspective for the focus group participants. Many of them though had strong views on adolescent males as Fathers. There was a general group consensus that adolescent males are not willing to commit to parenting. A perception however, that was not necessarily based on clinical experience but personal opinion.

and I think they [adolescent males] start off quite positive like with good intentions, but then they don't know how to make it work possibly cause all the other stuff gets in the way you know whether it be poverty or drugs.

Participant F, Social Worker [Education]

"Well they turn 18 and they've got freedom".

Participant C, Community Midwife

"Who wants to be home with the baby when they could be out partying with their mates".

Table 5 Focus on fatherhood

	Codes	Categories	Theme
• Young men want to be fathers too • We need to support our young dads • We need to teach them how to be dads	Support them as fathers	Fatherhood	Focus on Fatherhood
• Young mums can be at risk of domestic violence • Many young couples have complex legal issues • We need to protect the young mothers	Violence	Partners needs	
• Adolescent males do not commit to parenting • Successful teen couples are a minority	Young males don't commit		

Participant B, Sexual-Health Nurse

Several of the participants whose services provided assistance for adolescent mothers expressed that often exclusion of the male partner was due to their concern for the safety of the young women in their care.

> *The relationships are so volatile aren't they, they're in love one minute a week later and they're in court getting an intervention order and then you know they've moved on to the next partner.*
>
> Participant F, Social Worker [Education]

> *The cycle of violence is, such as it is, I'm assuming everyone understands probably better than I do and um you know that's another reason why we are pretty protective around the mums.*
>
> Participant A, Social Worker.

The final discussion point relating to adolescent males as fathers saw the group participants recognise that there is very limited support available to any adolescent males who do intend to stay involved in the pregnancy and take on the role of fatherhood.

> *You [females] go to your maternal and child health nurse and you learn you know certain techniques and things you can do to settle, but the guys don't learn that, so they need to be included in that process as well, so they can feel confident because I think a lot of it is also confidence.*
>
> Participant G, Social Worker

> *Even to the point where um men can get, I think its two weeks paid leave that's it. You know we don't as a society or a government or whatever value the male's role in that parenting anyway, so you know it's from the top down really.*
>
> Participant C, Community Midwife

> *It's also about the need for organisational and cultural change, so as service providers, we're thinking about adolescents as parents, adolescent males as parents rather than the focus that is on the females all the time. As service providers we actually start that conversation to get it more mainstream.*
>
> Participant D, Community Midwife.

Discussion

This purpose of this study was to explore Health Care Professionals and Educators perspectives on the male adolescents' role in unintended pregnancy and pregnancy prevention in a rural Victorian region.

There are several limitations to this study, including the small sample size, with only eight participants in the focus group. However the authors believe that the participants were a fair representation of the health care professionals within this rural community and quality data was obtained. Another limitation is that whilst one Health Care Professional was working in the education sector, no educators attended. This in itself it not a considerable issue as all Health Care Professionals act in the role of educators when providing client care. Furthermore, six of the eight participants were female and only two males. While this is representative of the gender balance within the health sector, having more males involved in the focus group may have given the data broader gender perspectives.

While it is self-evident that adolescent males are an important link in preventing unintended pregnancies, the findings of this focus group discussion clearly indicated that, health care professionals and educators in this rural region, do not consider them to be relevant in this context and that their focus is neither on male adolescents nor on prevention but mostly on supporting the adolescent mothers with unintended pregnancies.

There was a strong perception amongst the focus group participants that despite current discourse around gender equity, traditional gender roles play a role in the increasing number of unintended adolescent pregnancies. Traditional masculinity socialises young men to project strength and dominance, particularly over women [24, 25]. The focus group participants observed that the behaviour of the adolescent males in this rural region was typically 'boys being boys' who were 'sowing their wild oats'. Not only does this traditional masculinity seem to be accepted as normal in this rural region but the focus group participants did not believe that it was within their power to positively impact on this ideology. The young females in contrast are seen to be control of their own choices and bodies. The focus of care provision for the participants is with the adolescent females who are unintentionally pregnant.

Much of the published literature refers to adolescent males as invisible and hard to reach [8–10, 26]. The findings of this research project appear to substantiate this data. The health care professionals and educators involved in the focus group discussion, all identified adolescent males as a cohort that is very difficult to engage in any kind of health care strategy let alone one that is focused on pregnancy prevention and unintended pregnancy. This lack of interaction with health care, correlates with traditional masculinity norms that reinforce beliefs around the male body being strong [24, 25]. In contrast to this, the same participants were not consciously aware prior to participating, that adolescent males were not present within the context of the adolescent unintended pregnancies they came into contact with. This raises questions as to how health care professionals and educators can change their practices to include adolescent males in the care of their partners when experiencing unintended pregnancies.

The issue of adolescent males, pregnancy prevention and unintended pregnancy is clearly complex. The focus group participants identified a multitude of contributing factors, some such as confidentiality and access to family planning services, are related to the rurality of the region [27]. Others such as, male risk-taking behaviours and ambivalence, are further related to traditional masculinity [24, 27]. While all participants agreed strongly that these factors were real and important, they felt disempowered to address these issues in any significant way. The participants also had difficulty considering these issues from the adolescent male perspective. With the exception of risk –taking behaviours, all issues were only discussed from the perspective of the adolescent female who is unintentionally pregnant. This again serves to illustrate the limited contact with adolescent males that the participants have.

A significant positive change the focus group participants discussed, was potentially increasing support for adolescent males who unexpectedly found themselves as prospective fathers. Some participants still held reservations around the apparent suitability of the adolescent males to be involved with the mother and child, citing cycles of violence and lack of commitment on the males' part as worrying issues. Interestingly both violence towards partners and lack of commitment are seen as components of traditional masculinity, which once again reinforces the accepted stereotype in this rural region [24, 27]. The greater majority of participants however felt that benefits could be gained for all concerned if they were able to provide greater level of support to adolescent males who choose to remain involved in the pregnancy and play a role in fatherhood. This ideal is supported by Bunting & McCauley [8], Osborn [9] and Paranjothy et al. [10], who all identified that many young fathers, rather than being invisible and hard to reach, actually feel excluded from being involved in the pregnancy and fatherhood by Health Care Professionals.

Conclusion

In order to prevent and reduce unintended adolescent pregnancy, health care professionals and educators need to acknowledge that adolescent males are an integral part of this complex issue. Acceptance of traditional masculinity behaviours as an explanation for perceived adolescent male behaviour only serves to perpetuate gender stereotypes and does not help to solve the problem.

Further research to gain an understanding of adolescent males' perceptions of their own masculinity may be helpful in providing health care workers and educators enhanced understanding of the decisions that these young men make and work towards dispelling the gender stereotypes.

The responsibility for finding these invisible and hard to reach young men, rests in the professional duty of the health care professionals and educators. These professionals need to alter their current thinking and begin to develop more inclusive practices so that the significant issue of prevention of adolescent unintended pregnancy can be addressed.

Abbreviations

STI's: Sexually transmitted infections

Authors' contributions

SC facilitated the focus group discussion supported by KE and ES who took comprehensive field notes. SC conducted the analyses in collaboration with KE and ES. SC drafted the manuscript with input from KE and ES, all authors contributed to ongoing revisions of the manuscript and approved of definitive version. All authors accept responsibility for submitted manuscript.

Competing interests

The authors declare that they have no competing interests.

Author details

[1]Department of Rural Nursing & Midwifery, La Trobe Rural Health School, Vic, Mildura 3500, Australia. [2]Judith Lumley Centre, School of Nursing and Midwifery, La Trobe University, Vic, Bundoora 3086, Australia. [3]Department of Clinical Sciences, Obstetrics and Gynecology, Umeå University, 901 87 Umeå, SE, Sweden. [4]Department of Public Health, La Trobe Rural Health School, Mildura, Vic 3500, Australia.

References

1. World Health Organization. Adolescent Pregnancy, [Internet]. 2017. Available from: http://www.who.int/mediacentre/factsheets/fs364/en/. Accessed 10 Sept 2016.
2. Australian Bureau of Statistics. Media release – new data from the 2011 census reveals Victoria's most advantaged and disadvantaged areas. [internet]. Australian bureau of Statistics (2015). Births Australia, 2015 (Catalogue No 3301.0). Canberra: ABS; 2015. Available from: http://www.abs.gov.au/ausstats/abs@.nsf/Lookup/by%20Subject/2033.0.55.001~2011~Media%20Release~2011%20Census%20(SEIFA)%20for%20Victoria%20(Media%20Release)~3. Accessed 16 Oct 2016.
3. Boulden K. What it takes supporting pregnant and parenting young people The Association of Women's Educators National Symposium. Brisbane. [Internet]. 2009. Available from: http://www.awe.asn.au/drupal/sites/default/files/what_it_takes.pdf. Accessed 4 Oct 2016.
4. Marino J, Lewis LN, Bateson D, Hickey M, Skinner SR. Teenage mothers. Australia Family Physician. 2010;45(10):712–7.
5. Department of Prime Minister and Cabinet. A stronger, fairer Australia National statement on Social Inclusion. Canberra: Commonwealth of

Australia; 2009. Available from: http://www.voced.edu.au/content/ngv%3A45844. Accessed 6 Sept 2016.
6. Australian Bureau of Statistics. 2016 Census Community Profiles (Code SSC21671 (SCC)). Canberra: ABS; 2016. Available from: http://www.censusdata.abs.gov.au/census_services/getproduct/census/2016/communityprofile/036?opendocument. Accessed 16 Oct 2016.
7. Australian Bureau of Statistics. Labour Force, Australia, Detailed – Electronic Delivery (Catalogue No 6291.0.55.001). Canberra: ABS; 2013. Available from: http://www.abs.gov.au/ausstats/abs@.nsf/mf/6291.0.55.001. Accessed 16 Oct 2016.
8. Bunting L, McAuley C. Research Review: Teenage pregnancy and parenthood: the role of fathers, Child and Family Social Work [Internet]. [2004]; 9, 295–303. Available from: https://doi.org/10.1111/j.1365-2206.2004.00335.x.
9. Osborn M. Young fathers: unseen but not invisible. Families, Relationships and Societies [Internet] [2015]: 4, 2, pg. 323–329. Available from: https://doi.org/10.1332/204674315X4352272532129.
10. Paranjothy S, Broughton H, Adappa R. Teenage pregnancy: Who suffers? Archive of Disease in Childhood, [Internet]. 2009;94(3):239–45. Available from: https://doi.org/10.1136/adc.2007.115915
11. Ayton J, Hansen E. Complex young lives: a collective qualitative case study analysis of young fatherhood and breastfeeding. Int Breastfeed J, Work [Internet]. [2016]; 11(1):6. Available from: https://doi.org/10.1186/s13006-016-0066-9.
12. Fagan J, Bernd E, Whiteman V. Adolescent Father's parenting stress, social support, and involvement with infants. J Res Adolesc. 2007;17(1):1–22.
13. Schneider Z, Whitehead D, LoBiondo-Wood G, Haber J. Nursing & midwifery research, methods & appraisal for evidenced-based practice. 5th ed. Chatswood: Elsevier; 2013.
14. Sandelowski M. Focus on Research Methods Whatever Happened to Qualitative Description? Research in Nursing & Health, 23[2000], 334–340. [Internet]: Available from: https://doi.org/10.1002/1098-240X(200008)23:4%3C334::AID-NUR9%3E3.0.CO;2-G.
15. Sandelowski M. what's' in a name? Qualitative description revisited, Research in Nursing health, 33, 77–84. [Internet] [2010]: Available from: https://doi.org/10.1002/nur.20362.
16. Vaismoradi M, Turunen H, Bondas T. Content analysis and thematic analysis: implications for conducting a qualitative descriptive study. Nursing Health Sci[2013], 15, 398–405; [Internet] Available from: https://doi.org/10.1111/nhs.12048.
17. Curtis E, Redmond R. Focus groups in nursing research. Nurse Researcher. 2007;14(2):25–37.
18. Krueger RA. Is it a focus group? Tips on how to tell. J Wound, Ostomy Continence Nurses. 2006;33(4):363–6.
19. Lane P, McKenna H, Ryan A, Flemming P. Focus group methodology. Nurse Researcher. 2001;8(3):45–59.
20. Parahoo K. Nursing research principles, process and issues. 2nd ed. New York: Palgrave Macmillan; 2006.
21. Minichiello V, Sullivan G, Greenwood K. In: Axford R, editor. Research methods for nursing and health science. 2nd ed. Australia: Prentice-Hall; 2004.
22. Braun V, Clarke V. Using thematic analysis in psychology. Qual Res Psychol. 2006;3(2):77–101. [Internet]: Available from. https://doi.org/10.1191/1478088706qp063oa.
23. Tong A, Sainsbury P, Craig J. Consolidated criteria for reporting qualitative research (COREQ): a 32-item checklist for interviews and focus groups. Int J Qual Health Care. 2007;19(6):349–57.
24. Courtenay WH. Constructions of masculinity and their influence on men's well-being: a theory of gender and health. Social Sci Med. 2000;50:1385–401.
25. Lohan M, Cruise S, O'Halloran P, Alderdice F, Hyde A. Adolescent men's attitudes in relation to pregnancy and pregnancy outcomes: A systematic review of the literature from 1980–2009. J Adolesc Health [Internet] [2010]: 47: 327–345. Available from: https://doi.org/10.1016/jsocscimed.2011.02.044.
26. Quinton D, Pollock S, Golding J. The transition to fatherhood in young men: influences on commitment. ESRC, Brighton: London; 2002.
27. Brown S. 'They think it's all up to the girls': gender, risk and responsibility for contraception, Culture, Health & Sexuality[2015], 17: 3, 312–325. [Internet]: Available from: https://doi.org/10.1080/1369058.2014.950983.

6

The impact of FSH receptor polymorphism on time-to-pregnancy

Birute Zilaitiene[1*], Marius Dirzauskas[1], Rasa Verkauskiene[1], Rytas Ostrauskas[1], Joerg Gromoll[2] and Eberhard Nieschlag[2]

Abstract

Background: Single nucleotide polymorphism of the follicle-stimulating hormone (FSH) receptor (FSHR) is an important marker of ovarian function. However, its role in female fecundity remains debatable. The aim of the study to assess the relationship of FSHR polymorphism of *Serine/Serine*, *Asparagine/Asparagine* and *Asparagine/Serine* variants directly against the time-to-pregnancy (TTP) in women.

Methods: Data were collected from 291 consecutive selected post-partum Caucasians using this criterion: ethnicity, age between 21 and 34-year-old new mothers and, 0–3 days after delivery of newborns in the Klaipeda University Hospital, Lithuania. Questionnaires on factors associated with conception were given to patients, and blood samples were collected for genomic *DNA* extractions as well as for analysis of follicle-stimulating hormone receptor gene polymorphism. Odds ratios (OR) and 95% confidence intervals (CI) for time-to-pregnancy were estimated by multivariate logistic regression. Women with unplanned pregnancies and those who received assisted reproductive technologies were not included in the study.

Results: After adjustment for other possible factors, increased risk for time-to-pregnancy of 12 or more months was associated with: *Serine/Serine* polymorphism variant (OR = 1.38, 95% CI 1.56–2.71, $p = 0.007$), age of 30 or more years (OR = 1.95, 95% CI 1.25–2.71, $p = 0.015$), gynaecological diseases in the past (OR = 2.21, 95% CI 1.12–5.74, $p = 0.027$), prior contraception use (OR = 1.87, 95% CI 1.14–3.64, $p = 0.016$), and fertility problems in the past (OR = 1.57, 95% CI 1.16–4.76, $p = 0.019$).

Conclusion: The results suggest a possible relationship of FSH receptor gene *Serine/Serine* variant for the lower possibility of conception during the first 12 months of planned conception.

Keywords: Time to pregnancy, FSH receptor haplotypes, FSH receptor polymorphism

Background

Fecundity is the wonderful biological ability to produce abundant healthy offspring and is affected by genetic and environmental factors [1]. If pregnancy is planned, fertility may be expressed as time-to-pregnancy (TTP) [2]. TTP is defined as the number of contraceptive-free cycles needed to conceive [3]. A TTP greater than 12 months allocates the infertility status [4, 5]. Usually trying to conceive in the first year succeeds for ~ 85% of cases [6].

Impaired fertility is inherited and may be due to inactivating mutations in the gonadotropin and gonadotropin receptor genes [7, 8]. Recent genetic studies have revealed that the pathogenesis of subfertility or infertility can be due to mutations in the follicle-stimulating hormone receptor (FSHR) gene [9]. While mutations affecting FSHR are sporadic; polymorphism of the FSHR gene seems to be a common phenomenon [9]. FSHR inactivating mutations may cause primary or secondary amenorrhea, infertility, and premature ovarian failure [10]; whereas activating mutations can predispose to ovarian hyperstimulation syndrome,

* Correspondence: birute.zilaitiene@lsmuni.lt
[1]Institute of Endocrinology, Lithuanian University of Health Sciences, 50009 Kaunas, Lithuania

as a consequence of exogenous FSH administration, or to a spontaneous onset [10–12].

In-vitro studies have shown that the A allele at the 29th position in the 5′ untranslated region of the FSHR gene is associated with impaired transcriptional activity [13]. The polymorphism at position 29 in the promoter of the FSHR gene may contribute to the reduced receptor expression [14]. The FSHR shows nucleotide polymorphisms in the promoter and in exon 10 [15]. The single nucleotide polymorphisms in exon 10 results in four discrete allelic variants characterized by the amino acid combinations: *threonine (Thr)307-asparagine (Asn)680, alanine (Ala)307-Serine* (Ser)680, *Ala307-Asn680* and *Thr307-Ser680* [15]. The first two allelic variants are very frequent in the Caucasian population [15]. At position 680, three FSH receptor variants are possible: *Asn/Asn, Asn/Ser,* and *Ser/Ser;* however, *Ser/Ser-680* predominates in the studied infertile population [16].

The studies on FSHR polymorphism, performed on patients undergoing in-vitro fertilisation procedures show that women homozygous for the *Ser680* variant have higher follicular FSH levels and longer follicular phase length, which suggest a lower sensitivity to FSH. Thus the homozygous *Ala307-Ser680* variant is associated with a higher amount of FSH required for ovarian stimulation in women undergoing assisted reproduction [15]. This suggests that the FSHR genotype can influence the ovarian response to FSH stimulation [17, 18]. However, there are studies where this association was not confirmed [19, 20].

FSH is responsible for follicular maturation and for the length and stability of the menstrual cycle [21]. A longer cycle may be associated with more difficulties in conception; women who have the FSHR gene *Asn (Asparagine)* exchanged for *Ser (Serine)* at codon 680 have statistically proven longer menstrual cycles [22].

Despite the numerous publications on the FSHR polymorphism impact on women's reproductive function; an FSHR polymorphic relationship to TTP has not yet been studied. Here we aimed to assess the relationship of the FSHR polymorphism Serine/Serine, Asparagine/Asparagine and Asparagine/Serine variants on TTP in a sample of Lithuanian women.

Methods

Subjects

Klaipeda is the third largest city in Lithuania and has one obstetric department that performs approximately 3500 deliveries per year from all parts of the west region of Lithuania. Between March 2008 and May 2008, 291 consecutive selected 21–34-year-old (mediana [25–75%] – 27.0 [24.0–31.0] years) women who conceived naturally and delivered babies at the Klaipeda University Hospital were invited to participate in the study 0–3 days after delivery. This time interval was chosen because it allowed for the accurate recall of the time period preceding conception, and it was a time point at which the delivery outcome was already known. All selected women had planned pregnancies that were achieved without using assisted reproductive technologies. In 49.17% of cases women were nulliparous, the rest of them - multiparous. Prior to pregnancy planning, 67 (22.26%) women used hormonal contraception. Women were asked to complete a standardised questionnaire. It included questions concerning age, height, weight before pregnancy, the menstrual cycle, socioeconomic factors, lifestyle, sexual behaviour, and some other factors. The regular menstrual cycle was defined as 28 ± 7 days and this definition was explained to study participants. Women with irregular menstrual cycles were asked to report if the majority of their cycles are < 21 days or > 35 days. Only one participant reported irregular cycles < 21 days, so, she was excluded from the final analysis. The questions regarding gynaecological diseases were asked separately for non-infectious and infectious diseases. Women with unplanned pregnancies and those who received assisted reproductive technologies were not included in the study. However, women who get another infertility treatment, e.g. ovulation induction, treatment of infections - were enrolled into the study.

DNA sampling

A venous blood sample was drawn for DNA extraction from all 291participants.

DNA extraction was performed in a certificated "SORPO" laboratory of Thermo Fisher Scientific Inc. in Vilnius, Lithuania. *DNA* samples froze at-20 °C; were sent to the University of Munster in Germany. There are two known polymorphisms of clinical relevance in the hormone (FSH) receptor exon 10: *Ala* or *Thr* at position 307 (dbSNP numbers 6165), and *Asn* or *Ser* at position 680 (dbSNP numbers 6166). These give rise to two discrete allelic variants: Thr^{307}/Asn^{680} and Ala^{307}/Ser^{680}. The allelic variants at codon 307 and 680 are almost invariably associated, therefore codon 680 was assessed, and all women were classified as homozygous (*Ser/Ser* or *Asn/Asn*) or heterozygous (*Asn/Ser*).

Genomic *DNA* was extracted from peripheral blood using a FlexiGene *DNA* extraction kit (QIAGEN, Hilden, Germany) according to the manufacturer's instruction. All samples were screened for the single nucleotide polymorphism (SNP) at position 2039 (codon 680) of exon 10 by the TaqMan allelic discrimination assay while using the ABI Prism 7000 sequence detection system (Applied Biosystems, Darmstadt, Germany). The probes (SNP indicated in *bold lower case letters*) were 5′-*AGAGTCACC A**g**TGGTT*-3′ (6-carboxyfluorescein fluorescence) and 5′-*AGTCACCA**a**TGGTTC*-3′ (VIC fluorescence). The primers were 5′-*AAGGAATGGCCACTGCTCTTC*-3′ (forward) and 5′-*GGGCTAAATGACTTAGAGGGACAA* -3′ (reverse). Each polymerase chain reaction (PCR) (25 μl) contained: 2 μl DEPC-treated water, 12.5 μl Universal master mix, 0.25 μl of each probe, and 4.5 μl of each primer (5 pmol). Using the TaqManassay, PCR was performed in two steps: absolute quantification and allelic discrimination. For absolute quantification, the cycles were as follows: stage 1: Probe binding at 50 °C for 2 mins (1 cycle); stage 2: denaturation at 95 °C for 10 mins (1 cycle), followed by 35 cycles at 95 °C for 15 s; stage 3:60 °C for 1 min. Whereas the allelic discrimination assay took 1 min at 60 °C.

Statistical analysis

Analyses were performed using SPSS 17.0 software. Women who conceived after ≥12 months of trying were classified as the risk group. The normality of distribution was tested using the Kolmogorov-Smirnov test. Student's (t) criterion was used for comparison of means for normal distributions, and the Mann-Whitney (U) test was used in skewed distributions. In order to determine the difference between more than two groups; parametric and nonparametric dispersive analysis with ANOVA and Kruskal-Wallis test was performed. Bonferroni test was performed by comparing multiple pairs. For evaluating dependence between qualitative features χ^2 criterion was used. Results were presented as mean (M) ± standard deviation (SD) or n (%). Biological, social, demographic, economic, sexual behaviour, genetic, living, working and environmental confounders variables were retaining in models. Univariate analysis of the OR for each variable was taken initially. Multivariate logistic regression step-wise enter method model was used to estimate the most important relationship factors. Odds ratios (OR) and 95% confidence intervals (CI) for time-to-pregnancy was calculated. The limit of significance was defined as a two-sided p-value of< 0.05.

The study was approved by the Lithuanian Bioethics Committee (21/12/2006 No. 59/2). The aim of the survey protocol was carefully explained to each subject of study entry, and a written informed consent was obtained.

Results

FSHR genetic variants

The mean TTP in the study group of 291 woman was 5.3 ± 10.9 (mediana [25–75%]: 1.0 [1.0–5.0]) months. The main demographic, social, lifestyle and other characteristics of the participants are shown in Table 1.

During FSH receptor genotype analysis three groups of *Asn*^{680} and *Ser*^{680} variation were detected: 101 (34.7%) of cases were found to be homozygous for *Asn*^{680} (*Asn/Asn* -group), 148 (50.9%) heterozygous for *Asn*^{680} and *Ser*^{680} (*Asn/Ser* -group), and 42 (14.4%) homozygous for *Ser*^{680} (*Ser/Ser* -group). Median TTP in the *Asn/Asn* participant group was 1.0 [95% CI 1.0–4.0] months, in the *Asn/Ser* group: 1.0 [1.0–3.75] months, and in the *Ser/Ser* group: 7.0 [1.0–15.25] months. Furthermore, these differences of were significant ($p < 0.03$).

Women having the *Ser/Ser* polymorphism variant had significantly longer TTP compared to those bearing variants *Asn/Asn* and *Asn/Ser* ($p = 0.01$ and p = 0.01 respectively) (Fig. 1). When comparing *Asn/Asn* and *Asn/Ser* groups, no significant differences in TTP were found.

In the comparison between the *Ser/Ser* and the *Asn/Asn* FSHR genetic variants, the risk for a TTP of 12 months or longer is higher for those women with the variant *Ser/Ser* (Table 2). The highest sensitivity and positive prognostic value, along with the lowest false positive rate α, occur when comparing the Ser/Ser genetic variant to *Asn/Asn*. Thus this combination has the highest effect size for estimating TTP (Table 3).

Women with the *Ser/Ser* polymorphism had irregular menstrual cycles (> 35 days) more frequently when compared to other genetic variants ($\chi^2 = 20.2$; df = 2; $p < 0.001$) (Table 1). The highest odds ratio is found when comparing *Ser/Ser* and *Asn/Ser* FSHR genetic variants, and the risk for having irregular menstrual cycle is 4 times higher in women with the *Ser/Ser* variant.

Risk factors for a TTP of 12 or more months for the women in the study group

Logistic regression methods were used to explore potential risk factors for longer TTP. Proportional differences were analysed to compare data of women who conceived up till 12 months with data of women who conceived at 12 or more months. Meanwhile, other factors possibly having an influence on TTP were also checked in this study. Most of the study participants were living in the city, in their own residences, as couples had higher education, higher monthly salary, worked, didn't smoke, and drank coffee (Table 1). Only a few of cases were obese (5.50%), had previous gynaecological diseases (15.46%), or fertility problems (5.84%). Respondents with alcohol consumption reported stress during pregnancy planning and pregnancy quantity; both divided up equally. The use of folic acid or other food supplements was surprisingly low (24.40 and 33.33% respectively). TTP of ≥12 months was reported significantly more often by women whose age was 30 years or more ($p = 0.048$), who had irregular menstrual cycles ($p < 0.001$), previous fertility problems and/or gynaecological diseases (p < 0.001 both), used any contraception prior to pregnancy planning ($p = 0.004$), drank coffee (p = 0.048), consumed other food supplements (p = 0.004), lived within < 10 km from factories (p = 0.04), had low physical activity ($p = 0.044$), and the SER/SER polymorphism variant ($p < 0.001$). Unadjusted univariate OR and 95% CI for

Table 1 Main characteristics of study participants

Criteria	FSHR genetic variant					
	Asn/Asn		*Asn/Ser*		*Ser/Ser*	
	n	% or Median (25–75% CI)	n	% or Median (25–75% CI)	n	% or Median (25–75% CI)
Participants	101	34.7	148	50.9	42	14.4
Mean age (years)		27.4 ± 5.9		27.2 ± 5.5		27.9 ± 5.0
Median body mass index (kg/m^2)		21.4 (19.8–24.1)		22.3 (20.0–24.1)		21.5 (20.1–23.1)
Median TTP (month)		1.0 (1.0–4.0)*		1.0 (1.0–3.8)*		7.0 (1.0–15.3)
TTP < 12 month	92	91.1*	133	89.9*	27	64.3
TTP ≥ 12 month	9	8.9	15	10.1	15	35.7
Nuliparous	48	47.5	75	50.7	25	59.5
Multiparous	53	52.5	73	49.3	17	40.5
Living in the city	76	75.3	115	77.7	35	83.3
Living in the country	25	24.7	33	22.3	7	16.7
Education lower than college	37	36.6	63	42.6	14	33.3
College education and higher	64	63.4	85	57.4	28	66.7
Salary < 560 Euro/month	34	33.7	36	24.3	11	26.2
Salary ≥560 Euros/month	67	66.3	112	75.7	31	73.8
Smoking	28	27.7	28	18.9	6	14.3
Alcohol consumers	51	50.5	74	50.0	20	47.6
Coffee consumption	27	26.7*	37	25.0*	32	76.2
Folic acid use	24	23.8	36	24.3	11	26.2
Use of other food additives	32	31.7	50	33.8	14	33.3
Physical activity/sports	28	27.7	48	32.4	16	38.1
Prior hormonal contraception use	26	25.7	31	20.9	10	23.8
Regular menstrual cycle	68	67.3*	113	76.4*	17	40.5
Irregular menstrual cycle	33	32.7*	35	23.6*	25	59.5
Sexual intercourse one time/week	18	17.8	27	18.2	7	16.7
Sexual intercourse 2 times and more/week	83	82.2	121	81.8	35	83.3
Past fertility problems	8	7.9	6	4.0	3	7.1
Gynaecological diseases in the past	3	3.0	4	2.7	1	2.4
Working status	93	92.1	141	95.3	39	92.9
Stress	60	59.4	55	37.2	21	50.0
Use of pesticides	2	1.9	1	0.7	1	2.4

n – number of study participants; $^*p < 0.05$ compared with the *Ser/Ser* group. For quantitative variables p value by non-parametric ANOVA (Kruskal Wallis), for qualitative variables *p* value by χ^2 test

conceiving after 12 or more months with the presence of previously mentioned factors are presented in Table 4.

Coffee consumption and low physical activity correlated significantly with fertility problems in the past ($r = 0.2$; $p = 0.001$ and $r = 0.23$; $p = 0.013$ respectively); meanwhile, irregular menstrual cycles correlated with FSHR gene Ser/Ser variant ($r = 0.17$; $p = 0.008$); a ≥ 560 EURO monthly salary and the use of other food additives – with older age ($r = 0.17$; $p = 0.008$ and $r = 0.27$; $p = 0.03$ respectively); as well as living < 10 km from factories, which correlated with gynaecological diseases ($r = 0.18$; $p = 0.009$); therefore, these factors were excluded from further analysis. The use of contraception prior to pregnancy planning showed no correlation to other factors

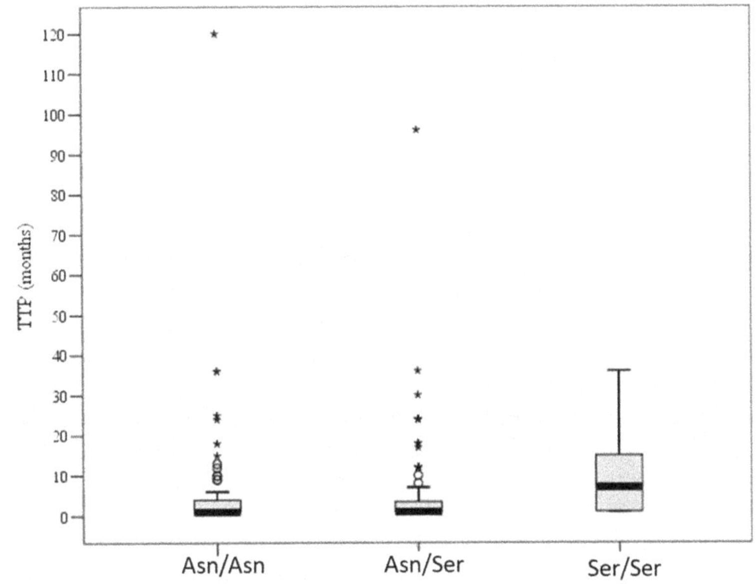

Fig. 1 Distribution of the FSHR polymorphism in TTP groups

from the univariate regression model. The evaluation of significant correlations was done using the Forward Stepwise likelihood ratio method and was referenced to the database. This algorithm converged through 3 steps; selecting: older age (≥30 years), the use of any contraception prior to pregnancy planning, previous fertility problems, gynaecological diseases, and the *Ser/Ser* polymorphism. These were the most significant factors that correctly predicted TTP of 12 or more months (positively classified prognosis was 91.1%). The combination of these factors formed the multivariate logistic regression model (Table 5). All independent variables were included in the analysis (older age, irregular menstrual cycle, past fertility problems, gynaecological diseases, use of contraception prior to conception, living < 10 km from factories, and having *Ser/Ser* polymorphism variant); however, the Forward Stepwise Likelihood ratio method selected the 5 most significant ones (stated above). Accordingly, older age (≥30 years), use of any contraception prior to conception, and having gynaecological diseases increased the OR of conceiving after 12 or more months almost by double; having fertility problems in the past: 1.5 times, and if *Ser/Ser* polymorphism is present: 1.7 times.

Table 2 Estimated odds ratios for TTP ≥12 months for FSHR genetic variants

	OR	95% CI	*P*-value
Ser/Ser vs. *Asn/Asn*	5.68	4.83–6.70	< 0.0001
Ser/Ser vs. *Asn/Ser*	4.93	4.28–5.68	< 0.0001
Ser/Ser vs. *Asn/Asn* + *Asn/Ser*	5.21	4.65–5.85	< 0.0001

OR – odds ratio, p – significance level

Discussion

The FSHR polymorphism's impact on women's reproductive function has been demonstrated in several studies [9, 11, 16, 17, 23]; particularly in some diseases, such as the polycystic ovary syndrome and amenorrhea [24–26]. Some investigations provide contradictory data on the relationship between single nucleotide polymorphisms, and their link to polycystic ovary syndrome and amenorrhea [27–29]. The main reported findings on changes of hormonal dynamics in women with homozygote mutated *Ser*^{680} throughout the menstrual cycle were with lower serum levels of estradiol, progesterone and inhibin A [22]. However, these women had significantly higher FSH levels, and longer menstrual cycles [12, 14, 18]. Patients with the *Ser*^{680}/*Ser*^{680} genotype are more resistant to FSH action and thus require a stronger stimulus for the same biological response [22]. This finding is important in infertility treatment; patients with the homozygous FSHR *Ser*^{680}/*Ser*^{680} polymorphism have double the chance of having a resistance to clomiphene citrate [30]. They require higher FSH dosages in order to show the same estradiol response during controlled ovarian stimulation [24]. Furthermore, it was also demonstrated that the frequency of *Ser*^{680}/*Ser*^{680} variation in the control population is lower than if compared to the infertile women's group [23]. Thus it may be hypothesised that the *Ser*^{680}/*Ser*^{680} genotype could be directly related to a women's fertility. To our knowledge, the FSHR polymorphism was never investigated in direct relation

Table 3 Prognostic value of FSHR polymorphism variants for TTP < 12 vs. ≥12 months

	Sensitivity (%)	Specificity (%)	Prognostic value		False rate	
			Positive (%)	Negative (%)	Positive (α)	Negative (β)
Ser/Ser vs. *Asn/Asn*	62.50	77.31	65.71	8.91	22.69	37.50
Ser/Ser vs. *Asn/Ser*	50.00	83.13	49.15	10.14	16.88	50.00
Ser/Ser vs. *Asn/Asn* + *Asn/Ser*	38.46	89.29	54.78	9.64	10.71	61.54

to TTP in a fertile population. In this study, women were considered to be fertile if they achieved pregnancy without using assisted reproductive technology methods. A large number of factors possibly affecting TTP were investigated along with the FSHR polymorphism in order to detect independent factors predicting longer TTP and to establish the role of FSHR polymorphism between other determinants of women's fertility.

Our data confirmed that higher age, previous gynaecological diseases, and/or fertility problems pose as risk factors for longer TTP. An association for the risk of longer TTP due to hormonal contraception use prior to conception is more questionable. However, an older age of women using contraception could be the reason for this finding.

The relationship of the FSHR polymorphism to the length of the menstrual cycle was demonstrated in our study, as well as in previous publications [22]. Differences in menstrual cycle length between the Ser^{680}/Ser^{680} and the Asn^{680}/Asn^{680} groups result in 12.5 vs. 13.5 menstrual cycles per year, respectively [22]. Assuming no difference in age at the time of menopause; women with the Ser^{680}/Ser^{680} genotype would experience 30–40 cycles fewer, than women with an Asn^{680}/Asn^{680} genotype during their reproductive life [22]. Some authors conclude that women with the Ser^{680}/Ser^{680} genotype have a lower chance to achieve pregnancy during the same time period if compared to the other variants [23, 30]. Therefore, menstrual periods are stressful events that have certain disadvantages; such as blood loss, menstrual discomfort, and the effects of hormone fluctuations on mood, breast and other oestrogen-dependent organs. This gives rise to some speculation that fewer menstrual cycles during the reproductive lifespan might represent an evolutionary advantage and might influence fertility positively [22]. Our data provide direct evidence that women with the Ser^{680}/Ser^{680} genetic variant had a lower chance of conception than females with Asn^{680}/Asn^{680} and Asn^{680}/Ser^{680} genetic variants.

We have demonstrated that the FSH receptor gene *Serine/Serine* variant polymorphism is associated with a fivefold lower likelihood to become pregnant during the first 12 months of attempts to conceive.

The other independent factors predicting a TTP of 12 or more months in the study group were older age, gynaecological diseases, fertility problems in the past, and the use of contraception prior to conception.

Some limitations of our study, especially related to the retrospective design, should be discussed. A retrospective design of the study was used in order to achieve a higher participation rate. Only one polymorphism in this region was evaluated, and furthermore, no replication in an independent cohort was attempted. However, it was previously demonstrated that immediately after delivery women can recall the period before conception very well, so data reported here can be treated as reliable [2]. Because of the selected study design, it was not possible to include women who had miscarriages, ectopic pregnancies, or an induced abortion; as well as, to collect information on other important factors that may affect TTP, such as basal FSH levels and semen quality. Moreover, the study was conducted in only one region of the country, which represents one quarter of the entire Lithuanian female population.

Table 4 Univariate odds ratios for TTP ≥12 months in the group of women analysed for FSHR polymorphism

Variables[a]	OR	95% CI	p
Past fertility problems	6.97	6.22–7.82	< 0.0001
Prior contraception use	6.43	5.74–7.22	0.0043
Irregular menstrual cycle	4.24	3.79–4.77	< 0.0001
Gynaecological diseases in the past	3.44	3.07–3.86	0.0009
Living 10 or less km from factories	2.06	1.84–2.32	0.0399
Age 30 years and older	1.31	1.17–1.47	0.0477
Ser/Ser polymorphism variant	5.20	2.45–11.05	0.0004

p – significance level, OR – odds ratio (unadjusted), CI – confidence intervals, [a] - only significative variables were presented in the table

Table 5 A multivariate stepwise Enter model describing significant factors for TTP ≥12 months in the group of women analysed for the FSHR polymorphism

Variables	OR	95% CI	*P*-value
Past fertility problems	1.568	1.16–4.76	0.019
Prior contraception use	1.871	1.14–3.64	0.016
Gynaecological diseases in the past	2.212	1.12–5.74	0.027
Age 30 years and older	1.952	1.25–2.71	0.015
Ser/Ser polymorphism variant	1.678	1.56–2.71	0.007

Constant = 3.741

Strengths and limitations of this study

- The FSH receptor gene polymorphism may affect human reproduction by causing menstrual cycle disorders.
- The present study demonstrates the effect of FSH receptor gene polymorphism on time to pregnancy* that has not been investigated till now.
- The relationship of FSHr *Serine*^{680}/*Serine*^{680} variant polymorphism to lower fecundity can have clinical relevance; e.g. more conservative infertility management can be suggested for women with unexplained infertility having this genetic variant.
- Further studies including prospective studies on the impact of genetic factors on women's fertility are needed.

Conclusions

Further studies including prospective studies on the impact of genetic factors on women's fertility are needed. Comprehensively study the effects of FSHR polymorphisms on various reproductive traits, the most studied rs6166 SNP should be evaluated together with the rs1394205 in the 5'UTR and with the SNPs in the FSHB locus [31]. However, it is already clear that the relationship of FSHR *Ser*^{680}/*Ser*^{680} variant polymorphism to lower fecundity can have clinical relevance; e.g. more conservative infertility management can be suggested for women with unexplained infertility whose have this genetic variation.

Abbreviations

5' UTR: 5' untranslated region; *Ala*: *Alanine*; *Asn*: *Asparagine*; CI: Confidence interval; FSH: Follicle-stimulating hormone; FSHB: Follicle-stimulating hormone beta subunit; FSHR: Follicle-stimulating hormone receptor; OR: Odds ratios; *Ser*: *Serine*; SNP: Single-nucleotide polymorphism; *Thr*: *Threonine*; TTP: Time-to-pregnancy

Acknowledgement

We hereby express sincere thanks to the staff of the Klaipeda University Hospital for affable conditions for our study. Susan Nieschlag, M.A. deserves special thanks for language editing of the manuscript. We appreciate the ultimate English grammar correction by Mr. Arnold Kincius.

Authors' contributions

MD, JG, EN, BZ, RV, and RO were involved in the concept and design. MD, JG, EN, and BZ performed the analyses and MD, JG, EN, RV, and RO contributed to the interpretation of the data. MD, BZ and RO drafted the manuscript, and JG, EN and RV provided critical revision. MD, JG, EN, BZ, RV, and RO were involved in the final approval. All authors read and approved the final manuscript.

Consent for publication

Not applicable.

Competing interests

All authors declare that they have no competing interest. The authors alone are responsible for the content and writing of the paper.

Author details

[1]Institute of Endocrinology, Lithuanian University of Health Sciences, 50009 Kaunas, Lithuania. [2]Center of Reproductive Medicine and Andrology, University of Münster, 48149Münster, Münster, Germany.

References

1. Caserta D, Mantovani A, Marci R, Fazi A, Ciardo F, La Rocca C, et al. Environment and women's reproductive health. Hum Reprod Update. 2011; 17(3):418–33. https://doi.org/10.1093/humupd/dmq061.
2. Joffe M. Feasibility of studying subfertility using retrospective self reports. J Epidemiol Community Health. 1989;43(3):268–74.
3. Baird DD, Wilcox AJ, Weinberg CR. Use of time to pregnancy to study environmental exposures. Am J Epidemiol. 1986;124(3):470–80.
4. Schmidt L, Holstein BE, Christensen U, Boivin J. Communication and coping as predictors of fertility problem stress: cohort study of 816 participants who did not achieve a delivery after 12 months of fertility treatment. Hum Reprod. 2005;20(11):3248–56.
5. Stanford JB, Dunson DB. Effects of sexual intercourse patterns in time to pregnancy studies. Am J Epidemiol. 2007;165(9):1088–95.
6. Gnoth C, Godehardt E, Frank-Herrmann P, Friol K, Tigges J, Freundl G. Definition and prevalence of subfertility and infertility. Hum Reprod. 2005; 20(5):1144–7. https://doi.org/10.1093/humrep/deh870.
7. Huhtaniemi IT, Themmen AP. Mutations in human gonadotropin and gonadotropin-receptor genes. Endocrine. 2005;26(3):207–17.
8. Latronico AC, Arnhold IJ. Gonadotropin resistance. Endocr Dev. 2013;24:25–32. https://doi.org/10.1159/000342496.
9. Levallet J, Pakarinen P, Huhtaniemi IT. Follicle-stimulating hormone ligand and receptor mutations, and gonadal dysfunction. Arch Med Res. 1999;30(6): 486–94. https://doi.org/10.1016/S0188-0128(99)00058-5.
10. Lussiana C, Guani B, Mari C, Restagno G, Massobrio M, Revelli A. Mutations and polymorphisms of the FSH receptor (FSHR) gene: clinical implications in female fecundity and molecular biology of FSHR protein and gene. Obstet Gynecol Surv. 2008;63(12):785–95. https://doi.org/10.1097/OGX.0b013e31818957eb.
11. Laan M, Grigorova M, Huhtaniemi IT. Pharmacogenetics of follicle-stimulating hormone action. Curr Opin Endocrinol Diabetes Obes. 2012; 19(3):220–7. https://doi.org/10.1097/MED.0b013e3283534b11.
12. Achrekar SK, Modi DN, Meherji PK, Patel ZM, Mahale SD. Follicle stimulating hormone receptor gene variants in women with primary and secondary amenorrhea. J Assist Reprod Genet. 2010;27(6):317–26. https://doi.org/10.1007/s10815-010-9404-9.
13. Achrekar SK, Modi DN, Desai SK, Mangoli VS, Mangoli RV, Mahale SD. Poor ovarian response to gonadotrophin stimulation is associated with FSH receptor polymorphism. Reprod BioMed Online. 2009;18(4):509–15. .
14. Desai SS, Achrekar SK, Pathak BR, Desai SK, Mangoli VS, Mangoli RV, et al. Follicle-stimulating hormone receptor polymorphism (G-29A) is associated with altered level of receptor expression in granulosa cells. J Clin Endocrinol Metab. 2011;96(9):2805–12. https://doi.org/10.1210/jc.2011-1064.
15. Simoni M, Nieschlag E, Gromoll J. Isoforms and single nucleotide polymorphisms of the FSH receptor gene: implications for human reproduction. Hum Reprod Update. 2002;8(5):413–21.
16. Falconer H, Andersson E, Aanesen A, Fried G. Follicle-stimulating hormone receptor polymorphisms in a population of infertile women. Acta Obstet Gynecol Scand. 2005;84(8):806–11.
17. de Koning CH, Benjamins T, Harms P, Homburg R, van Montfrans JM, Gromoll J, et al. The distribution of FSH receptor isoforms is related to basal FSH levels in subfertile women with normal menstrual cycles. Hum Reprod. 2006;21(2):443-6.
18. Altmäe S, Hovatta O, Stavreus-Evers A, Salumets A. Genetic predictors of controlled ovarian hyperstimulation: where do we stand today? Hum Reprod Update. 2011;17(6):813–28. https://doi.org/10.1093/humupd/dmr034.
19. Genro VK, Matte U, De Conto E, Cunha-Filho JS, Fanchin R. Frequent polymorphisms of FSH receptor do not influence antral follicle responsiveness to follicle-stimulating hormone administration as assessed by the follicular output RaTe (FORT). J Assist Reprod Genet. 2012;29(7):657–63. https://doi.org/10.1007/s10815-012-9761-7.
20. Klinkert ER, te Velde ER, Weima S, van Zandvoort PM, Hanssen RG, Nilsson PR, et al. FSH receptor genotype is associated with pregnancy but not with ovarian response in IVF. Reprod BioMed Online. 2006;13(5):687–95. https://doi.org/10.1016/S1472-6483(10)60660-8

21. Son WY, Das M, Shalom-Paz E, Holzer H. Mechanisms of follicle selection and development. Minerva Ginecol. 2011;63(2):89–102.
22. Greb RR, Grieshaber K, Gromoll J, Sonntag B, Nieschlag E, Kiesel L, et al. A common single nucleotide polymorphism in exon 10 of the human follicle stimulating hormone receptor is a major determinant of length and hormonal dynamics of the menstrual cycle. J Clin Endocrinol Metab. 2005; 90(8):4866–72.
23. Laven JS, Mulders AG, Suryandari DA, Gromoll J, Nieschlag E, Fauser BC, et al. Follicle-stimulating hormone receptor polymorphisms in women with normogonadotropic anovulatory infertility. Fertil Steril. 2003;80(4):986–92.
24. Simoni M, Tempfer CB, Destenaves B, Fauser BC. Functional genetic polymorphisms and female reproductive disorders: part I: polycystic ovary syndrome and ovarian response. Hum Reprod Update. 2008;14(5):459–84. https://doi.org/10.1093/humupd/dmn024.
25. Nakamura Y, Maekawa R, Yamagata Y, Tamura I, Sugino N. A novel mutation in exon8 of the follicle-stimulating hormone receptor in a woman with primary.amenorrhea. Gynecol Endocrinol. 2008;24(12):708–12. https://doi.org/10.1080/09513590802454927. .
26. Gu BH, Park JM, Baek KH. Genetic variations of follicle stimulating hormone receptor are associated with polycystic ovary syndrome. Int J Mol Med. 2010;26(1):107–12.
27. Du J, Zhang W, Guo L, Zhang Z, Shi H, Wang J, et al. Two FSHR variants, haplotypes and meta-analysis in Chinese women with premature ovarian failure and polycystic ovary syndrome. Mol Genet Metab. 2010;100(3):292–5. https://doi.org/10.1016/j.ymgme.2010.03.018.
28. Unsal T, Konac E, Yesilkaya E, Yilmaz A, Bideci A, Ilke Onen H, et al. Genetic polymorphisms of FSHR, CYP17, CYP1A1, CAPN10, INSR, SERPINE1 genes in adolescent girls with polycystic ovary syndrome. J Assist Reprod Genet. 2009;26(4):205–16. https://doi.org/10.1007/s10815-009-9308-8.
29. Tong Y, Liao WX, Roy AC, Ng SC. Absence of mutations in the coding regions of follicle-stimulating hormone receptor gene in Singapore Chinese women with premature ovarian failure and polycystic ovary syndrome. Horm Metab Res. 2001;33(4):221–6.
30. Overbeek A, Kuijper EA, Hendriks ML, Blankenstein MA, Ketel IJ, Twisk JW, et al. Clomiphene citrate resistance in relation to follicle-stimulating hormone receptor Ser680Ser-polymorphism in polycystic ovary syndrome. Hum Reprod. 2009;24(8):2007–13. https://doi.org/10.1093/humrep/dep114.
31. Simoni M, Casarini L. Mechanisms in endocrinology: genetics of FSH action: a 2014-and-beyond view. Eur J Endocrinol. 2014;170(3):R91–107. https://doi.org/10.1530/EJE-13-0624.

7

Effect of different delivery modes on the short-term strength of the pelvic floor muscle in Chinese primipara

Yun Zhao[1], Li Zou[2], Mei Xiao[1*], Wan Tang[1], Hai-yi Niu[3] and Fu-yuan Qiao[3]

Abstract

Background: To investigate the effect of different delivery modes and related obstetric factors on the short-term strength of the pelvic floor muscle after delivery in Chinese primipara.

Methods: A total of 4769 healthy Chinese primiparas at postpartum 6–8 weeks were interviewed. According to the difference of delivery mode, the selected primiparas were divided into 2 groups, including cesarean delivery group containing 2020 and vaginal delivery group containing 2749. All the vaginal deliveries were further divided into 3 groups, including episiotomy group containing 2279, perineal laceration group containing 398, and forceps assisted group containing72. The scales of their pelvic floor muscle (PFM) strengths were examined by specially trained personnel using digital palpation (Modified Oxford scale:0–5 grade). According to participants' willingness, if the PFM strength was weak (0 or 1 grade), at-home PFM training would be recommended and an electrical stimulation combined with biofeedback therapy would be conducted for them in hospital. Twelve weeks after delivery, the PFM strength would be measured again. For statistical analysis, *t*-test, one-way variance analysis, Chi-square analysis, Kruskal-Wallis test H, Mann-Whitney U test and Wilcoxon test were carried out.

Results: The PFM strength in cesarean delivery group was higher than in vaginal delivery group ($p < 0.05$). Among 3 vaginal delivery groups, the PFM strength in perineal laceration group was the highest ($p < 0.05$); however, there was no difference in PFM strength between episiotomy group and forceps assisted group ($p>0.05$). After accepting PFM training at home and therapy in hospital, 305 women showed increased PFM strength ($p < 0.05$).

Conclusions: Vaginal delivery is an independent risk factor causing the damage of PFM, and episiotomy may cause injury of PFM. Through PFM training at home and therapy in hospital, those damage will resume as soon as possible in the short-time period after delivery.

Keywords: Pelvic floor muscle strength, Cesarean delivery, Episiotomy, Perineal laceration, Forceps, Eletrical stimulation, Biofeedback

Background

Pelvic floor disorders (PFDs) are common and prevalent in adult women, which negatively affect women's self-perception of their body image and life quality [1] and bring great economic burden to patients and society. PFDs has become a public health problem attracting worldwide attention. According to recent epidemiological studies, pregnancy and childbirth are two independent factors causing PFDs [2]. Can cesarean delivery really protect pelvic floor function of women? Some studies have shown that the selective cesarean delivery may have a protective effect for the pelvic floor, but others have shown that the protective effect is very limited in the long term postpartum period [3]. How do different delivery modes affect female Pelvic Floor Muscle(PFM) and what are the effects of these delivery modes on Chinese primiparas in the short-term postpartum? This study was conducted to estimate the effect of different delivery modes on the PFM strength at postpartum 6–8 weeks and the refection of PFM training on the weak PFM strength in the short-time

* Correspondence: xiaomei971203@163.com
[1]Department of Obstetrics, Maternal and Child Health Hospital of Hubei Province, No 745 Wuluo Road, Wuhan City, People's Republic of China

period after delivery. The scale of PFM strength was examined by specially trained personnel using digital palpation.

Methods

Ethical approval

The study protocol was approved by the Ethics Committee of Maternal and Child Health Hospital of Hubei Province(201301) and all included women signed written informed consent.

Selection of patients and study design

Women who had delivered in the obstetric department at the Maternal and Child Health Hospital of Hubei Province from January 2013 to January 2014 and visited pelvic floor rehabilitation department in postpartum 6–8 weeks period were selected as research objects. All selected women were healthy Chinese primiparas, with age ranging from 20 to 35 years old. They had clean lochia without obstetric complications. Exclusion criteria included those with age less than 20 years old or more than 35 years old, non-Chinese nationality, multiple pregnancies, vaginitis and urinary tract infection, and mental incapacity. A total of 4959 women were selected in this study, excluding 39 for being non-Chinese nationality, 105 for having red lochia, 46 for not cooperative with specially trained personnel. According to delivery mode, 4769 cases were divided into 2 groups, including cesarean delivery group containing 2020 and vaginal delivery group containing 2749. Then, All vaginal deliveries were further divided into 3 groups, including episiotomy group containing 2279 (Left lateral episiotomy during vaginal delivery), perineal laceration group containing 398 (I, II degree natural perineal laceration during vaginal delivery), and forceps assisted group containing 72 (Left lateral episiotomy and forceps assisted operation during vaginal delivery). In our hospital, all instrument–assisted operations of vaginal delivery were carried out with the aid of forceps in place of vacuum-assisted delivery, and midwifery care was conducted during the antenatal period, labor and delivery period, and postnatal period according to The National Midwifery Guidelines. The evaluation of pelvic floor muscle strength and routine physical examination on maternal gynecological situation were performed by trained specialists. All the investigation and examination results were recorded truthfully, including patient characteristics, medical history, and pregnancy delivery data. All selected women had not accepted formal training of pelvic floor muscle during pregnancy and postpartum 6–8 weeks period (see Fig. 1).

According to participants' actual condition in the 6–8 postpartum weeks, if the PFM strength was weak (0 or 1 grade according to modified Oxford scale), at-home PFM training plus in-hospital electrical stimulation combined with biofeedback therapy would be recommended for them, that was guided by specialized medical personnel in our department. Twelve weeks after delivery, the PFM strength would be examined again. There were only 310 primiparas with weak PFM strength who were treated with at-home PFM training plus in-hospital electrical stimulation combined with biofeedback therapy. Among them, excluding 1 case having electrostatic proble phobia when accepting electrical stimulation for the first time, 3 cases showing irregular vaginal bleeding, 1 case failing to continue treatment, the remaining 305 cases were included in the study for observing the therapeutic effect of PFM training at home plus PFM therapy in hospital.

Determination of pelvic floor muscle strength

Pelvic floor muscle was determined by specialized medical personnel using digital palpation. Before the examination, women were told to empty the bladder and take lithotomy position. PFM contraction without any movement of the pelvis or visible contraction of the glutei, hip, or abdominal muscles was emphasized [4].

Digital palpation [5]. First put the index and middle fingers 2–3 cm deep into the vagina and identify the levator ani muscle. Then, separate the two fingers and fall on two sides of levator ani muscle, meanwhile, put the other hand on the abdomen to make sure the abdominal muscle was relaxed. The scale of pelvic floor muscle strength was described by Modified Oxford scale. On the basis of contraction strength and retraction capability, the PFM strength was divided into 0–5 grades and 6 classes. (Table 1).

PFM training [6]

When the scale of PFM during 6–8 weeks postpartum period was < 2 grades (0 or 1 grade), the specialists in our department of pelvic floor rehabilitation would teach them how to contract their PFM by demonstrating vaginal palpation. At first, the specialist placed her index finger into the vaginal and told the women to lift and squeeze around the finger. Then, the women took Kegel exercise 10 times a day at home, each exercise included 10 repetitions. After 12 weeks of postpartum, the woman was told to come back again for PFM strength examination.

Eletrical stimulation and biofeedback [7]

The PFM enforcement program consisting of biofeedback and electrical stimulation therapy, lasting 30 min, was implemented twice a week. A complete course of PFM enforcement program lasts for 5 weeks, which is 10 times as long as the program of biofeedback and electrical stimulation. MyoTrac infiniti (SA9800) device (Thought Technology Inc., Montreal, Canada) was adopted in this experiment. The biostimulation feedback system is based on biofeedback technology, bioformatics principles and bioengineering technology, and so on. Safe and effective electrical stimulation combined with biofeedback technology were conducted by vaginal sensor to record pelvic

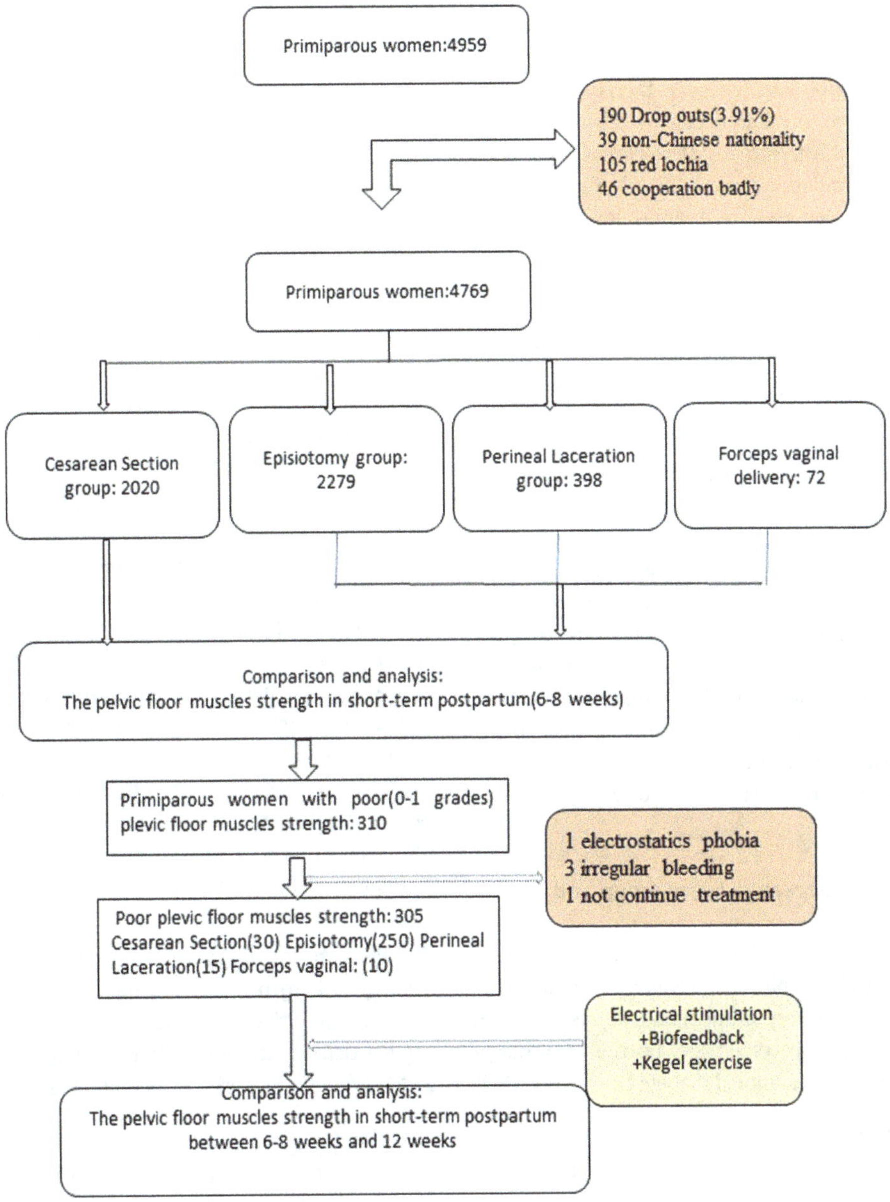

Fig. 1 Flowchart demonstrating. The number of Participants who attended and the reasons for lost to follow-up

Table 1 Modified Oxford scale for digital evaluation of pelvic floor muscle strength

Grade	Description
0	Nil
1	Flicker
2	Weak
3	Moderate, slight lift of the examiner's fingers, no resistance
4	Good, sufficient to elevate the examiner's fingers against light resistance
5	Strong, sufficient to elevate the examiner's fingers' against strong resistance

floor muscle activity and pelvic floor muscle contraction strength, based on which the strength of electrostimulation was controlled. The direct vagina low-voltage low-frequency electric stimulation including 3 reference electrodes on the iliac and two sides hypogastric skin was performed to prevent the abdominal or giuteus musles contraction. A separate proble was used for primiparas to prevent cross-infection. With the help of computer graphics, various parameters of the device was adjusted to make every primipara feel the PFM active and passive contraction and guarantee the primiparas not feel any pain or discomfort. The parameters of electrical stimulation were set as pulse width of 20–40 us and low voltage of 40-80 Hz. The electrostimulation included rapid contraction exercise of PFM (stimulation and interval time is 2 s:2 s) and continuous contraction exercise of PFM ((stimulation and interval time is 5–8 s:10 s). The electrical stimulation and biostimulation feedback therapies were applied alternatively based on the needs of primiparas with weak PFM strength. Each treatment of electrical stimulation combined with biostimulation lasted for 30 min, and was conducted two times per week, 10 times for a complete course of treatment.

Statistical analyses

All the statistical analyses were carried out using the Statistical Package of Social Sciences software (SPSS Version 13.0 Inc., Chicago, IL, USA). The values and variables were reported in the form of mean ± standard deviation. One-Way ANOVA and Student's test were performed to compare the variables in Gaussian distribution. Chi-square test was used to evaluate the categorical variables. Kruskal-Wallis H test was used to assess the difference of the PFM function and the variables in no Gaussian distribution among K independent samples. Mann-Whitney U test and Bonferroni's correction were conducted to assess further pairwise samples. Wilcoxon test was used to evaluate the difference of the PFM function before and after PFM training. The difference was considered statistically significant at $p < 0.05$.

Results

Demographic data of cesarean delivery group and vaginal delivery group

Through statistical comparison, it can be known that the difference is not statistically significant between cesarean delivery group and vaginal delivery group ($p > 0.05$). Samples in cesarean delivery group have older age, heavier new baby's weight, and higher rate of gestational diabetes mellitus(GDM) than that in vaginal delivery group ($p < 0.05$). The demographic data of two groups are list in Table 2.

The PFM strength of women in postpartum 6–8 weeks after accepting cesarean delivery or vaginal delivery

Table 3 shows that the PFM strength of women in cesarean delivery group is stronger than in vaginal delivery group, and the difference is statistically significant ($p < 0.05$).

Demographic data of the three groups of vaginal delivery

Through statistical comparison, it can be known that there are no differences in age, BMI of delivery, new baby's birth weight, gestational weight gain, gestational age at birth and the rate of GDM among episiotomy group, perineal laceration group, and forceps assisted group ($p > 0.05$). The median duration of the 2nd stage in forceps assisted group was 28 m(95%CI, 11-129 m), there was no statistical significance among the three groups ($p > 0.05$).The rates of 0, 1 and 2 degree of perineal lesions in perineal laceration group was 1.3, 26.4%(105/398) and 72.4%(288/398). The rates of 2 degree of perineal lesions in episiotomy group and in forceps assisted group were 100%, there was no 3 or 4 degree of perineal lesions in any of the three groups of vaginal delivery. There was common preineum local block anesthesia before episiotomy but no neuraxial labor anlagesia for vaginal delivery. The demographic data of 3 vaginal delivery groups are list in Table 2.

The PFM strength of women in postpartum 6–8 weeks among three groups of vaginal delivery

Table 4 shows that the PFM strength of women among three vaginal delivery groups is significant different ($p < 0.05$). The PFM strength in perineal laceration group is stronger than

Table 2 Comparison of demographic data among Cesarean delivery and three groups of vaginal delivery

	Cesarean delivery Group (2020)	Vaginal delivery Group (2749)	t or X^2	*p* value	Perineal laceration Group (398)	Episiotomy Group (2279)	Forceps assisted Group (72)	F or X^2	*p* value
Age(y) [mean ± sd]	28.3 ± 3.0	27.7 ± 2.9	7.017	0.000	27.7 ± 2.8	27.7 ± 2.9	28.1 ± 2.8	0.639	0.528
BMI of delivery (kg/m^2) [mean ± sd]	27.3 ± 2.6	27.5 ± 2.7	−1.658	0.098	27.5 ± 2.8	27.4 ± 2.7	27. 8 ± 2.6	0.656	0.519
Birth weight(g) [mean ± sd]	3322.0 ± 550.0	3252.6 ± 476.1	4.554	0.000	3226.3 ± 334.2	3254.8 ± 499.1	3329.2 ± 385.0	1.563	0.210
Gestational weight gain(kg)[mean ± sd]	15.9 ± 7.0	15.6 ± 7.2	1.470	0.142	15.6 ± 6.7	15.6 ± 7.3	14.6 ± 6.2	0.639	0.528
Gestational age at birth(w) [mean ± sd]	39.2 ± 1.4	39.3 ± 1.4	−0.638	0.523	39.2 ± 1.3	39.3 ± 1.4	39.7 ± 1.1	2.135	0.094
Rate of GDM (%)	30.0 (605/2020)	26.0 (714/2749)	9.009	0.003	24.1 (96/398)	26.0 (593/2279)	25 (18/72)	0.660	0.719
Duration of 2nd sta(m) [median(95%CI)]	/	26(7–110)	/	/	29(6–77)	25(7112)	28(11–129)	4.258	0.119

Student's test, One-Way ANOVA, Kruskal-Wallis H test and Chi-square analysis are performed; GDM: gestational diabetes mellitus

Table 3 The PFM strength of women in 6–8 weeks postpartum betwee the two delivery modes

	N	0	1	2	3	4	5
Cesarean secarean Group	2020	38	232	1364	366	20	0
Vaginal delivery Group	2749	223	1184	1195	140	7	0
Z	−27.861						
p value	0.000						

Mann-whitney U test is performed

Table 5 Comparison with the PFM strength before and after treatment

	n	0	1	2	3	4	5
Before	305	208	97	0	0	0	0
After	305	0	51	202	40	12	0
Z		−15.572					
p-value		0.000					

Wilcoxon test is used

that in episiotomy group and forceps vaginal delivery group, and the intergroup differences are statistically significant ($p < 0.025$). There is no significant difference in PFM strength of women between episiotomy group and forceps vaginal delivery group ($p>0.05$).

The weak PFM strength of women in postpartum 6–8 weeks

There were 305 cases with weak PFM willing to receive at-home PFM exercise plus electrical stimulation combined with biofeedback therapy in hospital twice a week (10 times for a complete course). Among them, there were 30 cases of cesarean delivery, 250 cases of were episiotomy, 15 cases of perineal laceration, and 10 cases of forceps vaginal delivery. By the last time of their treatment (nearly 12 weeks postpartum), their PFM strengths were examined again, and it could be found that their PFM strengths were improved ($p < 0.05$), as shown in Table 5.

Discussion

Pregnancy and childbirth are two important events in a women's life. The two phases of life have been proved to be associated with increased incidence of PFDs. Pregnancy and childbirth, especially vaginal childbirth, are two independent factors causing PFDs [8, 9]. Although severe morbidity of women from PFDs is rare, PFDs do seriously affect the quality of women's life. At present China, permanent damage of PFM in older women has attracted much attention and lots of money have been invested on this issue. However, the prevention and treatment of PFDs during pregnancy and childbirth have not been attached with sufficient attention. The postpartum period is the time during which the PFM damage of women may develop into the most serious condition (fortunately it is reversible). If a woman in postpartum cannot persist on accepting conservation treatment (pelvic muscle exercise, electrical stimulation, and biofeedback, and so on) for postnatal PFDs, permanent PFDs will gradually come into being [10, 11]. Paying attention to PFM damage and PFDs in recent postpartum period as well as finding effective method to guide restoration of pelvic floor function and improving the quality of women's life are the direction of our efforts in the future.

Table 4 The PFM strength of women in 6–8 weeks postpartum among the different vaginal delivery modes

	N	0	1	2	3	4	5
Perineal laceration Group①	398	21	151	192	30	4	0
Episiotomy Group②	2279	197	996	975	108	3	0
Forceps assisted Group③	72	5	37	28	2	0	0
	①②③		①-②	①-③		②-③	
X^2 or Z	18.736		−4.182	−2.550		−0.830	
p-value	0.000		0.000	0.032		1.000	

Kruskal-Wallis H test was used to assess the difference of the PFM function among the three vaginal delivery modes
Mann-Whitney U test and Bonferroni's correction were conducted to assess pairwise samples

At present, common detection methods of PFM strength include digital palpation, vaginal balloon, and surface electromyography (SEMG) and so on. Digital palpation can quantify the PFM strength directly, although it has always been questioned for its subjectivity. Vaginal balloon is more objective but not as precise as digital palpation. SEMG detects the electrical activity of PFM, yet its reliability in clinical application is still controversial. There is a strong correlation among the three methods in the assessment of the PFM strength [12–14]. Digital palpation is mainly used in the census, while SEMG is normally used in evaluation of therapeutic effect of the PFM strength [14]. In this study, through census of the PFM strength of women in postpartum 6–8 weeks, it can be known that the PFM strength of women having cesarean delivery is higher than that of women having vaginal delivery (including perineal laceration, episiotomy, and forceps assisted vaginal delivery), although t primiparas having cesarean delivery have older age, heavier baby's weight and higher rate of GDM than those having vaginal delivery. This shows vaginal delivery is one of the important factors causing PFM damage in recent postpartum, which is consistent with results of previous researches [15, 16]. This study shows that the PFM strength of primiparas having perineal laceration vaginal delivery is higher than that of primiparas having episiotomy vaginal delivery or forceps assisted vaginal delivery, which is mainly due to that the episiotomy may damage PFM and the integrity of pudendal nerve. It has always been a controversial topic to perform routine episiotomy on low-risk pregnant women during vaginal delivery [17–19]. Supporters think that routine episiotomy can protect the anal sphincter [18]. Opponents argue that routine episiotomy can increase the rates of postpartum bleeding, postpartum perineal incision infection, postpartum pain, urinary morbidity, and so on [19]. Our study suggests that routine episiotomy cannot protect the PFM from being damaged. The PFM damage is also related with PFDs, therefore the effective measure to reduce and prevent PFDs on low-risk pregnant women is to protect the perineal integrity and do not perform routine episiotomy during vaginal delivery. Many studies show that operation vaginal delivery by forceps or vacuums significantly damage the PFM strength and increase the risk of PFDs during both the recent and long term postpartum period [20–22]. But our study shows that there is no significant difference between episiotomy and forceps assisted vaginal delivery. This may be due to that the rate of forceps assisted vaginal delivery is very low in China, which is 1.51% (72/4769) in our hospital of primiparous women; for comparison, the percentage of operative vaginal delivery is 29.1% among primigrous women in Ireland [23]. The fetal head position will be lower or outlet when using forceps, and some difficult forceps vaginal deliveries have been replaced by cesarean delivery in our hospital. Vaginal delivery is an independent risk factor leading to PFDs of primiparous women in short-time postpartum period. Although cesarean delivery reduces the risk of pelvic floor trauma, it is not entirely protective [24]. Cesarean delivery is a protective delivery method for PFM of women in recent postpartum, but may be not useful for women in late postpartum [17]. Moreover, cesarean delivery may easily bring other severe complications. Episiotomy may cause injury of PFM in low risk vaginal delivery or forceps vaginal delivery. We should try our best to reduce the rate of episiotomy in order to protect PFM in primiparous women.

When the damage of PFM occurs, how to restore and exercise the weak PFM in the short-time postpartum period is the focus. Many studies show that the PFM training can prevent and treat pelvic floor disease in antenatal and postnatal women [25]. Our study shows that the combined treatment of at-home PFM exercise plus in-hospital electrical stimulation combined with biofeedback is an effective way to restore the PFM strength that is damaged by pregnancy and delivery in a short-time.

The limitation of our study

Our study is subjected to a few limitations. Firstly, the modified Oxford score is very simple and is not sensitive enough to describe accurate change of PFM strength of the postpartum women. Another limitation is that palpation does not provide global assessment of the levator ani muscle which can be measured by techniques such as ultrasound imaging, MRI, a predefined protocol [26], and so on. Lastly, due to lack of experience, it is difficult for postpartum women to properly cooperate with examination expert.

The high rate of cesarean delivery and low rate of operative vaginal delivery are the limitations of our study. In China, the high cesarean delivery rate is a social problem, nearly half of all newborns in China are delivered by cesarean approach [27]. From January 2013 to January 2014, there were 13,490 cases of Chinese s primiparas delivered in our birth centre, the overall rate of cesarean delivery was 43.1%(5809/13490) and the overall rate of operative vaginal delivery was 1.6%(220/13490). Many operative vaginal deliveries were replaced by cesarean delivery, and the rate of maternal request cesarean delivery was nearly 10.0%(1351/13490). There was common preineum local block anesthesia before episiotomy but no neuraxial labor anlagesia for vaginal delivery.

Conclusions

Vaginal delivery is an independent risk factor causing the damage of PFM in the short-term after delivery. Episiotomy may cause injury of PFM. Through PFM training at home plus electrical stimulation combined with biofeedback therapy in hospital, those damage will resume as soon as possible in the short-time period after postpartum.

Abbreviations

GDM: Gestational diabetes mellitus; PFDs: Pelvic floor disorders; PFM: Pelvic floor muscle; SEMG: Surface electromyography

Acknowledgments

Thank the postpartum women, students, midwives and nurses for their contribution to this study. Special thanks to Dr. Liyan Gong for the contributions to guide the PFM training at home and in hospital.

Funding

This work was supported by the Natural Science Foundation of Hubei Province, China (No.2009CDA064, No: 2011CDC098) and Foundation from Health and Family Planning Commission of Hubei Province (No: WJ2015MB121).

Authors' contributions

YZ, who was the assessor of the PFM strength, conceived the study, analyzed the data, interpreted the results, and drafted the manuscript. MX conceived the study and drafted the manuscript. WT, who was also the assessor of the PFM strength, guided the PFM training and analyzed the data. LZ, HN, FQ analyzed the data and revised the manuscript. All authors read and approved the final manuscript.

Competing interests

The authors declare that they have no competing interests.

Author details

[1]Department of Obstetrics, Maternal and Child Health Hospital of Hubei Province, No 745 Wuluo Road, Wuhan City, People's Republic of China. [2]Department of Obstetrics and Gynecology, Union Hospital of Tongji Medical

College, Huazhong University of Science and Technology, Wuhan City, People's Republic of China. [3]Department of Obstetrics and Gynecology, Tongji Hospital of Tongji Medical College, Huazhong University of Science and Technology, Wuhan City, People's Republic of China.

References

1. Jelovsek JE, Barber MD. Women seeking treatment for advanced pelvic organ prolapse have decreased body image and quality of life. Am J Obstet Gynecol. 2006;194(5):1455–61. PMID: 16647928
2. van Veelen GA, Schweitzer KJ, van der Vaart CH. Ultrasound imaging of the pelvic floor: changes in anatomy during and after first pregnancy. Ultrasound Obstet Gynecol. 2014;44(1):476–80. PMID: 24436146
3. Herrmann V, Scarpa K, Palma PC, Riccetto CZ. Stress urinary incontinence 3 years after pregnancy: correlation to mode of delivery and parity. Int Urogynecol J Pelvic Floor Dysfunct. 2009;20(3):281–8. PMID: 19020787
4. Tennfjord MK, Hilde G, Stær-Jensen J, Ellström Engh M, Bø K. Dyspareunia and pelvic floor muscle function before and during pregnancy and after childbirth. Int Urogynecol J. 2014;25(9):1227–35. PMID: 24687365
5. Chen X, Gong Y, Wu D, Li X, Li H, Tong X, et al. Pre- and postoperative evaluation of pelvic floor muscle function in POP patients using surface electromyography and digital palpation. Neurourol Urodyn. 2014;33(4): 403–7. PMID: 23754311
6. Zhao Y, Xiao M, Tang F, Tang W, Yin H, Sun GQ, et al. The effect of water immersion delivery on the strength of pelvic floor muscle and pelvic floor disorders during postpartum period: an experimental study. Medicine (Baltimore). 2017;96(41):e8124. PMID:29019880
7. Lee IS, Choi ES. Pelvic floor muscle exercise by biofeedback and electrical stimulation to reinforce the pelvic floor muscle after normal delivery. Taehan Kanho Hakhoe Chi. 2006;36(8):1374–80. PMID: 17215611
8. Yang S, Sang W, Feng J, Zhao H, Li X, Li P, et al. The effect of rehabilitation exercises combined with direct vagina low voltage low frequencyelectric stimulation on pelvic nerve electrophysiology and tissue function in primiparouswomen: a randomised controlled trial. J Clin Nurs. 2017;26(23–24):4537–47. PMID: 28252827
9. Shek K, Dietz H. Intrapartum risk factors of levator trauma. Br J Obstet Gynecol. 2010;117(12):1485–92. PMID: 20735379
10. Glazener CM, MacArthur C, Hagen S, Elders A, Lancashire R, Herbison GP, et al. Twelve-year follow-up of conservative management of postnatal urinary and faecal incontinence and prolapse outcomes: randomized controlled trial. BJOG. 2014;121(1):112–20. PMID: 24148807
11. Boyle R, Hay-Smith EJ, Cody JD, Mørkved S. Pelvic floor muscle training for prevention and treatment of urinary and faecal incontinence in antenatal and postnatal women. Cochrane Database Syst Rev. 2012;17(10):CD007471. PMID: 23076935
12. Peng Y, Miller BD, Boone TB, Zhang Y. Modern theories of pelvic floor support: a topical review of modern studies on structural and functional pelvic floor support from medical imaging, computational modeling, and electromyographic perspectives. Curr Urol Rep. 2018;19(1):9. PMID 29435856
13. Botelho S, Pereira LC, Marques J, et al. Is there correlation between electromyography and digital palpation as means of measuring pelvic floor muscle contractility in nulliparous, pregnant, and postpartum women? Neurourol Urodyn. 2012;32(5):420–3. PMID: 23023961
14. Riesco ML, Caroci Ade S, de Oliveira SM, Lopes MH. Perineal muscle strength during pregnancy and postpartum: the correlation between perineometry and digital vaginal palpation. Rev Lat Am Enfermagem. 2010; 18(6):1138–44. PMID: 21340279
15. Memon H, Handa VL. Pelvic floor disorders following vaginal or cecarean delivery. Curr Opin Obstet Gynecol. 2012;24(5):349–54. PMID: 22907482
16. Lavy Y, Sand PK, Kaniel CI, Hochner-Celnikier D. Can pelvic floor injury secondary to delivery be prevented? Int Urogynecol J. 2012;23(2):165–73. PMID: 21822710
17. Handa VL, Blomquist JL, McDermott KC, Friedman S, Muñoz A. Pelvic floor disorders after vaginal birth: effect of episiotomy, perineal laceration, and operative birth. Obstet Gynecol. 2012;119(2 Pt 1):233–9. PMID: 22227639
18. Heit M, Mudd K, Culligan P. Prevention of childbirth injuries to the pelvic floor. Curr Womens Health Rep. 2001;1(1):72–80. PMID: 12112955
19. Macleod M, Goyder K, Howarth L, Bahl R, Strachan B, Murphy DJ. Morbidity experienced by women before and after operative vaginal delivery: prospective cohort study nested within a two-centre randomized controlled trial of restrictive versus routine use of episiotomy. BJOG. 2013; 120(8):1020–6. PMID: 23464382
20. Barbosa Am MG, Piculo F, Rudge CV, Calderon IM, Rudge MV. Prevalence of urinary incontinence and pelvic floor muscle dysfunction in primiparas two years after cesarean section:cross-sectional study. Sao Paulo Med J. 2013; 131(2):95–9. PMID: 23657511
21. Friedman S, Blomquist JL, Nugent JM, McDermott KC, Muñoz A, Handa VL. Pelvic muscle strength after childbirth. Obstet Gynecol. 2012;120(5):1021–8. PMID: 23090518
22. Handa VL, Blomquist JL, Knoepp LR, Hoskey KA, McDermott KC, Muñoz A. Pelvic floor disorders 5-10 years after vaginal or cesarean childbirth. Obstet Gynecol. 2011;118(4):777–84. PMID: 21897313
23. Daly N, Bonham S, O'Dwyer V, O'Connor C, Kent E, Turner MJ. National variations in operative vaginal deliveries in Ireland. Int J Gynaecol Obstet. 2014;125(3):210–3. PMID: 24709535
24. Elenskaia K, Thakar R, Sultan AH, Scheer I, Beggs A. The effect of pregnancy and childbirth on pelvic floor muscle function. Int Urogynecol J. 2011;22(11): 1421–7. PMID: 21789660
25. Xing W, Zhang Y, Gu C, Lizarondo L. Pelvic floor muscle training for the prevention of urinary incontinence in antenatal and postnatal women: a best practice implementation project. JBI Database System Rev Implement Rep. 2017;15(2):567–83. PMID:28178026
26. Kruger JA, Budgett SC, Wong V, Nielsen PMF, Nash MP, Smalldridge J, et al. Characterizing levator-ani muscle stiffness pre- and post-childbirth in European and Polynesian women in New Zealand: a pilot study. Acta Obstet Gynecol Scand. 2017;96(10):1234–42. PMID:28664535
27. Xiong C, Zhou A, Cao Z, Zhang Y, Qiu L, Yao C, et al. Association of pre-pregnancy body mass index, gestational weight gain with cesarean secti on in termdeliveries of China. Sci Rep. 2016;6:37168. PMID 27872480

8

Underreporting of stillbirths in Pakistan: perspectives of the parents, community and healthcare providers

Muhammad Zakria Zakar[1], Rubeena Zakar[2], Mudasir Mustafa[1], Aisha Jalil[1] and Florian Fischer[3*]

Abstract

Background: Pakistan has the highest rate of stillbirths globally. Not much attention has been given so far to exploring the sociocultural factors hindering the reportage of stillbirths and the causes of death. Therefore, the aim of this study was to assess the perspectives of parents, communities and healthcare providers regarding the sociocultural practices and health system-related factors contributing to stillbirths and their underreporting.

Methods: This study used a qualitative approach including in-depth interviews and 14 focus group discussions to collect data from four districts of Pakistan. We conducted 285 in-depth interviews and 14 focus group discussions with health professionals – mainly active in the areas of maternal and child health – and parents who had experienced stillbirth. Constant comparative method and analytical induction method were performed to analyze the data.

Results: The results of this study show that stillbirth is frequently misclassified and, therefore, an underreported phenomenon in Pakistan. It is an outcome of sociocultural practices, such as the social meaning of stillbirth and their understanding about the conflict between cultural and medical anatomy. In addition to grief and psychological distress, it endangers the maternal identity and worth in society in contrast to the mothers of live-born children.

Conclusion: The misclassification of stillbirth, especially by healthcare providers, is a significant impediment to designing preventive strategies for stillbirth. We recommend that the reporting system for stillbirth should be aligned with the WHO definition of stillbirth to avoid its underreporting. Reporting procedures at a more administrative level need to be made uniform and simplified.

Keywords: Stillbirths, Pakistan, Gestational health, Cause of death, Underreporting

Background

The birth of child with no sign of life, such as breath, voluntary muscle movement and heartbeat, after 28 weeks of pregnancy is known as stillbirth [1, 2]. The main causes of stillbirths are hypertension, eclampsia, abruptio placenta, birth asphyxia, preterm labor, inadequate antenatal care and suboptimal intrapartum [3]. It is important to distinguish among the pregnancies which does not result in a live child to improve the registration of fetal deaths as a vital part of global newborn survival efforts [4]. Global health statistics showed that around 2.6 million stillbirths occur annually, of which 75% takes place in low- and middle-income countries [5, 6]. Pakistan was the country with the highest stillbirth rate (43.1 stillbirths per 1000 total births compared to a global estimate of 18.4) globally in 2015 [7]. Despite the relevance of stillbirths, it remains an unrecognized issue in several countries, including Pakistan.

High stillbirth rates may be attributed to the lack of proper gynecological and obstetric care, poor maternal health, inadequate modes of delivery, violence in gestation and sociocultural practices [8, 9]. Additionally, the risk of stillbirth is high for low- or overweight fetuses [10]. Empirical evidence revealed that 2.6 million stillbirths take place annually in rural areas away from health facilities [11]. Similarly, the high incidence of stillbirth in Pakistan can be attributed to the delayed healthcare-seeking

* Correspondence: f.fischer@uni-bielefeld.de
[3]Department of Public Health Medicine, School of Public Health, Bielefeld University, Bielefeld, Germany

behavior, especially in rural areas due to the lack of accessible and quality healthcare facilities [12].

Research has revealed that stillbirths are not reported to hide the errors in healthcare provision [13]. Effective reporting depends on accurate knowledge regarding stillbirth, specifically how it is distinguishable from neonatal deaths. The records of child mortality and causes of death (COD) are maintained through vital statistics reporting systems in developed countries. However, the COD is mostly not recorded for stillbirths, particularly in developing countries. The vital registration data of Pakistan, for example, did not include COD for approximately 97% of perinatal deaths [14]. In addition, the District Health Information System (DHIS) and Lady Health Workers Management Information System are used to record child health- and mortality-related information in Pakistan. The DHIS report for 2013 lacks any kind of information on stillbirths and related COD [15].

The identification of the contextual and maternal factors leading to potentially preventable stillbirths can help to control the occurrence of stillbirths [16]. Stillbirths may lead to parental depression and sometimes condemnation for mothers by the community [15]. Moreover, a growing body of literature on stillbirths highlighted that statistics about stillbirths are not accurate and lead mostly to an underreporting in developing countries. This is due to various reasons, including the stigma associated with stillbirths [16–18]. Given this backdrop, the aim of this study is to understand sociocultural- and health system-related factors hindering the timely reporting of stillbirths.

Methods

Study design and data collection

This study used a qualitative approach including focus group discussions (FGDs) and in-depth interviews (IDIs) to collect data from four districts of Pakistan (Nowshehra, Mardan, Tando Allah Yar and Thatta) from the two provinces of Sindh and Khyber Pakhtunkhawa (KPK). The participants were recruited using purposive and snowball sampling. At initial stage, the researchers contacted with district healthcare officer/ manager to get access to district coordinators, and Lady Health Workers (LHW) or Community Midwives (CMWs) and Traditional Birth Attendants (TBAs). The LHWs, CMWs, and TBAs provided further access to couples and women who had experienced stillbirths in past 5 years.

The FGDs were conducted at first and the participants who were found to be more informative were also recruited for IDIs. The participants of FGDs provide referrals to more women and men for IDIs. A total 14 FGD (7 with men and 7 with women) were conducted in both provinces of Pakistan (see Table 1). In each FGD, around 6 to 8 participants were recruited, thus, a total 42 women and 46 men – who had experienced stillbirth – participated in FGDs.

After FGDs, a total of 285 IDIs were conducted with a variety of stakeholders. Of which, 10 IDIs were conducted with District Health Coordinators, 124 with staff from the Health Facility in Charge, 65 with LHWs or CMWs and TBAs (Table 1). Each IDI was conducted at the desired place of the participants. All district health coordinators and in-charge of health facility, LHWs, CMWs, and TBAs provided interviews at health facility. However, more than half of the participating women also requested to provide the interview at the health facility as they found it to be a comfortable place to talk. Thus, the researchers took more than half of the interview at the health facility, while the rest was taken at the respective home of the women.

Both IDIs and FGDs are conducted in their native or mother language, Sindhi and Pashto. For this, a total of 10 female and two male researchers, who spoke the native language as well as were able to speak and write national and official language of Pakistan, Urdu and English respectively, were hired to conduct the IDIs and FGDs. A two-day training was organized for them. The IDIs and FGDs were recorded after the consent of the participants had been granted. Healthcare providers who had had more than 1 year of work experience and women and men participants who had experienced at least one stillbirth were included in the study.

The study followed ethical issues throughout research. The participation in study was voluntarily and the study participants were told that they can drop at any point of the study. The privacy and confidentiality of the participants were maintained, thus, the name and addresses of the participants were neither asked nor recorded at paper or audio-recorded. In addition, the security concerns of researchers and study participants were also catered and the IDIs and FGDs were conducted at health facility, which were considered safest by study participants. In case, when the study participants were requested to provide interview at their homes, then, the trustworthy LHWs and CMWs accompany the female researcher, while the health-facility in-charge or male dispenser of the health facility accompany the male researchers.

Data analysis

The data collected through IDIs and FGDs were transcribed into verbatim Urdu (when the conversations were in Sindhi and Pushto [local languages], they were first translated into Urdu with the help of native speakers) and then translated into English. It was ensured throughout the process of translation that the contextual meaning intended by the participant's statements did not get lost. We used the constant comparative method [19] and analytical induction method of data analysis [20] to generate causal

Table 1 Participants, sample size and methods of data collection

	Participant categories	Methods of data collection	Number of interviews	Province
1	Health facility in charge, Lady Health Visitor, Medical Technician	In-depth interview	124	Sindh: 62 KPK: 62
2	Lady Health Worker, Community Midwife	In-depth interview	65	Sindh: 32 KPK: 33
3	Women who experienced a stillbirth	In-depth interview	50	Sindh: 21 KPK: 29
4	Traditional Birth Attendants	In-depth interview	36	Sindh: 19 KPK: 17
5	Coordinators (e.g. for LHW, District Health Information System, Maternal Neonatal Child Health program)	In-depth interview	10	Sindh: 6 KPK: 4
6	Men and women who experienced stillbirth	Focus group discussion	14	Sindh: 7 KPK: 7

explanations of phenomena. In this regard, we studied a few cases of the phenomenon to be explained initially and looked for similar factors. The explanation for further cases was established after developing a hypothetical explanation based on the primary analysis. The researchers read the translated data thoroughly and moved back and forth in the transcripts. The themes were identified from the data based on the similarities and differences of the views/responses of the participants. Subsequently, various sub-themes were identified under each theme based on the frequency of the codes. The data validity and triangulation of findings were ensured by frequent meetings and analysis by the researchers.

Results

The findings are presented under four main themes: community views on the nature of pregnancy and stillbirth, women's experiences of stillbirth reporting, stillbirth causation and the reasons for underreporting. Each theme has more than two sub-themes which are presented as follows.

Community views on the nature of pregnancy and stillbirth

Sociocultural practices

It was found that women's access to health facilities was restricted due not only to their unavailability in their vicinity, but also to the cultural inhibitions and reliance on male family members (such as a brother, father or husband). Healthcare accessibility is controlled mainly by the male head of the household and mothers-in-law. It is usual cultural practice that the mother-in-law decides about healthcare utilization for her daughter in-law. In most cases, the mother-in-law is not in favor of seeking emergency services, and this may lead to the death of the fetus. Women related that they were not taken to the hospital when a complicated pregnancy arose. Poverty was one reason cited for such undesirable situations, yet some women blamed themselves for the negligence:

> *Poverty devastated me; I had four stillbirths in a row. Most people are illiterate and poor here. They are conservative; they do not allow their women to go for check-ups. But rich women do not face such issues; they have more freedom than us.*

A TBA reported similar experiences:

> *Women are not allowed to visit the health facility center without being accompanied by a male relative or an older woman of the house. For this reason, I went for irregular antenatal check-ups.*

Stoicism and sorcery

Most community members and parents referred to the causes of stillbirths that were rooted in the local religious and cultural context. People believe that stillbirths are an outcome of the evil eye, black magic, curses and *taweez* (an amulet or locket usually containing verses from the Quran or other prayers and symbols) which is inflicted by jealous relatives. A feeling of fear and helplessness was observed from the discourse of participants in this regard. A male FGD participant said:

> *Taweez and black magic are the reasons for child deaths before birth and often these are performed by other female relatives.*

By contrast, another very consistent response was that the life and death are at the sole discretion of Allah (God) and it was his will that caused the stillbirth:

> *You cannot stand before the will of Allah. Each second of our life is predetermined and these cases (stillbirths) are essentially a test by Allah to check our faith and patience.*

In some cases, women were not allowed to carry the babies of other women because the former were ill-fated and, thereby, considered to be untouchables:

> *My sister-in-law did not allow me to hold her newborn baby. She said that I killed (lost) my two babies and she did not want to have such misfortune.*

Mothers of stillborn babies were also not allowed to attend celebrations to welcome the unborn baby. Women are not invited to such happy occasions as a reminder of their lost child. However, most participants refuted this proposition and argued that women were not invited simply because they were considered "sinful child-killers." A woman described such a situation:

> *I was not allowed to place fruit in my sister's lap (a ritual) at her* gaud bharai *(a celebration to congratulate an expecting mother in the seventh month of her pregnancy). I cannot explain the pain of such a rejection by my own family members.*

As a response to social discrimination, some women consulted religious and traditional healers to avoid stillbirth in the future. These healers give the women either *taweez* (amulets) to wear around the neck or some kind of 'holy' water to drink.

Indigenous terminology and understanding about stillbirth

The terminology used for stillbirth varies by sociocultural milieu among the regions in Pakistan. The data analysis demonstrated that the meaning of stillbirth was unclear and vague to the parents, community and healthcare providers. Labelling the reality by a local word may not be the issue, but it becomes a matter of concern by the virtue of connotations attached to it. The parents and families not only had a misplaced understanding of the concept of stillbirth, but the healthcare providers also wrongly defined and, thus, erroneously classified it in a certain category. Most of the time, for example, they were unclear about the difference between miscarriages, stillbirths and neonatal deaths, which resulted consequently in the underreporting of the cases of stillbirth. Hence, stakeholders were asked to clarify the meanings of stillbirth to assess the validity of reporting.

Male and female participants of FGDs exhibited a deficient understanding about stillbirth. Of the 14 FGDs conducted, there were only two such discussions where the participants defined the concept of stillbirth correctly. It is also significant to note that there were no marked differences between the knowledge of male and female FGD participants regarding stillbirths. In addition, the discussion about stillbirths was judged as useless:

> *Why are you people wasting time discussing things which are not in our hands? If a fetus dies in the abdomen of mother, who knows the cause? Who knows the time? It is by the will of Allah. He knows better.*

In addition, male and female participants during the FGD used the word *batcha* for a fetus whether it was dead or alive. The place of *batcha* in the uterus was also culturally defined and understood; some mothers thought that the *batcha* is positioned somewhere in the abdomen, while others considered it was in the *bitcha-e-dani* (the lower abdomen/uterus). Keeping such folk anatomy in mind, women were advised to drink hot milk with ghee (butter with the fat removed) so that a slippery situation in the *bitcha-e-dani* facilitates the delivery. Any action of women which deviates from such cultural understanding was considered to be a cause of stillbirth. Thus, we found that a lack of understanding about stillbirth was augmented because of inconsistent terminologies (a wide gap between biomedical and local terminologies).

The entire process of delivery, its method, competence of the care provider, correct temperature maintained at the place of delivery, appropriate method of delivery, handling of mother and child at the time of delivery and afterwards (e.g. massage of the abdomen, position of the mother, type of food given to the mother at the time of delivery) were all comprehensively defined by the local culture with appropriate language and terminology. Additionally, the local culture had a readily available 'tool-kit' for all these steps, processes and procedures, which was shared by the local population. The phenomenon of stillbirth was conceived, interpreted and reported with this cultural understanding of the entire reproductive process.

Women's experiences of stillbirth reporting

Threat to maternal identity

The participants reported the perception that any disability or weakness, such as stillbirth, needs to be kept secret, at least as far as possible. This is because no one wants to be stigmatized with any disability, primarily because of its negative implications regarding one's image in society. A common belief is that a woman brings her fortune and misfortune with her to her in-laws. If something adverse happens, women are blamed as ill-omened. A woman is threatened with a second marriage of her husband by the in-laws. Therefore, mothers experiencing stillbirths have to face dehumanization, humiliation and sometimes social exclusion. The healthcare system in Pakistan often tends to reveal the identity of patients, though the government has been providing training to healthcare staff (particularly community-based healthcare staff and providers) to maintain the confidentially of the patients. However, the community healthcare workers often reveal the identity of the women who have experienced stillbirths. Therefore, mothers do not report a stillbirth to avoid any associated threats.

Avoidance of isolation and shame

The findings revealed that stillbirths are less reported by women to avoid getting blamed and being stigmatized. The LHWs highlighted adverse social consequences for women who experienced stillbirth. They pointed out that in the case of one stillborn baby, some families who were educated and knowledgeable took it as "Allah's will" and did not blame the woman or anyone else for this happening. In fact, they analyzed the situation resulting in stillbirth and, thereby, started to take care of the mother and followed the appropriate treatment. In cases of repeated stillbirths, women reported becoming dishonored and stigmatized as ominous or unfortunate. In addition, they frequently reported neglect and mistreatment by their husband and his family. In extreme situations in the case of repeated stillbirths, women were even divorced.

It was noted during the male FGDs that women were often blamed for not taking care of their pregnancy. Contrary to the views expressed by the female interviewees, men believed that it was the responsibility of the woman to manage her dietary habits and health issues during pregnancy. Maternity-related issues were considered by some male participants as an exclusively female domain where the women should discuss any problems with other females at home or with female neighbors:

> *We (males) remain outside the home for most of the day. Females understand these issues better and they should deal with them at their own level.*

Another male participant provided the following statement:

> *Both, family and women are responsible for stillbirth, but it is obvious that the woman is to be blamed more for her carelessness.*

Women who had experienced stillbirth stated that they were not only ostracized by their men but also by other women of the family.

Not a single woman who experienced stillbirth in the sample confirmed that they reported the stillbirth to DHIS or vital registration. The disconnect between government health facilities and private clinics/hospitals for DHIS-based data collection was frequently reported as a cause of lower stillbirth reporting.

Stillbirth causation

Social mobility and healthcare accessibility

The qualitative data analysis revealed that the long distances between the house of the pregnant woman and the nearest health facility, lack of availability of transport, restricted mobility of (pregnant) women, delayed healthcare-seeking behavior and irregular antenatal visits contributed significantly to the occurrence of stillbirths. One TBA, for example, endorsed this issue by stating:

> *After feeling labor pains, waiting for a male guardian to come home sometimes extends for hours, which increases the intensity of the complexity of the delivery.*

Several babies were reported to have died in their mothers' wombs before reaching the nearest health facility. In most of the cases, public health facilities were located far away from the residence of the expectant mothers, which constrained their ability to use the facility. Another woman shared similar experiences:

> *My doctor told me that my baby's position was abnormal, so I had to report to doctor when pains came. Unfortunately, my husband was not at home at that time, so delayed contact to the doctor resulted in the death of my baby.*

The participants frequently mentioned in the FGDs that healthcare accessibility varies between women depending on their financial resources. The socioeconomic dependence on husbands was also found to be linked with pregnancy problems. Women could not spend money on their health during pregnancy, which was related as follows:

> *Women cannot spend money on their health. Male members of family say that it is useless to go to the doctor both before and at the delivery.*

It was implicit in the comments of some women that their families or husbands were responsible for not taking care of them:

The doctor advised me to take multivitamins and calcium tablets, but I was not able to go to the pharmacy alone.

> *I had been having severe pains since the early morning that day, but my husband came home late from work. I think it was all over by the time he took me to the hospital.*

Major deficiencies and diseases

Regarding medical grounds, nutritional deficiency, anemia, and high or low blood pressure were cited as frequent medical problems experienced during pregnancy by the women who had had a stillbirth. Most of the women attributed the cause of the stillbirth to lack of proper food at the proper time. Others considered propriety not in food itself, but also in the process of cooking:

> *When I was pregnant, my mother in-law always gave me inappropriate food. My husband said that beef was not good during pregnancy, but my in-laws never cared about this. They frequently cooked beef. Since nothing else was available at home, I used to have beef and you can see its result [referring to the stillbirth.*

The TBAs agreed that anemia, malnutrition, dehydration and high blood pressure were the most common reasons for the occurrence of stillbirths. They used complex local terminology mixed with biomedical concepts while expanding such reasons. Sometimes they tried to converge and connect the meaning of both medical systems by using their own culture-specific knowledge. One TBA, while explaining high blood pressure as the cause of adverse pregnancy outcomes, narrated:

> *A child is very tender and vulnerable in the womb. It can die with the pressure and excessive heat. When the mother has blood pressure and she also works in the kitchen for long hours, it creates a double burden and heat on the fetus. If mother is then denied cold and fresh food, the child will die.*

Women also used different terminologies when talking about the causes of stillbirth, and the mother was usually blamed for the baby's death. It was observed that the women were frequently not informed about the cause of stillbirths by the healthcare professionals:

> *The doctor did not tell us (about the cause of stillbirth), neither did we ask. I do not know anything more than that. I lost my child before his birth.*

> *I strongly believe that my child was born alive and I could feel movement until the last moment. I do not know why it was a stillbirth.*

Mishandling of pregnancy-related complications

Some women stated that the health professionals initially told them that their case was normal, but when they went to the health facility, they were operated on. These women considered that an unwarranted operation was the cause of the stillbirth:

> *Half of the child was out and they were trying to pull it. Then it was pushed back and they operated. This was why the baby died.*

It was also reported that there was a deep distrust between the care provider and the mother. One reason for this distrust was that the care providers never took the mother or her relatives into their confidence when making the decisions. A male participant recorded his strong suspicions about the unnecessary medical procedures recommended or even carried out by care providers in order to make money:

> *Doctors have stories to tell each patient. Firstly, they create fear by saying that there is not enough fluid, the baby's movement is low or the cord is around the neck. Then they start preparing for a major operation (referring to caesarean section). They just fool people. This was how they killed my brother's unborn son.*

Reasons for underreporting

Understanding of healthcare providers about stillbirth

The findings showed that about two-thirds of the LHWs were unable to differentiate clearly between stillbirths and other adverse pregnancy outcomes and neonatal deaths. It may be assumed that they would not be reporting stillbirth cases accurately. One LHW with several years of experience as a community care provider said:

> *Stillbirth refers to either the death of the child within one to one days after birth or the death of the child in the mother's womb.*

Although, according to this definition, she considered perinatal death as a stillbirth, it was interesting to note that she had not observed a stillbirth in her area. Since management information systems rely on the reporting of Lady Health Workers Management Information Systems for the collection of primary data, the restricted ability of any LHW to differentiate between various kinds of child mortalities obscures the credibility of the whole process of the information systems in place. Another LHW stated her confusion about the reporting of stillbirths:

> *It is very confusing to define stillbirth. I have asked the Lady Health Supervisor about the difference between a stillbirth and a neonatal death. She said, it's almost the same, so we can report it any way we want.*

It was also noted that some LHWs did not consider it necessary to understand a clear distinction between miscarriage, fetal death and stillbirth. Like the general public, they used local terminology to explain the reality; the problem with the local terminology was that it was very vague and embedded in the cultural anatomy, which is the cultural understanding of the body. However, this cultural anatomy may not correspond to the biomedical understanding of the human body and its functioning. For example, in the local culture, Stillbirth, for example, is understood in the local culture as a fetus who has died in the *pait* (means literally "abdomen") of the mother. Technically, the fetus is not positioned in the abdomen but in the uterus. When health care providers, especially non-doctors, use local terminology and subscribe to the local world view, it distorts the accurate information.

Mistrust of healthcare providers

Poverty, sociocultural practices, lack of adequate services/staff availability at government facilities and transport problems were the reasons for using the services of TBAs as birth attendants. The magnitude of relying on the TBAs can be assessed by the claim of one TBA who reported having conducted 3000 deliveries in 11 years. Since the role of TBAs has a cultural connotation in many villages, it was noted that some interviewees showed of mistrust of healthcare providers and were more confident with the proficiency of TBAs – such as Dais – than skilled health care providers:

> *The Dai in our village is very experienced. If she could not save my baby, it was Allah's will. There is no need to report it to anyone.*

Missing capacity and competency for reporting

The capacity and competency of the medical officers and other administrational support staff for handling and maintaining the health information system's data including the stillbirths was a matter of serious concern. It was reported that most of the staff members, such as medical technicians, dispensers, nurses and even medical officers, were not adequately trained to handle different formats of registers and reports for retrieving and compiling information on stillbirths. The task was delegated to one or two staff members who had some relevant competency for recording and retrieving data from different sources and compiling it for preparing monthly reports for timely submission to the district management. The absence of systematic mechanisms for monitoring and quality assurance was claimed; staff members themselves were responsible for ensuring the accuracy of the information. In the case of their leaving or being absent from duty, the data was not maintained and updated by other staff members due to a lack of relevant expertise.

Lack of institutionalized coordination among healthcare providers

Healthcare providers at the community level include LHWs, TBAs and CMWs. The LHWs have the primary role of collecting and recording stillbirth-related information. Additionally, TBAs and CMWs contribute by reporting stillbirths under the maternal, newborn and child health (MNCH) program. Data gathered from IDIs with LHWs, CMWs and TBAs revealed that all these functionaries belonged to the same local communities where they worked. Most of them knew one another and shared information on mother and child health-related issues routinely, including the cases of stillbirths. However, they did not have any institutionalized and structured mechanism for sharing such information. They could only receive such information as a matter of chance during their occasional interactions while moving around in the community.

Some of the LHWs opined that collecting and reporting information on different registers, cards and reports was a merely futile exercise, because they did not see that these reports could be of any use to higher authorities. They were also of the view that nobody bothered to check the reports and act accordingly; it was mere waste of time and money. They were convinced that information and monthly reports could only be of importance if the government started programs for controlling stillbirths. This was accentuated by one LHW as follows:

> *Preparing monthly reports on stillbirths is merely a formality and nothing more than that. Nobody is interested why this is happening. When the government does not do anything to control stillbirths, then why we are pressurized to submit reports every month?*

Perceived uselessness of reporting

The TBAs included in the study were asked to give insights into the community trends about reporting stillbirths. Almost two-thirds of the TBAs agreed that the women or members of their households did not share information about stillbirths:

> *If the stillbirth occurred at a private hospital or through home delivery, then the families did not bother to inform us and considered it unnecessary.*

TBAs thought that people considered reporting unnecessary because it could not bring their babies back. Some TBAs were themselves critical of the usefulness of reporting:

> *When nobody, neither managers nor families, care to take or adopt any preventive measures to avoid*

stillbirths or adverse pregnancy outcomes, then it is a useless activity.

In addition, the community perception about the lower prevalence of stillbirths undermines the reporting of stillbirth cases. The outcomes of the FGDs revealed that the prevalence of stillbirth was considered to be very rare.

Discussion

The data analysis demonstrated that the reporting behavior of stillbirths was associated with stigma [11, 21]. Another significant factor was the inaccurate understanding about the meaning of stillbirth by both healthcare providers and the community [22]. Previous research has already shown that mothers were frequently not sure whether their child was stillborn and what caused the death of their child [14]. We noted restrictions on women mobility and their dependency on males regarding the utilization of health services was a major factor contributing to poor pregnancy outcomes such as stillbirths. Our findings are aligned with research previously conducted in other developing countries including Pakistan [23, 24].

In addition, the local terminologies used for stillbirth in the four districts selected were inconsistent, vague and indicated misperceptions about its definition and causes. Women were stigmatized and blamed for delivering a stillborn child in all four districts. Women experiencing repeated stillbirths felt discriminated against and socially excluded by the community. In addition to maltreatment by their husbands, the other female members of the family also ostracized the women who experienced stillbirths. Consequently, women had low self-esteem and a sense of dejection, which may increase the likelihood of further adverse health outcomes [25].

There was absence of acceptance of caesarean section and women did not realize that the occurrence of stillbirths can be reduced through the provision of emergency obstetric services. By contrast, many healthcare providers believed that stillbirths cannot be prevented [26]. Moreover, the fatalistic attitude of the parents contributes to the number of stillbirths, because many people believe that "the baby was not destined to live." We also found that the stillbirths leave psychosocial impacts on mothers who have experienced them, which has already been extensively studied and proven empirically [27]. It is considered the mother's fault due to inappropriate diet or lifestyle, and a consequence of their sins/evil spirits [9, 16].

This study fills the gaps in the literature by providing an understanding of health providers, male community members and women who have experienced stillbirth. Additionally, this study helps towards understanding the local context and circumstances influencing stillbirth and its reporting in Pakistan. Collection of data from all tiers of stakeholders and community members is the major strength of this study. The study is well triangulated by using multiple methods of data collection. However, this study has certain limitations. The scope of the study did not include the voice of the older women of the family who have a major say in decision-making regarding seeking medical care in pregnancy. Information on health-related issues was based on self-reports of women and were not clinically proven. Recall bias and socially desirable answers by the participants were some further limitations.

Conclusion

Comprehensive strategies are needed to improve community participation and understanding about stillbirth. The reporting system for stillbirths should be aligned with the WHO definition of stillbirth [28]. Early screening and identification of high-risk pregnancies can prevent stillbirths. Specialized training and refresher courses are needed for LHWs, CMWs and other healthcare providers to screen and refer the cases of high-risk pregnancies to the health facilities. There is a need for raising the awareness and knowledge of mothers and families about the causes and risk factors leading to stillbirths with scientific evidence [29]. Community awareness and advocacy programs for better maternal health should be organized by health departments through designing media-based customized information programs regarding MNCH, and displaying awareness posters at health facilities,

Since the attitude and behavior of men are one of the important factors, it is imperative to improve the health literacy of the communities by involving them, particularly local religious leaders and men in MNCH awareness programs. Cultural narratives about stillbirth and stigmatization of women who experience stillbirth are a major bottleneck in implementing effective responses against the issue [30]. It is important to challenge the societal stereotypes about stillbirth by enhancing the communities' awareness and improving health literacy about the causes of stillbirth and the significance of its reporting.

Abbreviations

CMW: Community Midwife; COD: Cause of death; DHIS: District Health Information System; FGD: Focus group discussion; IDI: In-depth interview; KPK: Khyber Pakhtunkhawa; LHW: Lady Health Worker; MNCH: Maternal neonatal child health; TBA: Traditional Birth Attendant; WHO: World Health Organization

Acknowledgements

We acknowledge support of the publication fee by Deutsche Forschungsgemeinschaft and the Open Access Publication Funds of Bielefeld University.

Funding

The study was conducted with the financial support of Care International in Pakistan.

Authors' contributions

MZZ, RZ, MM contributed to the study design and data collection. MZZ, RZ, MM, AJ and FF contributed to data analysis and interpretation. MZZ drafted the manuscript, supported by RZ. MM, AJ and FF contributed to the writing of the manuscript and revised it critically for important intellectual content. All authors have read and approved the final version of this manuscript.

Competing interests

The authors declare that they have no competing interests.

Author details

[1]Department of Sociology, Institute of Social and Cultural Studies, University of the Punjab, Lahore, Pakistan. [2]Department of Public Health, Institute of Social and Cultural Studies, University of the Punjab, Lahore, Pakistan. [3]Department of Public Health Medicine, School of Public Health, Bielefeld University, Bielefeld, Germany.

References

1. World Health Organization. Maternal, newborn, child and adolescent health. Geneva: World Health Organization; 2017.
2. Hemenway HB, Davis WH, Chapin CV. Definition of stillbirth. Am J Public Health Nations Health. 1928;18(1):25–32.
3. Korde-Nayak Vaishali N, Gaikwad Pradeep R. Causes of stillbirth. J Obstet Gynecol India. 2008;58(4):314–8.
4. Lawn JE, Blencowe H, Pattinson R, Cousens S, Kumar R, Ibiebele I, Gardosi J, Day LT, Stanton C. Lancet's stillbirths series steering committee. Stillbirths: Where? When? Why? How to make the data count? Lancet. 2011;377(9775): 1448–63.
5. The Lancet Ending Preventable Stillbirths study group. Ending preventable stillbirths. An executive summary for The Lancet Series Lancet 2016 http://www.thelancet.com/pb/assets/raw/Lancet/stories/series/stillbirths2016-exec-summ.pdf
6. Baqui AH, Choi Y, Williams EK, Arifeen SE, Mannan I, Darmstadt GL, Black RE. Levels, timing, and etiology of stillbirths in Sylhet district of Bangladesh. BMC Pregnancy Childbirth. 2011;11(1):25.
7. Blencowe H, Cousens S, Jassir FB, Say L, Chou D, Mathers C, Hogan D, Shiekh S, Qureshi ZU, You D, Lawn JE, for the lancet stillbirth epidemiology investigator group. National, regional, and worldwide estimates of stillbirth rates in 2015, with trends from 2000: a systematic analysis. Lancet Global Health. 4:e98–108.
8. Chuwa FS, Mwanamsangu AH, Brown BG, Msuya SE, Senkoro EE, Mnali OP, Mazuguni F, Mahande MJ. Maternal and fetal risk factors for stillbirth in northern Tanzania: a registry-based retrospective cohort study. PLoS One 2017;12(8):e0182250.
9. Stephens L, Navin C, Thomas S, Sripada S, Church E, Tower C, Heazell A. Improving quality of care in pregnancies after stillbirth- an improvement science project in two UK maternity hospitals. BMC Pregnancy Childbirth. 2017;17(1):1–47.
10. Avachat S, Phalke DB, Phalke VD. Risk factors associated with stillbirth in the rural area of western Maharashtra, India. Arch Med Health Sci. 2015;3(1):1–4.
11. Engmann C, Garces A, Jehan I, Ditekemena J, Phiri M, Mazariegos M, Chomba E, Pasha O, Tshefu A, McClure EM, Thorsten V. Causes of community stillbirths and early neonatal deaths in low-income countries using verbal autopsy: an international, Multicenter Study. Am J Perinatol. 2012;32(8):585–92.
12. Mustufa MA, Kulsoom S, Sameen I, Moorani KN, Memon AA, Korejo R. Frequency of stillbirths in a tertiary care hospital, Karachi. Pak J Med Sci. 2016;32(1):91–4.
13. Earle S, Komaromy C, Layne L. Understanding reproductive loss: perspectives on life, death and fertility. New York: Routledge; 2016.
14. Jehan I, McClure EM, Salat S, Rizvi S, Pasha O, Harris H, Moss N, Goldenberg RL. Stillbirths in an urban community in Pakistan. Am J Obstet Gynecol. 2007;197(257):e1–8.
15. District Health Information System Punjab. MIS Director General Health Services Punjab, Lahore, Pakistan. 2013. http://www.phispb.com/dhis/
16. Froen FJ, Cacciatore J, McClure EM, Kuti O, Jokhio AH, Islam M, Shiffman J. Stillbirths: why they matter. Lancet. 2011;377(9774):1353–66.
17. Heazell AE, Siassakos D, Blencowe H, Burden C, Bhutta ZA, Cacciatore J, Dang N, Das J, Flenady V, Gold KJ, Mensah OK. Stillbirths: economic and psychosocial consequences. Lancet 2016;12;387(10018):604–616.
18. Sather M, Fajon AV, Zaentz RCE. The GAPPS review group. Global report on preterm birth and stillbirth: advocacy barriers and opportunities. BMC Pregnancy Childbirth. 2010;10(Suppl1):S5.
19. Boeije H. A purposeful approach to the constant comparative method in the analysis of qualitative interviews. Qual Quant. 2002;36(4):391–409.
20. Strauss A, Corbin J. Basics of Qualitative Research: Grounded Theory Procedures and Techniques. Newbury Park: Sage Publications; 1990.
21. Brierley-Jones L, Crawley R, Lomax S, Ayers S. Stillbirth and stigma: the spoiling and repair of multiple social identities. Omega – J Death Dying. 2015;70(2):143–68.
22. Olagbuji BN, Igbarumah S, Akintayo AA, Olofinbiyi BA, Aduloju PO, Alao OO. Maternal understanding of fetal movement in third trimester: a means for fetal monitoring and reducing stillbirth. Niger J Clin Pract. 2014;17(4):489–94.
23. McClure EM, Saleem S, Pasha O, Goldenberg RL. Stillbirth in developing countries: a review of causes, risk factors and prevention strategies. J Matern-Fetal Neonatal Med. 2009;22(3):183–90.
24. Hamid SA, Malik U, Richard F. Stillbirth – a neglected priority: understanding its social meaning in Pakistan. J Pak Med Assoc. 2014;64:3.
25. Goudar SS, Somannavar MS, Clark R, Lockyer JM, Revankar AP, Fidler HM, Sloan NL, Niermeyer S, Keenan WJ, Singhal N. Stillbirth and newborn mortality in India after helping babies breathe training. Pediatrics. 2013; 131(2):e344–52.
26. de Bernis L, Kinney MV, Stones W, ten Hoope-Bender P, Vivio D, Leisher SH, Bhutta ZA, Gülmezoglu M, Mathai M, Belizán JM, Franco L. Stillbirths: ending preventable deaths by 2030. Lancet. 2016;387(10019):703–16.
27. Säflund K, Sjögren B, Wredling R. The role of caregivers after a stillbirth: views and experiences of parents. Birth. 2004;31(2):132–7.
28. Da Silva FT, Gonik B, McMillan M, Keech C, Dellicour S, Bhange S, Tila M, Harper DM, Woods C, Kawai AT, Kochhar S. Stillbirth: case definition and guidelines for data collection, analysis, and presentation of maternal immunization safety data. Vaccine. 2016;34(49):6057.
29. Flenady V, Wojcieszek AM, Middleton P, Ellwood D, Erwich JJ, Coory M, Khong TY, Silver RM, Smith GC, Boyle FM, Lawn JE. Stillbirths: recall to action in high-income countries. Lancet. 2016;387(10019):691–702.
30. Horton R, Samarasekera U. Stillbirths: ending an epidemic of grief. Lancet. 2016;387(10018):515–6.

9

Risk factors of premature rupture of membranes in public hospitals at Mekele city, Tigray

Natnael Etsay Assefa*, Hailemariam Berhe, Fiseha Girma, Kidanemariam Berhe, Yodit Zewdie Berhe, Gdiom Gebreheat, Weldu Mamu Werid, Almaz Berhe, Hagos B Rufae and Guesh Welu

Abstract

Background: The incidence of premature rupture of membranes ranges from about 5% to 10% of all deliveries. A woman with premature rupture of membranes is at risk of intra-amniotic infection, postpartum infection, endometritis, and death. A neonate born from premature rupture of membranes mother is at high risk of respiratory distress syndrome, sepsis, intraventricular hemorrhage and death. Little is known regarding the risk factors in Ethiopia. Therefore, this study was conducted to identify risk factors of premature rupture of membranes among pregnant women admitted to public hospitals in Mekelle city, Tigray, Ethiopia.

Methods: Hospital based unmatched case control study design was implemented on 240 samples (160 controls and 80 cases) from pregnant mothers admitted to public hospitals in Mekelle city from February – April/2016. Data was collected by interviewer administered Structured questionnaire and checklist. Binary logistic regression model was used to see the association between dependent and independent variables and multivariable logistic regression was used to identify the independent predictors of premature rupture of membranes.

Results: A total of 160 controls and 80 cases were enrolled in the study. Multivariable logistic regression showed that history of abortion [AOR 3.06 (CI: 1.39, 6.71)], history of PROM [AOR 4.45 (CI: 1.87, 10.6)], history of caesarean section [AOR 3.15(CI: 1.05, 9.46)] and abnormal vaginal discharge in the index pregnancy [AOR 3.31(CI: 1.67, 6.56)] were positively associated with premature rupture of membranes.

Conclusions: Past obstetric history and risks in the index pregnancy have an association with premature rupture of membranes. The finding of the study suggests early identification and treatment of genitourinary infection.

Keywords: PROM, Risk factors, Case control, Public hospitals, Ethiopia

Background

Premature rupture of the membranes (PROM) is usually defined as rupture of membranes at any time before the onset of uterine contractions. PROM which occurs prior to 37 weeks of gestation is referred as preterm premature rupture of membranes (PPROM), whereas; PROM which occurs after 37 weeks of gestation is referred as term premature rupture of membranes. The latent period is defined as the duration from rupture of the membranes until the onset of true labor [1].

The fetal membrane is composed of the inner amnion and the outer chorion. At term, the amnion is a tough and firm but pliable membrane. This innermost avascular fetal membrane is contiguous with amniotic fluid and occupies a role of incredible importance in human pregnancy. The amnion provides almost all tensile strength of the fetal membranes. Thus, development of its components that protect against its rupture or tearing is vitally important to successful pregnancy outcome [2].

Worldwide, there is a slight difference in the prevalence of premature rupture of membranes and this could be due to the difference in the population studied. The incidence of PROM ranges from about 5% to 10% of all deliveries, and PPROM occurs in approximately 3% of all pregnancies. Approximately 70% of cases of PROM occur in pregnancies at term, but in referral centers,

* Correspondence: natty416@gmail.com
Adigrat University College of Health Sciences, Adigart, Tigray, Ethiopia

more than 50% of cases may occur in preterm pregnancies. PROM is the cause of about one third of all preterm births [1].

PROM is a significant cause of perinatal morbidity and mortality. The burden of PROM ranges from maternal and neonatal mortality and morbidity to national economic loss due to drug expense, hospitalization, absence from the workplace and expense to the health professionals [3].

Analysis of cost endured by PROM in Mexico showed a total cost for maternity and baby stay of 244,565 dollars and 496,3 97.8 dollars respectively. In addition to other costs, the total cost was 1,029,698.8 dollars. In USA hospital 16,500 dollars was incurred [4, 5].

Premature rupture of membranes results in maternal, infant and neonatal risks. Regarding Maternal risks; Infection of the amniotic cavity is the most common complication after PROM. Endometritis and Abruptio placenta occurs in approximately 2 to 29% and15–25% of cases respectively. Uncommon but serious complications of PROM managed conservatively include retained placenta and hemorrhage requiring dilation and curettage (12%), maternal sepsis (0.8%), and 0.14% maternal death [1, 3].

Fetal complications after membrane rupture include infection and fetal distress due to umbilical cord compression or placental abruption. Because of these factors, women with PROM have a higher risk of cesarean delivery for non-reassuring fetal heart rate. Fetal death occurs in 1 to 2% of cases of conservatively managed PROM. Respiratory distress syndrome (10–40%) is the most common serious acute morbidity after preterm PROM. Necrotizing enterocolitis, and intraventricular hemorrhage are also common. Serious perinatal morbidity can lead to long-term consequences such as chronic lung disease, visual or hearing difficulties, intellectual disabilities, developmental and motor delay, cerebral palsy, or death. Pulmonary hypoplasia is a serious fetal complication which occurs following PROM. (1,3,).

A study conducted in Adis Ababa at Tikur Anbesa Hospital on feto-maternal outcome found the prevalence of PROM to be 1.4%. Intraamnioutic infection was found in 31.5% of the women. Regarding perinatal outcome, 23.6% of them were delivered by c/s, whereas 12 perinatal deaths occurred [6].

So far neonatal and maternal mortality in the nation has declined from 49 per 1000 and 871 per 100,000 in 2000 GC to 28 and 420 in 2014 GC respectively. Despite the achievements, neonatal and maternal mortality is still among the highest in the globe. PROM is one of the major causes of prematurity and infection, which in turn are the leading cause of neonatal death. Consequences of PROM; preterm labour, Low birth weight and neonatal infection are common and significant health problem in Ethiopia [1, 7, 8].

In Ethiopia training manuals and guidelines like Basic Emergency Obstetric & Newborn Care were prepared to make health professionals competent in managing a woman with obstetric emergencies including PROM. Other Strategies were also developed to address the problem including referring women with pre-term prolonged rupture of membranes (longer than 12 h) to a referral-level facility for assessment and Use of prophylactic antibiotics and steroid following pre-labour rupture of membranes [9].

Prediction and prevention of PROM would offer the best opportunity to prevent its complications. The risk factors of PROM include prior preterm birth, cigarette smoking, polyhydramnios, urinary and sexually transmitted infection, prior PROM, work during pregnancy, low Body Mass Index, bleeding, low socioeconomic status [3].

Previous studies to identify the risk factors of PROM were done at different country and different time. Even though, a study was carried out to assess the feto-maternal outcome of PROM, information about the risk factors of PROM in Ethiopia is not available. Hence, this study was conducted to fill this gap by identifying the risk factors.

Methods

The study was conducted in Mekelle city from December/2015 – June/2016. Mekelle is the capital city of Tigray Region. There are three public hospitals and eight health centers along with many private health institutions [10].

Hospital based unmatched case control study design was implemented. The Study population was pregnant mothers who came to labour ward at public hospitals in mekelle city during the data collection period. Pregnant Women with PROM and without PROM beyond 28 weeks of gestation were included in this study. In Ethiopia, Rupture of membrane before 28 weeks gestation is regarded as abortion.

EPI INFO version 3.5.1 statistical software was used to calculate the sample size using the Double population formula for unmatched case control study by considering the proportion of abnormal vaginal discharge in controls 36.8% with Odds Ratio 2.30 in a previous study done in Uganda [11]. With assumption of 95% CI, 80% power, control to case ratio 2:1 the sample size was 228. By adding 5% non-response rate the total sample size becomes 240 (160 control and 80 cases).

There are three public hospitals in Mekele city. The sample size was allocated to the study hospitals proportionally based on a case flow in the preceding three months. Women with premature rupture of membranes who met the inclusion criteria were recruited consequently until the calculated sample size was attained.

Women without premature rupture of membranes who met the inclusion criteria and admitted following the cases was selected using simple random sampling technique as controls and interviewed in the study period.

A Structured questionnaire and checklist developed by the Authors after reviewing different literatures was used. Data was collected by three midwifes. The questionnaire was prepared in English, and translated to Tigrigna, and back to English to ensure consistency. The Data collection was supervised. The collected data was checked for completeness, consistency and clarity.

Data was entered using EpiData version 3.1and exported to SPSS version 20 for analysis. Frequency and percentage was used for categorical variable. Median and inter quartile range was computed. Odds ratio with 95% confidence interval was used to measure strength of association. Bivariate logistic regression model was performed to determine the crude association of the independent variables with the dependent variable. Variables with P-value < 0.25 at the bivariate logistic regression were exported to multivariable logistic regression model (backward stepwise) to control confounding factors and to see the independent predictors of PROM. Statistical significance was declared at $P < 0.05$. Efforts were made to confirm the fulfillment of major assumption of logistic regression. Absence of multicolinarity was found to be satisfied. Goodness of fit was checked by Hosmer and Lemeshow test and Omnibus test of model coefficients.

Results

Socio-economic and demographic factors

Two hundred forty participants ($n = 80$ for cases and $n = 160$ for controls) were enrolled in the study. The median age of the women for the case and control were 27 (IQR = 5) and 26 (IQR = 7) respectively. More than half of cases and controls were housewives, and the majority of cases and controls have attended more than secondary Education. Regarding residence, majority of cases and controls were living in urban. Majority of cases and controls belong to Tigray ethnicity. The proportion of participants earning < 1000 Ethiopian birr (1 us dollar = 27 birr) was higher in the cases than controls. Proportion of partner job, as a daily laborer is higher in cases than controls (Table 1).

Physical activity habits

The majority of the participants have no history of carrying heavy objects. Regarding to sleep more than two third of cases and controls reported that they sleep less than 8 h per day. Two in ten of women in cases and 15% of controls use transportation daily. It was observed that low proportion of cases and controls have a maid (Table 2).

Past obstetric and gynecologic history

Twenty-five (31.2%) of cases and 10.6% of controls had an abortion. Among the women who had an abortion, almost quarter of cases and 1 out of 10 controls had two abortions. One hundred two controls and 77.8% of cases have no history of preterm delivery. With regard to PROM one third of pregnant women in the case group and a small number of pregnant women in the control group have history of PROM. A few women in both case and control groups had cervical operation and cerclage. More than half of pregnant women, in case group and almost two third of pregnant women in control group has used modern contraceptive; the injectable being the commonly used one. Lower proportion of women had caesarean section in both case and control groups (Table 3).

Risks in the index pregnancy

The median gestational age of the pregnant women was 37.25 (IQR = 3.4) and 38.4(IQR = 2.8) for cases and controls respectively. Proportions of Primigravida and Nullipara mothers were higher in the control group than cases. A small number of cases and controls had mid-upper arm circumference below 23 cm. Abnormal vaginal discharge was reported by almost half of cases and 15.6% controls. The proportion of mothers who had antenatal care follow up in the cases, and controls was high. More than half of cases and controls had intercourse during third trimester. With regard to smoking, the number of active and passive smokers was few. The proportion of women who had vaginal bleeding in case and control group was low. The majority of cases and controls had no history of accident. Majority of women in both case and control groups had cephalic presentation. Number of PIH, Polyhydramnious and Multiple pregnancies were very few in both groups (Table 4a and b).

Risk factors of premature rupture of membranes (bivariate and multivariate analysis)

The bivariate analysis showed that only 13 variables were with a P- value less than 0.25. The 13 variables with a P-value less than 0.25 have been exported to the multivariable logistic regression. The multivariable analysis showed that only four variables have shown a significant association.

Accordingly, History of Abortion was found significantly associated with PROM. Those who had abortion were 3.06 times more likely to develop premature rupture of membranes with AOR 3.06 (CI: 1.39, 6.71). History of C/S also showed a significant association with the AOR 3.15(CI: 1.05, 9.46). Previous premature rupture of membrane was the strongly associated risk factor than the others. The odds of developing premature rupture of membranes among women who had previous PROM was 4.45 times higher than who had not history of PROM. Furthermore, abnormal vaginal discharge in

Table 1 Socio-demographic characteristics of cases and controls attending public hospitals of Mekelle city, Tigray, Ethiopia 2016

VARIABLES	CATEGORY	Cases N = 80(%)	Controls N = 160(%)	Total N = 240(%)
AGE	15–19	1(1.2)	10(6.2)	11(4.6)
	20–34	73(91.2)	132(82.5)	205(85.4)
	35–49	6(7.5)	18(11.2)	24(10)
Educational level	No formal Education	13(16.2)	29(18.1)	42(17.5)
	Primary	18(22.5)	30(18.8)	48(20)
	Secondary	19(23.8)	52(32.5)	71(29.6)
	More than secondary	30(37.5)	49(30.6)	79(32.9)
Mothers occupation	House wife	47(58.8)	90(56.2)	137(57.1)
	Merchant	14(17.5)	27(16.9)	41(17.1)
	Employee	15(18.8)	31(19.4)	46(19.2)
	Others[a]	4(5)	12(7.5)	16(6.7)
Residence	Urban	68(85)	133(83.1)	201(83.8)
	Rural	12(15)	27(16.9)	39(16.2)
Monthly Income[b]	< 1000	18(22.5)	24(15)	42(17.5)
	1001–2000	13(16.2)	39(24.4)	52(21.7)
	2001–3000	18(22.5)	31(19.4)	49(20.4)
	> 3000	31(38.8)	66(41.2)	97(40.4)
Marital status	Unmarried	4(5)	11(6.9)	15(6.2)
	Married	76(95)	149(93.1)	225(93.8)
Ethnicity	Tigray	76(95)	153(95.6)	229(95.4)
	Non Tigray	4(5)	7(4.4)	119(4.6)
Partner Educational level	No formal education	12(15)	29(18.1)	41(17.1)
	Primary	9(11.2)	29(18.1)	38(15.8)
	Secondary	22(27.5)	39(24.4)	61(25.4)
	More than secondary	37(46.2)	63(39.4)	100(41.7)
Partner job	daily laborer***	11(13.8)	21(13.1)	32(13.3)
	merchant	18(22.5)	30(18.8)	48(20.0)
	employee	44(55)	89(55.6)	133(55.4)
	others[a]	7(8.8)	20(12.5)	27(11.2)

[a] E.g. farmer, student
[b] = Ethiopian Birr
***Daily laborer- Daily laborer means someone who doesn't have a formal training, profession or employment, and does whatever job comes its way with a minimum and daily wage for a living

the index pregnancy was also significantly associated risk factor with AOR 3.31(CI: 1.67, 6.56). Whereas, carrying heavy objects, monthly income, sleep < 8, smoking, chronic cough, sexual intercourse, gravidity and parity, and accident were not associated with PROM (Table 5).

Discussion

The aim of this unmatched case control study was to identify the risk factors of premature rupture of membranes. This study identified that history of abortion, history of C/S, previous PROM and abnormal vaginal discharge to be significantly associated with PROM.

In our study, socio-demographic factors have no significant association with the occurrence of premature rupture of membranes though it was observed that a higher proportion of women below 1000 Ethiopian Birr (45 US dollar) per month in case group than the control. The result is in discordant with findings from Canada, USA, Brazil, Lithuania, Australia, Pakistan and India [12–18]. However, the finding is in line with researches

Table 2 Distribution of Risky physical activity habits among women in the case and control groups attending Public Hospitals of mekelle city, Tigray Ethiopia, 2016

Variable	Category	PROM status		Total
		Case n = 80(%)	Control n = 160(%)	
Carry heavy objects	Yes	28(35)	34(21.2)	62(25.8)
Sleep < 8 hours	Yes	25(31.2)	35(21.9)	60(25)
Daily transportation	Yes	17(21.2)	24(15)	41(17.1)
Help at home	I don't have	20(25)	61(38.1)	81(33.8)
	My husband	18(22.5)	20(12.5)	38(15.8)
	Maid	16(20)	41(25.6)	57(23.8)
	Family	26(32.5)	38(23.8)	64(26.7)

Table 3 Past obstetric and gynecologic history of women among cases and controls attending public hospitals of mekelle city, Tigray Ethiopia

Variable	Category	PROM status		Total
		Case n = 80(%)	Control n = 160(%)	
Abortion	Yes	25(31.2)	17(10.6)	42(17.5)
Number of Abortion	1	17(68)	15(88.2)	32(76.2)
	2	6(24.0)	2(11.8)	8(19)
	3	2(8)	0(0)	2(4.8)
Type of Abortion	Spontaneous	18(72)	13(76.5)	31(73.8)
	Induced	5(20)	4(23.5)	9(21.49)
	Both	2(8)	0(0)	2(4.8)
Preterm delivery	Yes	6(7.5)	18(11.2)	24(10)
Previous PROM	Yes	27(33.8)	10(6.2)	37(15.4)
Cervix operation	Yes	4(5)	3(1.9)	7(2.9)
Cervical cerclage	Yes	3(3.8)	4(2.5)	7(2.9)
Modern contraceptive	Yes	48(60)	101(63.1)	149(62.1)
Contraceptive type	IUCD	2(4.2)	4(4)	6(4)
	Pill	7(14.6)	19(18.8)	26(17.4)
	Injectable	36(75)	64(63.4)	100(67.1)
	Implant	3(6.2)	14(13.9)	17(11.4)
C/S	Yes	13(16.2)	7(4.4)	20(8.3)

Table 4 Risks in the index pregnancy of women among cases and controls attending public hospitals of mekelle city, Tigray Ethiopia

Variable	Category	PROM status		Total
		Case $n = 80(\%)$	Control $n = 160(\%)$	
GA	< 37	33(42.3)	18(11.8)	51(22.2)
	37–42	42(53.8)	128(84.2)	170(73.9)
	> 42	3(3.8)	6(3.9)	9(3.9)
Gravidity	1	19(23.8)	60(37.5)	79(32.9)
	1–4	50(62.5)	84(52.5)	134(55.8)
	≥ 5	11(13.8)	16(10)	27(11.2)
Parity	0	25(31.2)	65(40.6)	90(37.5)
	1	28(35)	51(31.9)	79(32.9)
	2–4	22(27.5)	34(21.2)	56(23.3)
	≥ 5	5(6.2)	10(6.2)	15(6.2)
Hemoglobin level	< 11	4(5.1)	4(2.5)	8(3.4)
	≥ 11	75(94.9)	155(97.5)	230(96.6)
MUAC	< 23	11(13.8)	24(15)	35(14.6)
	≥ 23	69(86.2)	136(85)	205(85.4)
Abnormal Vaginal discharge	Yes	39(48.8)	25(15.6)	64(26.7)
ANC	Yes	78(97.5)	158(98.8)	236(98.3)
Number of Visit	1	1(1.3)	6(3.8)	7(3)
	2	1(1.3)	3(1.9)	4(1.7)
	> 2	76(97.5)	149(94.3)	225(95.3)
Chronic cough	Yes	28(35)	44(27.5)	72(30)
Third trimester intercourse	Yes	49(61.2)	84(52.5)	133(55.4)
Smoking/active or passive	yes	8(10)	13(8.1)	21(8.8)
Coffee intake	No	17(21.2)	8(5)	25(10.4)
	≤ two cup	32(40)	72(45)	104(43.3)
	>two cup	31(38.8)	80(50)	111(46.2)
Vaginal bleeding	Yes	7(8.8)	9(5.6)	16(6.7)
Accident	No	73(91.2)	151(94.4)	224(93.3)
	Fall	7(8.8)	9(5.6)	16(6.7)
Alcohol	Yes	24(30)	24(15)	48(20)
Presentation	Cephalic	71(88.8)	150(93.8)	221(92.1)
	Breech	8(10)	8(5)	16(6.7)
	Others	1(1.2)	2(1.2)	3(1.2)
PIH	Yes	5(6.2)	5(3.1)	10(4.2)
Polyhdramnious	Yes	1(1.2)	0(0)	1(0.4)
Multiple pregnancy	Yes	2(2.5)	4(2.5)	6(2.5)

done in Egypt and Uganda [19, 20]. The reason might be due to the participants sharing similar background.

In this study history of abortion was found to be a risk factor for PROM. Participants who had a history of abortion were 3.06 times more likely to develop PROM than who had no abortion. The number and type of abortion were not significant. This is supported by researches done in USA, Lithuania, India, China and Uganda [18, 19, 15, 21, 22]. Unlike our study Kaya in Uganda found a significant association between two and more induced abortions and PROM [19]. This difference might be due to low prevalence of induced abortion in our study.

Literatures from USA and China revealed that history of preterm birth to be a risk factor for premature rupture of membranes [21, 22]. This study however revealed no significant association between history of preterm birth and premature rupture of membranes. This is in line with other researchers from Lithuania, India, Pakistan and Uganda [15, 17–19].

Several studies from USA, Sweden, India, Thailand, Egypt, Nigeria and Uganda revealed that previous PROM was a significant risk factor for premature rupture of membranes [18–21, 23]. This study also showed that previous PROM to be the strongest risk factor for premature ruptures of membranes. Women who had previous PROM were 4.45 more likely to develop PROM with AOR 4.45 (CI: 1.87, 10.6). This might be due to untreated genitourinary infection and a short cervical length. In addition, obstetric problems are recurrent by nature.

Cervical cerclage was found to be a risk factor for PROM in the literatures of India and Uganda. This study failed to detect a significant association between a cervical cerclage and PROM since the factor was low in both groups [18, 19]. Similarly, our study revealed no significant association between history of operation on the cervix and PROM. This is supported by a study from India and Uganda [18, 19].

A study from Uganda revealed that caesarean section was a significant risk factor for premature rupture of membranes [19]. Our study also found the caesarean section to be a significant risk factor. Participants with history of C/S were 3.15 times more likely to develop PROM than who hadn't history of c/s. This might be due to the increased risk of rupture of C/S scar in the subsequent pregnancy.

Abnormal vaginal discharge has shown a significant association with the occurrence of PROM. Women who had an abnormal vaginal discharge in the index pregnancy were 3.31 times more likely to develop PROM. This is in line with a study conducted in Uganda and Egypt [19, 20]. Abnormal vaginal discharge is indicative of infection. Infection causes inflammation of the membranes leading to the rupture. Some genital bacteria elaborate enzymes such as proteases, phospholipases, and collagenases which cause membrane weakness and rupture [1].

In a study conducted in India and Uganda Antenatal care less than two follow up was found associated with PROM. During ANC visit there is a period

Table 5 Bivariate and multivariable logistic regression (final model) analysis result for significant variables ($p \leq 0.25$) in bivariate analysis in Mekelle City Public Hospitals, North Ethiopia, 2015

Variable	Category	COR (95% CI)	AOR (95% CI)
Monthly income	< 1000	1	1
	1001–2000	0.44(0.18,1.07)	0.37(0.13, 1.05)
	2001–3000	0.77(0.33, 1.80)	0.57(0.21, 1.53)
	> 3000	0.63(0.30, 1.32)	0.63(0.26, 1.52)
Carrying heavy objects	No	1	1
	Yes	1.99 (1.10, 3.62)[a]	1.63(0.81, 3.30)
Sleep < 8	No	1	1
	Yes	1.62(0.89, 2.97)	1.25(0.59, 2.64)
Abortion	No	1	1
	Yes	3.82 (1.91, 7.62)[a]	3.06 (1.39, 6.71)[a]
Previous PROM	No	1	1
	Yes	7.64 (3.47, 16.8)[a]	4.45 (1.87, 10.6)[a]
CS	No	1	1
	Yes	4.24 (1.62, 11.1)[a]	3.15(1.05, 9.46)[a]
Abnormal Vaginal discharge	No	1	1
	Yes	5.13 (2.78, 9.47)[a]	3.31(1.67, 6.56)[a]
Chronic cough	No	1	1
	Yes	1.42(0.80, 2.53)	0.75(0.36, 1.56)
Third trimester sexual intercourse	No	1	1
	Yes	1.43(0.83, 2.47)	1.44(0.75, 2.76)
Alcohol Intake	No	1	1
	Yes	2.42 (1.27, 4.63) [a]	1.93(0.91, 4.08)
History of accident	No	1	1
	Yes	4.33 (1.26,14.8) [a]	2.27(0.69, 7.40)
Gravidity	1	1	1
	1–4	1.88 (1.01, 3.51) [a]	1.80(0.30,10.6)
	> 5	2.17 (0.86, 5.48)	2.76(0.20, 36.8)
Parity	0	1	1
	1	1.48(0.77, 2.82)	0.66(0.29, 1.48)
	2–4	1.60(0.78,3.28)	0.50(0.19, 1.32)
	> 5	1.30(0.40, 4.18)	0.29(0.06, 1.45)

COR = Crude odds ratio, *AOR* = adjusted odds ratio
[a]Significant association

for counseling and health Education. This component helps pregnant women to keep their personal hygiene and avoid risky habits. In our study ANC was not found significantly associated with PROM. The reason might be ANC coverage in both groups was similarly high. Therefore, the study couldn't identify a significant difference [18, 19].

Several researchers found sexual intercourse during late pregnancy to be a risk factor to develop PROM. However, in this research association was not found between sexual intercourse and PROM. This is supported by a finding from Egypt [18–20, 24].

Nicotine, which is found in cigarette, causes constriction of arteries leading to ischemia of the decidua. Studies done in USA, India and Uganda revealed that smoking increases the risk of developing premature rupture of membranes. In this study there was no significant association found between smoking and PROM. This might be due to the low prevalence of the smoking in the study participants. Similarly, chronic cough and alcohol intake were not significant. This is comparable with a study done in Nigeria and Uganda [18–21, 24].

Vaginal bleeding, Accident, gestational age, Gravidity, parity, presentation, Polyhydramnious, multiple pregnancy, Anemia and Pregnancy Induced Hypertension were not found to be a significant predictor of premature rupture of membranes. This is discordant with findings from a research conducted in Sweden, Lithuania and India [18, 19, 15, 25].

Conclusion

In conclusion, this study found that past obstetric history and factors in the index pregnancy have association with premature rupture of membranes. The study revealed history of abortion, previous premature rupture of membranes, history of caesarean section and abnormal vaginal discharge in the index pregnancy to be a risk factor for premature rupture of membranes.

Abbreviations

ANC: Ante-natal care; IUCD: Intra uterine contraceptive device; MDGs: Millennium development Goals; OR: Odds ratio; PPROM: Preterm premature rupture of membranes; PROM: Premature rupture of membranes

Acknowledgements

We would like to thank Mekelle University for the approval of ethical clearance and technical support. Our deepest gratitude goes also to the respective hospitals for providing us the necessary information. Last but not least we would like to acknowledge data collectors, supervisor and study participants for their commitment.

Authors' contributions

NE, HB, and FG designed the study. NE, HBR, FG, KB, YB, GG, WW and AB made substantial contribution in data collection and analysis. NE, YB, KB, GW and HB draft the manuscript and revise it critically for important intellectual content. All authors given final approval of the final draft to be published.

Competing interests

The authors declare that they have no competing interests.

References

1. Gibbs R, Karlan B, Haney A, Nygaard I. Danforth's obstetrics and gynecology. 10th ed. Philadelphia: Lippincott Williams & Wilkins; 2008.
2. Cunnigham FGLK, Bloom SL, Hauth JC. Williams's obstetrics. 23th ed. USA: McGraw-Hill Companies; 2010.
3. Gabbe SG, Niebyl JR, Simpson JL. Obstetrics: Normal and problem pregnancies. 5th ed: Ed: Churchill Livingstone; 2007.
4. Nava Flores JEMM, Hernández-Valencia M. Maternal and fetal morbidity in patients with premature rupture of the membrane after 27-week gestation. Causes and Costs.
5. Wanda NKF, Neil P. Economic burden of hospitalizations for preterm labor in the United States. American College of obstetricians and Gynecologists. 2000;96(1):97–8.
6. Sirak B, Mesfin E. Maternal and perinatal outcome of pregnancies with PROM at Tikur Anbesa specialized teaching hospital. Ehtiop Med J. 2014;(4):52.
7. Ministry of Finance and Economics. Ethiopia MDGs report; 2012. p. 23–9.
8. Agency ECS, ICF International. Ethiopia demographic and health survey. Addis Ababa E, and Calverton. Central Statistical Agency and ORC Macro: Maryland, USA; 2014.
9. Addise M. Maternal and Child Health Care: Lecture note: University of Gondar; 2003.
10. Agency FDRoECS. Population Projection of Ethiopia for All Regions at Wereda Level from 2014–2017. 2013.
11. Sarah N, Dan K, Freddie B, Nazarius M, Florence M. Genital infections and risk of premature rupture of membranes in Mulago Hospital,Uganda: a case control study. BMC Res Notes. 2015.
12. Fergusun SE, Smith GN, Salenieks ME, Windrim R, Walker MC. Preterm premature rupture of membranes; nutritional and socio demographic factors. Obstet Gynecol. 2002;100(6):1250–6.
13. A S, Nicola S, Piazzi G, Ghazal K, Colonna L, Baltaro F. Epidemiological correlates of preterm premature rupture of membranes. Int J Gynaecol Obstet. 1994;47(1):7–15.
14. Arnildo A, Elaine P, Tania M. Preterm premature rupture of the fetal membranes: association with socio-demographic factors and maternal genitourinary infections. J De Pediatrica. 2014;90(2).
15. Daiva V, Stafan B, Vidaa M. Antenatal risk factors associated with PPROM. Acta Medica Litutania. 2002;9(3).
16. Sarah J. Demographic, clinical and environmental risk factors for PROM in western Australia: University of western Australia; 2008.
17. Shehla N, Ali F, Rubina B, Ruqqia S. Prevalance of PPROM and its outcome. J Ayub Med College. 19(4):15–6.
18. Choudhary M, Rathore SB, Chowdhary J, Garg S. Pre and post conception risk factors in PROM. Int J Res Med Sci. 2015;3(10).
19. Kaye D. Risk factors for preterm premature rupture of membranes at Mulago Kampala Uganda. East Afr Med J. 2001;78(2):65–9.
20. Tarek KA, Sahar NM, Hamida AE, Amal AA, et al. Cervicovaginal Infection during Pregnancy and Its Relation to Preterm Pre-Labour Rupture Of Membranes. J Am Sci. 2012;8(12).
21. Edem E, Carol A, Robert W, Atef M. Risks for premature rupture of amniotic membranes. Int J Epidemiol. 1993;22(3).
22. Zhou Q, Zhang W, Xu H, Liang H, Ruan Y, Zhou S, et al. Risk factors for preterm premature rupture of membranes in Chinese women from urban cities. Int J Gynecol Obstet. 2014;127:3–5.
23. Ekachai K, Patipan S. Risk factors related to premature rupture of membranes in term pregnant womens. Aust N Z J Obstet Gynaecol Zoao. 2000;40(1).
24. Emechebe CI, Njoku CO,KA, Udofia U. Determinants and complications of pre-labour rupture of membranes (PROM) at the University of Calabar Teaching Hospital (UCTH), Calabar, Nigeria. Scholars J Applied Med Sci. 2015;3(3B):2–4.
25. Lars L. Clinical and epidemiological studies: premature rupture of membranes. Br J Obstet Gynaecol. 1998;103(28):13.

10

Vaginal birth after caesarean birth in Italy: variations among areas of residence and hospitals

Paola Colais[1], Katia Bontempi[1], Luigi Pinnarelli[1*], Carlo Piscicelli[2], Ilenia Mappa[2], Danilo Fusco[1] and Marina Davoli[1]

Abstract

Background: The rates of caesarean section (CS) are increasing globally. CS rates are one of the most frequently used indicators of health care quality. Vaginal Birth After Caesarean (VBAC) could be considered a reasonable and safe option for most women with a previous CS. Despite this fact, in some European countries, many women who had a previous CS will have a routine CS subsequently and VBAC rates are extremely variable across countries. VBAC use is inversely related to caesarean use. The objective of the present study was to analyze VBAC rates with respect to caesarean rates and the variations among areas of residence, hospitals and hospital ownership types in Italy.

Methods: This study was based on information from the Hospital Information System (HIS). We collected data from all deliveries in Italy from January 1, 2010 to December 31, 2014 and we considered only deliveries with a previous caesarean section. Applying multivariate logistic regression analysis, the adjusted proportions of VBAC for each Local Health Units (LHU), each hospital and by hospital ownership types were calculated. Cross-classified logistic multilevel models were performed to analyze within geographic, hospitals and hospital ownership types variations.

Results: We studied a total of 77,850 deliveries with a previous caesarean section in Italy between January 1, 2010 and December 31, 2014. The proportion of VBAC in Italy slightly increased in the last few years, from 5.8% in 2010 to 7.5% in 2014. Proportions of VBAC ranged from 0.29 to 50.05% in Italian LHUs. The LHUs with lower proportions of VBAC deliveries were characterized by higher values for primary caesarean deliveries. Private hospitals showed the lowest mean of crude VBAC proportions but the highest variation among hospitals, ranging from 0 to 47.1%.

Conclusions: Hospital rates of caesarean section for women with at least one previous caesarean section vary widely, and only some of the variation can be explained by case-mix and hospital-level factors, suggesting that additional factors influence practices. Identifying disparities in VBAC may have important implications for health services planning and targeted efforts to reduce overall rates of caesarean deliveries.

Keywords: Caesarean section, VBAC, Health information systems, Hospital care

Background

The rates of caesarean section (CS) are increasing globally. CS rates rose throughout Europe between 2004 and 2010. In 2010, the Italian CS rate (38.0%) was among the highest in the world and only the Netherlands, Slovenia, Finland, Sweden, Iceland and Norway had rates below 20% [1]. The growth of Italian CS rates slowed down over the last few years, both for women who had not had a previous caesarean delivery (primary) [2] and for women who had undergone a previous caesarean delivery (repeated) [3].

Higher rates could be considered inappropriate, and maternal and neonatal benefits may no longer outweigh the costs and risks associated with this procedure [4]. Primary caesarean deliveries, which comprise two-thirds of the overall CS rate, are an important target for reduction because they lead to increased risk for a repeat caesarean delivery [5–7]. However, repeated CS following previous CS is a significant factor contributing to overall increased CS rates [8].

* Correspondence: l.pinnarelli@deplazio.it
[1]Department of Epidemiology, Lazio Regional Health Service, Via Cristoforo Colombo 112, 00142 Rome, Italy

Furthermore, most women with a previous CS could have a Vaginal Birth After Caesarean (VBAC) [9] on the basis of randomized controlled trials that compared outcomes for women planning a repeated elective caesarean with women planning a vaginal birth [10]. There is a clear evidence of an association between VBAC and lower rates of maternal deaths or complications for mothers and babies [10]. Nevertheless, VBAC rates are extremely variable across European countries [1]. The variation in CS rates across Europe might reflect national, regional and individual clinicians' attitudes to clinical decision-making and the use of caesarean section is not related to patient's clinical risk factors and pregnancy characteristics, but it could be ascribed to differences in clinical practices [1, 11].

In general, VBAC use is inversely related to caesarean use such that higher VBAC rates are associated with lower caesarean rates. Previous studies showed that variation in hospital caesarean rates is not related to a patient's clinical risk factors, but it could be ascribed to differences in practice patterns [12].

The Italian National Health System provides health-care services through public and private hospitals that are reimbursed by different systems:

- "Public hospital" have a global budget with a fixed amount of money for health care spending;
- "Teaching hospitals" and "Classified hospitals" (hospitals owned by religious congregations) are partially reimbursed by the Diagnosis Related Groups (DRG) system and have a budget to cover the remaining health care spending;
- "Private hospitals" are totally paid by the DRG system.

The types of hospital ownership, such as whether it is a private or public hospital, teaching or nonteaching hospital, are associated with different CS and VBAC rates. In general, public hospitals and teaching hospitals have lower rates of caesarean delivery and higher VBAC rates in respect to private hospitals [13–16].

Patient factors and patient-specific clinical characteristics have been studied as risk factors for both caesarean delivery and VBAC. Maternal age, race/ethnicity, prematurity, pre-eclampsia, twins, more than one caesarean and previous vaginal birth are the most commonly studied [17, 18].

The objective of the present study was to analyze VBAC rates with respect to caesarean rates and the variations among areas of residence, hospitals and hospital ownership types in Italy.

Methods

Data sources

This study was based on information from the Hospital Information System (HIS). The HIS collects data on hospital discharges in Italy and contains patient demographic data (gender, age, place of residence), admission and discharge dates, discharge diagnoses and procedures (International Classification of Diseases, 9th Revision, Clinical Modification ICD-9-CM), and the regional code of the admitting facility.

Data were collected within the framework of the National Outcome Program, active from 2010 in the Italian Health System. The program measures more than 150 outcome indicators with the aim of comparing primary and hospital care in Italy [19]. The results provided by the National Outcome Program are updated every year and are publicly available [2].

Study population

We collected data from all deliveries in Italy from January 1, 2010 to December 31, 2014. To identify deliveries from the Hospital Information System, three different sources of information were used: diagnosis-related group, procedure codes and diagnosis codes.

We considered only deliveries with a previous caesarean section. Previous caesarean deliveries were defined on the basis of the diagnosis code during hospitalization for delivery, or the diagnosis-related groups or diagnosis codes or procedure codes reported in hospitalizations occurred during the previous 5 years. Details and ICD-9-CM codes are reported in Additional file 1.

Moreover, we excluded the following from the analysis:

- all deliveries of mothers who were not residents of Italy;
- mothers under the age of 10 years or over the age of 55 years;
- hospital discharges with a diagnosis of abortion (diagnosis codes ICD-9-CM: 634–639);
- stillborn cases (diagnosis codes ICD-9-CM: 656.4, V27.1, V27.4, V27.7);
- admissions not remunerated by the National Health Service (e.g., admission remunerated by private insurance or by out-of-pocket fee).

We cannot exclude women < 37 weeks of gestation (potentially not eligible for VBAC) because the information about week of gestation is not completely available in the Italian Hospital Information System.

Outcomes

The proportion of VBAC was calculated as the ratio of vaginal births to the total number of deliveries by women with a previous caesarean section. Vaginal deliveries were defined as deliveries without a caesarean section.

Exposure

The results were calculated for each Local Health Unit (LHU) (a body delegated by the National Health System to provide health care to a specific area), and hospital and by hospital ownership types (public hospital, teaching hospitals, classified hospitals, and private hospitals).

Comorbidities

Data on maternal and neonatal clinical factors, potentially associated with the outcome under study, were collected based on primary and secondary discharge diagnoses from the HIS; information was retrieved from the index hospital admission and all hospital admissions in the previous two years. Details and ICD-9-CM codes are reported in Additional file 1. Maternal age was classified as ≤ 24, 25–28, 29–33, 34–38, and $\geq$ 39 years. We also considered as risk factors the mother's citizenship, the number of previous caesarean sections (1, ≥ 2) and previous vaginal deliveries.

Moreover, we evaluated the proportion of factors that usually contraindicate a VBAC (placenta praevia 0.7%, > = 2 previous CS 2.6%, podalic 2.3%). Considering the low proportion of these factors in the study population and the fact that sometimes a VBAC was performed in women with these factors, according to previous studies [20–22], we preferred to include them in the adjusted model in order to evaluate their impact on the likelihood of VBAC.

Statistical analysis

The proportions of VBAC for each LHU, each hospital and by hospital ownership types were calculated. We used multivariate regression analysis to assess the effect of each exposure under study on the likelihood of a VBAC, adjusting for other factors (maternal age and comorbidities) that could affect the outcome under study. Among all factors potentially associated with the outcome under study, maternal age was considered an a priori risk factor; the others were selected using a stepwise bootstrap procedure to assign an importance rank of predictors in the logistic regression analysis. In this approach, the logistic regression with all predictors was run 100 times on random samples drawn with replacement from the original data set. Only the risk factors identified as at least 30 times as significant ($p \leq 0.05$) were included in the predictive model.

To estimate the adjusted proportion of VBAC, a multivariate logistic regression analysis with no intercept, including centered covariates, was applied. This model estimates the log odds of VBAC with respect to Local Health Units and hospitals.

Adjusted proportions were obtained for each level of exposure by back-transforming parameter estimates with the following formula [23]:

$$\text{Adj proportion} = [\exp(\text{estimate})/(1+\exp(\text{estimate}))]^{*} k$$

where k is a correction coefficient introduced to consider the nonlinear nature of the logistic model (Additional file 2).

To estimate the adjusted OR of VBAC by hospital ownership types, a multivariate logistic regression analysis was applied.

Furthermore, maps of adjusted proportions of VBAC and primary caesarean deliveries were produced to compare each Italian Local Health Unit (ArcGIS 9.2 software). The classes used in the maps have been calculated applying the Jenks natural breaks optimization algorithm [24].

Finally, cross-classified logistic multilevel models were performed to analyze geographic, hospitals and hospital ownership type variations [25].

The variance components were expressed in terms of Median Odds Ratios (MORs) [26].

All analyses were undertaken using SAS Version 9.2.

The National Agency of Regional Health Services (Rome, Italy) gave approval for the study conducted within the broader scope of the National Outcome Program.

Results

We studied a total of 416,758 deliveries with a previous caesarean section in Italy between January 1, 2010 and December 31, 2014. The proportion of VBAC in Italy slightly increased in the last few years, from 5.8% in 2010 to 7.5% in 2014; in the same period, the total number of deliveries and primary caesarean sections decreased (Fig. 1).

The risk factors included in the predictive model are reported in the Additional file 3. The likelihood of VBAC was lower in women aged 35–55 years than women aged 29–33 years, in Italian women, in women with more than 2 previous caesarean sections, eclampsia/pre-eclampsia, multiple pregnancy, malposition and malpresentation of the fetus, fetopelvic disproportion/ excessive fetal growth affecting management of mother, intrauterine growth retardation and antepartum hemorrhage, abruptio placentae, and placenta previa and /or cord prolapse. On the other hand, the likelihood of VBAC was higher in women with previous vaginal deliveries, at-risk pregnancy, preterm labor, late pregnancy (over 40 weeks of gestation) and premature rupture of membranes. The strongest predictive factors for a VBAC were having a previous vaginal birth (OR = 8.76, $p < 0.001$) and late pregnancy (OR = 7.36, $p < 0.001$).

Figure 2 shows the adjusted proportion of VBAC and primary caesarean deliveries for each Italian LHU in 2014. Comparing the maps, we noted that areas with a lower proportion of VBAC deliveries were characterized by higher values of primary caesarean deliveries.

The geographic variation of VBAC proportions ranged from 0.29 to 50.05% (MOR = 3.37) and was higher than

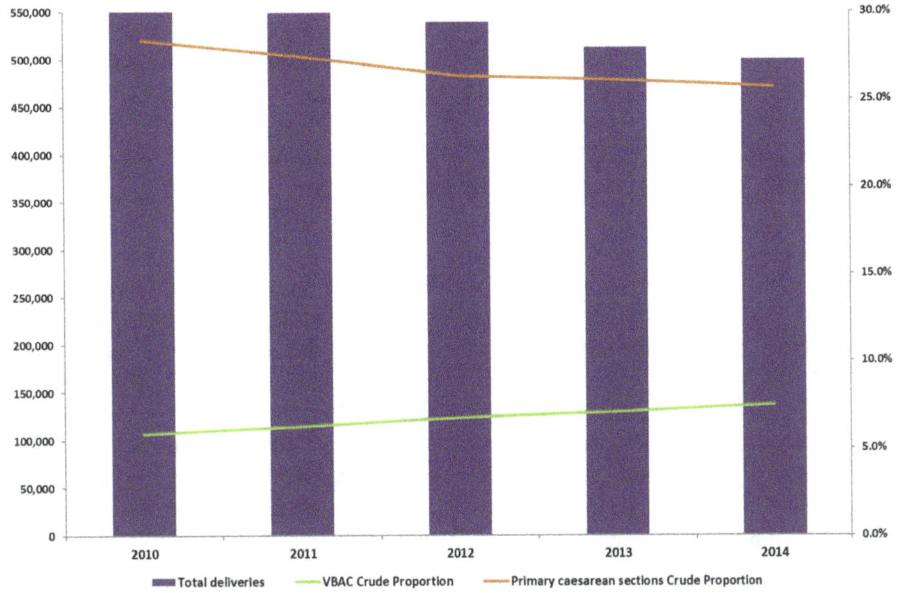

Fig. 1 Crude proportion of VBAC deliveries, Italy 2010–2014

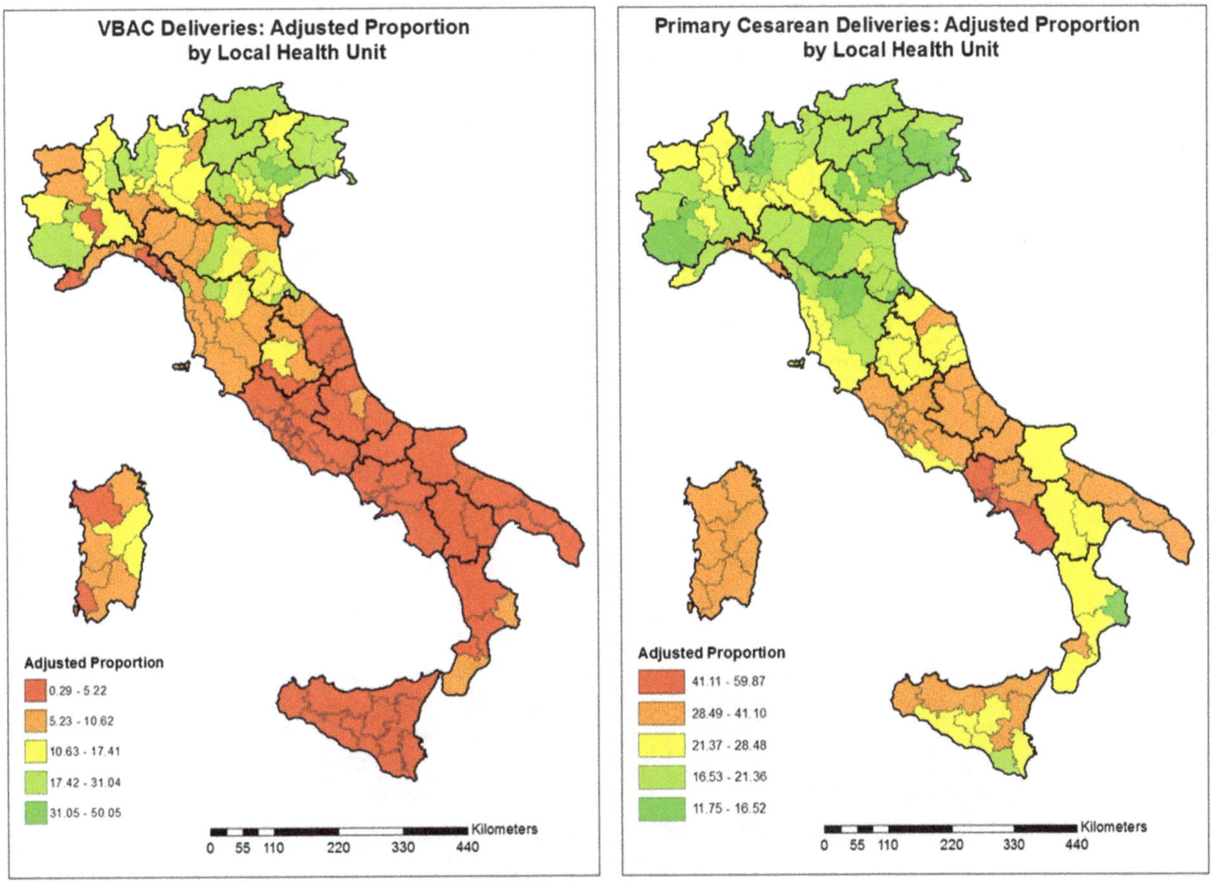

Fig. 2 Adjusted proportion of VBAC and caesarean deliveries for Italian Local Health Units, 2014

the geographic variation of primary caesarean deliveries, ranging from 11.75 to 59.87% (MOR = 1.69).

A similar relationship between VBAC and primary caesarean deliveries could be found at the hospital level. Figure 3 shows that hospitals with a lower proportion of VBAC deliveries were characterized by higher values of primary caesarean deliveries. The VBAC proportion showed a higher variation between hospitals compared to primary caesarean deliveries (MOR = 7.01 vs MOR = 2.37, respectively).

Private hospitals showed the lowest crude VBAC proportion, whereas Public and Teaching hospitals showed the highest (Table 1). We observed a higher adjusted probability of VBAC in Public and Teaching hospitals (adjusted OR = 2.75 and adjusted OR = 2.75 respectively). However, the private category had a relevant variation between hospitals, ranging from 0 to 47.1% (MOR = 12.03), compared to the other types of hospital ownership.

Discussion

The study evaluated VBAC rates with respect to caesarean rates and the variations among areas of residence, hospitals and hospital ownership types in Italy. We found that VBAC use is inversely related to caesarean use such that higher caesarean rates are associated with lower VBAC rates. There is clear evidence of this inversion relationship at the hospital level, but it can also be appreciated at the LHU level. Moreover, we found high geographic and hospital variations for both VBAC and primary caesarean deliveries. Although it was higher for VBAC, it was independent of the considered risk factors. Private hospitals showed the lowest mean of crude VBAC proportion with respect to Public and Teaching hospitals, but it had the highest variation among hospitals. These results are in line with previous studies [13–15, 27].

Our data suggested that younger women had higher VBAC success rates. Knight HE et al. found that women of non-white ethnicity and those who lived in deprived areas had a higher rate of attempted VBAC, but women of white ethnicity had a higher success rate [28]. We found that Italian women had a lower likelihood of success compared to women from Eastern Europe and developing countries citizenship but also compared to women coming from developed countries different from Italy. These results may reflect different preferences for modes of delivery or choice of hospital type for Italian women with respect to women from other countries.

Consistent with other studies and according to the Royal College of Obstetricians and Gynaecologists, we found that a prior vaginal delivery is the strongest predictive factor for a vaginal birth after caesarean [18, 29].

Although differences in the case mix may be important in explaining variation in hospital caesarean rates, these findings suggest that hospital planned repeat caesarean section rates vary markedly for reasons other than the individual's characteristics.

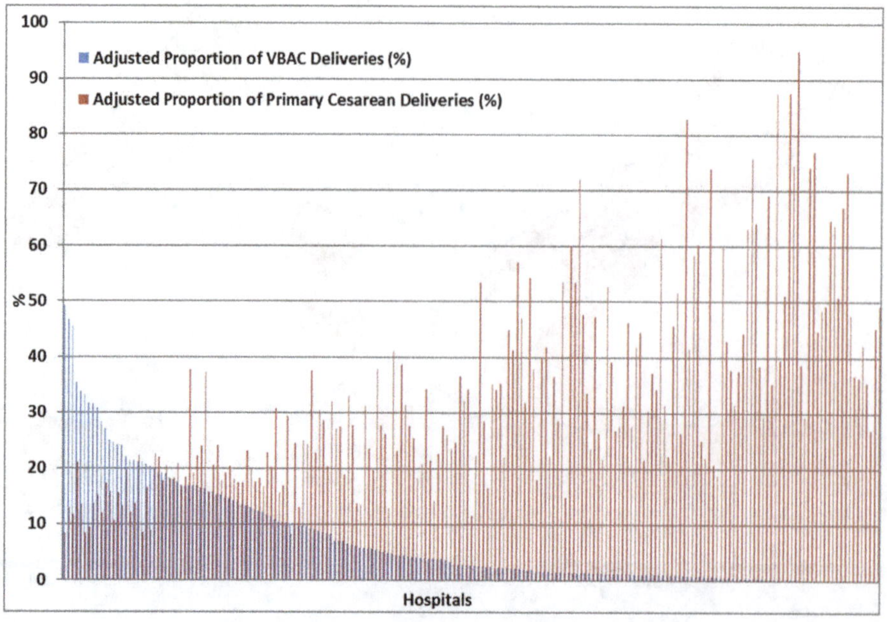

Fig. 3 Adjusted proportion of caesarean and VBAC deliveries by hospital, 2014

Table 1 Adjusted OR of VBAC by hospital ownership types, 2014

Hospital ownership	n	Crude proportion			Crude OR	Adj OR	*p* value	Median OR
		%	% min	% max				
Public	49,353	8.69	0.00	41.86	3.35	2.75	<.0001	5.62
Teaching	10,332	8.68	0.89	37.75	3.34	2.76	<.0001	3.83
Classified	4382	5.48	0.68	20.30	2.04	1.87	<.0001	3.71
Private	13,783	2.76	0.00	47.12	1.00	1.00	–	12.03

Despite the existence of Italian national guidelines regarding the choice of caesarean section [30], our results suggest that its adoption is still very poor and heterogeneous and there is a need for interventions to change physicians' attitudes and promote women's empowerment. A wider implementation strategy for the existing clinical guidelines for the management of pregnant women should be promoted.

The main limitation of our study is the lack of information on personal patients' data, i.e., height, body mass index, obstetric history and individual patient attitudes and physician decision-making processes.

However, this study is the first to compare VBAC rates respect to caesarean rates and the variations among areas of residence, hospitals and hospital ownership types in Italy in the recent past, using a large national dataset and routinely collected data on hospital admissions. Moreover, the hospital discharge data, even if have a value as a source for healthcare research, have several limitations that have been recognized [31]. On the other hand, this study uses a large data sample, a validated algorithm for the selection of patients and measures robust outcomes [31, 32].

Conclusions

In Italy, VBAC use is inversely related to caesarean use such that higher caesarean rates are associated with lower VBAC rates at the hospital and LHU level. The geographical similarity between high CS and low VBAC rates is striking as is the wide range of rates for both. Hospital rates of caesarean sections for women with at least one previous caesarean section vary widely, and only some of the variation can be explained by case-mixes and hospital-level factors; other factors such as structural peculiarities and organizational and professional preferences seem to influence the use of caesarean section more strongly than women's health conditions and pregnancy characteristics.

Identifying disparities in VBAC may have important implications for health services planning and targeted efforts to reduce overall rates of caesarean deliveries.

Additional files

Additional file 1: List of codes used for selection of study population, outcome and comorbidities used for risk adjustment. The document contains the list of ICD-9-CM codes used for selection of study population, outcome and comorbidities used for risk adjustment

Additional file 2: Correction coefficient. The document contains the formula of correction coefficient (k) used to consider the nonlinear nature of the logistic model.

Additional file 3: Comorbidities included in a model to predict VBAC. The document contains the list of comorbidities included in the regression model and the associated Crude OR, adjusted OR and *p*-value.

Abbreviations

CS: Caesarean Section; DRG: Diagnosis Related Groups; HIS: Hospital Information System; ICD-9-CM: International Classification of Diseases, 9th Revision, Clinical Modification; LHU: Local Health Units; MOR: Median Odds Ratio; OR: Odds Ratio; VBAC: Vaginal Birth After Caesarean

Authors' contributions

PC: study conception and design, data analysis, interpretation of data. KB: data analysis. LP: study conception and design, interpretation of data. DF: study conception and design, interpretation of data. CP: study conception and design, interpretation of data. IM: study conception and design, interpretation of data. MD: study conception and design, interpretation of data. All authors read and approved the final manuscript.

Competing interests

The authors declare that they have no competing interests.

Author details

[1]Department of Epidemiology, Lazio Regional Health Service, Via Cristoforo Colombo 112, 00142 Rome, Italy. [2]Cristo Re Hospital, Via delle Calasanziane, 25, 00167 Rome, Italy.

References

1. EURO-PERISTAT. European perinatal health report: the health and care of pregnant women and babies in Europe in 2010. 2013. [http://www.europeristat.com/reports/european-perinatal-health-report-2010.html]. Accessed 23 May 2015.
2. The Italian outcome program. website at http://95.110.213.190/PNEed15/.
3. Di Martino M, Fusco D, Colais P, Pinnarelli L, Davoli M, Perucci CA. Differential misclassification of confounders in comparative evaluation of hospital care quality: caesarean sections in Italy. BMC Public Health. 2014;14:1049.
4. Betran AP, Torloni MR, Zhang JJ, Gülmezoglu AM. WHO statement on caesarean section rates. WHO Working Group on Caesarean Section BJOG. 2016 Apr;123(5):667–70.

5. Royal College of Obstetricians and Gynaecologists. Birth after previous caesarean birth. In: London (UK): RCOG Press; Green-top guideline n°45; 2007.
6. Robson MS. Can we reduce the caesarean section rate? Best Pract Res Clin Obstet Gynaecol. 2001;15:179–94.
7. Meikle SF, Steiner CA, Zhang J, Lawrence WL. A national estimate of the elective primary caesarean delivery rate. Obstet Gynecol. 2005;105(4):751–6.
8. Cheng Y, Eden K, Marshall P, Pereira L, Caughey A, Guise J-M. Delivery after prior caesarean: maternal morbidity and mortality. Clin Perinatol. 2011;38(2):297–309.
9. Guise J-M, Eden K, Emeis C, Denman MA, Marshall N, Fu R, et al. Vaginal birth after cesarean: new insights. Evidence Reports/Technology Assessments. 2010;191:1–397.
10. Dodd JM, Crowther CA, Huertas E, Guise JM, Horey D. Planned elective repeat caesarean section versus planned vaginal birth for women with a previous caesarean birth. Cochrane Database Syst Rev. 2013;12:CD004224.
11. Hanley GE, Janssen PA, Greyson D. Regional variation in the caesarean delivery and assisted vaginal delivery rates. Obstet Gynecol. 2010;115(6):1201–8.
12. Schemann K, Patterson JA, Nippita TA, Ford JB, Roberts CL. Variation in hospital caesarean section rates for women with at least one previous caesarean section: a population based cohort study. BMC Pregnancy Childbirth. 2015;19(15):179.
13. Bailit JL, Dooley SL, Peaceman AN. Risk adjustment for interhospital comparison of primary cesarean rates. Obstet Gynecol. 1999;93:1025–1030, 1999.
14. MacDorman MF, Menacker F, Declerq E. Cesarean birth in the United States: epidemiology, trends, and outcomes. Clin Perinatalol. 2008;35:293–307, 2008.
15. EA DF, Rampersad R, Atkins KL, et al. Do vaginal birth after cesarean outcomes differ based on hospital setting? Am J Obstet Gynecol. 2007; 197(e1):2007400e6.
16. Colais P, Pinnarelli L, Fusco D, Davoli M, Braga M, Perucci CA. The impact of a pay-for-performance system on timing to hip fracture surgery: experience from the Lazio region (Italy). BMC Health Serv Res. 2013 Oct 7;13:393.
17. Algert C, Morris J, Simpson J, Ford J, Roberts C. Labor before a primary cesarean delivery: reduced risk of uterine rupture in a subsequent trial of labour for vaginal birth after cesarean. Obstetrics and Gynecology. 2008; 112(5):1061–6.
18. Cahill AG, Macones GA. Vaginal birth after cesarean delivery: evidence-based practice. Clin Obstet Gynecol. 2007;50(2):518–25.
19. Agabiti N, Davoli M, Fusco D, Stafoggia M, Perucci CA. Comparative evaluation of health services outcomes. Epidemiol Prev. 2011;35(2 Suppl. 1):1–80.
20. De Franco EA, Rampersad R, Atkins KL, Odibo AO, Stevens EJ, Peipert JF, Stamilio DM, Macones GA. Do vaginal birth after cesarean outcomes differ based on hospital setting? Am J Obstet Gynecol. 2007 Oct;197(4):400.e1–6.
21. Misra A. Impact of the HealthChoice program on cesarean section and vaginal birth after C-section deliveries: a retrospective analysis. Matern Child Health J. 2008;12(2):266–74 Epub 2007 Jun 5.
22. Cheng ER, Declercq ER, Belanoff C, Iverson RE, McCloskey L. Racial and ethnic differences in the likelihood of vaginal birth after cesarean delivery. Birth. 2015;42(3):249–53 Epub 2015 Jun 19.
23. Zhao D, Anderson N: Poisson Regression Adjustment of Event Rates And Its Macro Procedure ADJ_POIS. SAS Conference Proceedings: SAS Users Group International 24 April 11-14, 1999, Miami Beach, Florida: SUGI24.
24. Jenks George F. The data model concept in statistical mapping. Int Yearb Cartography. 1967;7:186–90.
25. Hox J. Multilevel Analysis: techniques and Applications. Mahwah, NJ: Lawrence Erlbaum Associates; 2002. p. 123.
26. Larsen K, Merlo J. Appropriate assessment of neighborhood effects on individual health: integrating random and fixed effects in multilevel logistic regression. Am J Epidemiol. 2005;161:81–8.
27. Gregory KD, Fridman M, Korst L. Trends and patterns of vaginal birth after cesarean availability in the United States. Semin Perinatol. 2010;34(4):237–43.
28. Knight HE, Gurol-Urganci I, van der Meulen JH, Mahmood TA, Richmond DH, Dougall A, Cromwell DA. Vaginal birth after caesarean section: a cohort study investigating factors associated with its uptake and success. BJOG. 2014;121(2):183–92.
29. Royal College of Obstetricians and Gynaecologists (RCOG). Birth after previous caesarean birth. Green-Top Giudeline No. 45. London: RCOG, October 2015.
30. Taglio cesareo: una scelta appropriata e consapevole Seconda parte. Sistema nazionale per le linee guida dell'Istituto superiore di sanità (SNLG-ISS). http://percorsonascita.ats-bg.it/documenti_istituzionali/LG_Cesareo_finaleL.pdf.
31. Iezzoni LI. Assessing quality using administrative data. Ann Intern Med. 1997;127:666–74.
32. Colais P, Di Martino M, Fusco D, Perucci CA, Davoli M. The effect of early surgery after hip fracture on 1-year mortality. BMC Geriatr. 2015 Oct 28;15:141.

11

Foetal weight prediction models at a given gestational age in the absence of ultrasound facilities: application in Indonesia

Dewi Anggraini[1,2*], Mali Abdollahian[1] and Kaye Marion[1]

Abstract

Background: Birth weight is one of the most important indicators of neonatal survival. A reliable estimate of foetal weight at different stages of pregnancy would facilitate intervention plans for medical practitioners to prevent the risk of low birth weight delivery. This study has developed reliable models to more accurately predict estimated foetal weight at a given gestation age in the absence of ultrasound facilities.

Methods: A primary health care centre was involved in collecting retrospective non-identified Indonesian data. The best subset model selection criteria, coefficient of determination, standard deviation, variance inflation factor, Mallows C_p, and diagnostic tests of residuals were deployed to select the most significant independent variables. Simple and multivariate linear regressions were used to develop the proposed models. The efficacy of models for predicting foetal weight at a given gestational age was assessed using multi-prediction accuracy measures.

Results: Four weight prediction models based on fundal height and its combinations with gestational age (between 32 and 41 weeks) and ultrasonic estimates of foetal head circumference and foetal abdominal circumference have been developed. Multiple comparison criteria show that the proposed models were more accurate than the existing models (mean prediction errors between − 0.2 and 2.4 g and median absolute percentage errors between 4.1 and 4.2%) in predicting foetal weight at a given gestational age (between 35 and 41 weeks).

Conclusions: This research has developed models to more accurately predict estimated foetal weight at a given gestational age in the absence of ultrasound machines and trained ultra-sonographers. The efficacy of the models was assessed using retrospective data. The results show that the proposed models produced less error than the existing clinical and ultrasonic models. This research has resulted in the development of models where ultrasound facilities do not exist, to predict the estimated foetal weight at varying gestational age. This would promote the development of foetal inter growth charts, which are currently unavailable in Indonesian primary health care systems. Consistent monitoring of foetal growth would alleviate the risk of having inter growth abnormalities, such as low birth weight that is the most leading factor of neonatal mortality.

Keywords: Fundal height, Gestational age, Estimated foetal head circumference, Estimated foetal abdominal circumference, Regression analysis, Foetal weight estimation, Absence of ultrasound facilities, Primary health care centre, Prediction accuracy, Indonesia

* Correspondence: dewi.anggraini@rmit.edu.au; dewi.anggraini@ulm.ac.id
[1]School of Science (Mathematical and Geospatial Sciences), College of Science, Engineering, and Health, RMIT University, GPO BOX 2476, Melbourne, VIC 3001, Australia
[2]Study Program of Statistics, Faculty of Mathematics and Natural Sciences, University of Lambung Mangkurat (ULM), Ahmad Yani Street, Km. 36, Banjarbaru, South Kalimantan 70714, Indonesia

Background

Birth weight is a primary measurement and significant indicator to ensure the optimal growth, survival, and future well-being of new-borns. Deviation from normal delivery weights (2500–3999 g), such as low birth weight (LBW) (< 2500 g) and macrosomia (> 4000 g) could lead to some negative consequences on neonatal health [1–3]. While macrosomia may cause neonatal and maternal morbidity [4], LBW is well-documented to be one of the most contributing factors to the neonatal mortality [1]. LBW is defined as weight less than 2500 g at birth regardless of gestational age (GA) and can be caused by preterm birth or intrauterine growth restriction [5]. In this paper, LBW includes both preterm and term new-borns of appropriate for GA.

Routine and reliable estimates of foetal weight at a given GA throughout pregnancy are vital. These estimates could create evidence-based track records/analysis to assist medical practitioners to detect the signs of potential LBW during pregnancy and provide the appropriate interventions. Although a wide range of simple and advanced multivariate weight prediction models based on clinical and ultrasonic measurements has been developed, most are only based on maternal or foetal factors [6–25]. Less is known about the combinations of these characteristics to estimate foetal weight during pregnancy despite the fact that birth weight is significantly associated with characteristics of both mother and foetus [1, 26].

Several models based on combined maternal and neonatal characteristics have been developed and reviewed, these existing models were mostly developed based on the information available at delivery time [27, 28]. In most developing countries, the availability of foetal biometric measurements during pregnancy is low, particularly in rural areas due to limited access to ultrasound machines and skilled personnel [29]. Westerway et al. (2000), Loughna et al. (2009), and Papageorghiou et al. (2014) have used a large number of ultrasonic measurements to develop formulas that estimate foetal biometric characteristics at a given GA [30–32]. These formulas then could be used to fill the foetal database gaps during pregnancy when ultrasound facility is absent.

The present research develops foetal weight prediction models based on combined maternal and estimated foetal biometric characteristics to estimate foetal weight at any given GA. The proposed models can be simply implemented in low-resource primary health care centres where ultrasound machines and trained ultra-sonographers are not always available. The predicted foetal weight will assist in the development of foetal growth charts for Indonesia. No such charts currently exist for the Indonesian population.

Methods

Study design and setting

A quantitative and analytic study based on a retrospective pregnancy cohort analysis was carried out. Unidentified secondary quantitative data were collected and analysed to (1) assess the adequacy of the existing ultrasonic models in estimating foetal biometric characteristics, (2) develop new foetal weight prediction models based on both maternal and estimated foetal biometric characteristics, (3) assess the accuracy of the proposed models in predicting foetal weight between 35 and 41 weeks of GA, and (4) carry out a comparison study between the proposed and commonly used models. The study was conducted in a primary health care centre in South Kalimantan province, Indonesia. The locality was selected because it is one of the five provinces with the highest neonatal mortality in the country [33–35].

Conceptual framework

Figure 1 shows the framework used in this study, along with the selected possible predictors of foetal weight estimation.

Data source

Study data were sourced primarily from a paper-based pregnancy register of pregnant women who received antenatal care (ANC) services and gave birth in the selected primary health care centre from January 2013 to August 2015. Prior to delivery, GA, fundal height (FH), foetal head engagement/foetal station (FS), and recorded foetal weight estimation (EFW_r) at a given GA were measured and recorded by the assigned midwives. At delivery time, actual birth weight (ABW), neonatal head circumference (HC), and neonatal abdominal circumference (AC) were also measured and recorded.

Data management

Data was recorded in Microsoft Excel and the statistical analyses were performed using Minitab version 17 and R. The ordinary least square (OLS) and robust regression (the weighted likelihood estimation) were carried out by using ***lm*** function and ***wle.lm*** function, respectively in R [36–39].

Statistical analysis

The adequacy assessment of existing ultrasonic models to estimate foetal biometric characteristics during pregnancy

The existing ultrasonic formulas to estimate foetal HC and foetal AC which were developed based on the Australian foetal biometry data (measured between 11 and 41 weeks), the UK foetal biometry data (measured between 13 and 42 weeks), and the international foetal biometry data (measured between 14 and 42 weeks or until birth) [30–32] (provided in Additional file 1: Table S1) were applied to estimate foetal HC and foetal AC at a given GA for Indonesian foetus ($n = 127$). A reliability analysis using intraclass correlation coefficient (ICC) [40, 41] was performed to assess the consistency of the ultrasonic

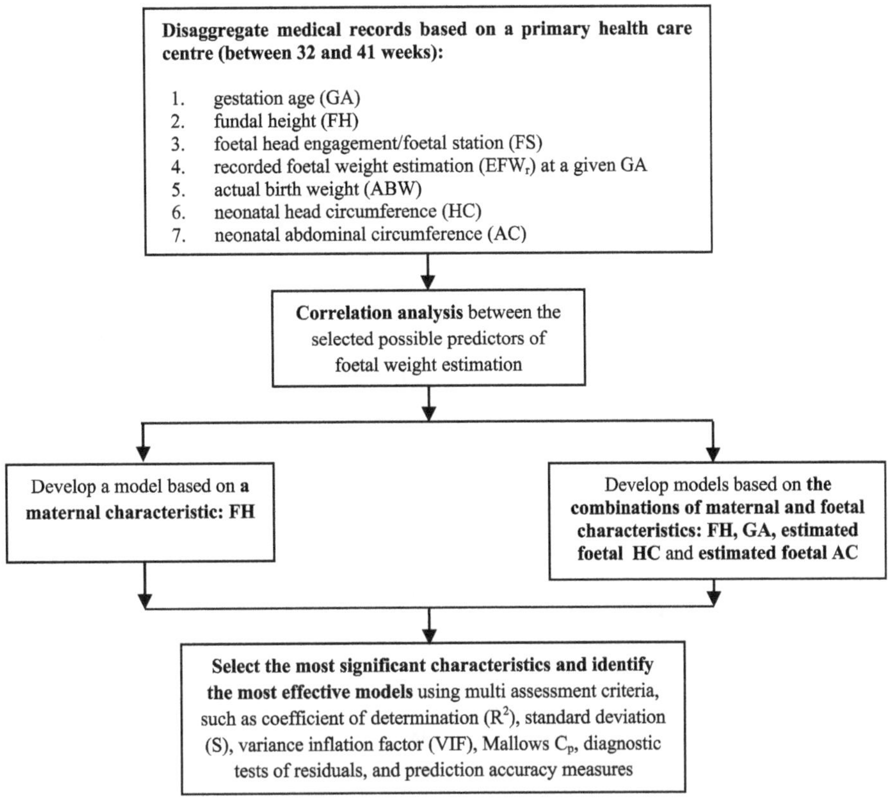

Fig. 1 Conceptual framework for factors influencing foetal weight estimation between 32 and 41 weeks of pregnancy

formulas for Indonesian population. The obtained ICC values (provided in Additional file 2: Table S2) were computed by single-rating, consistency, and two-way random effects models for the foetal biometrics with three raters (different ultrasonic formulas) across 127 subjects (pregnant women). Interclass (Pearson) correlation coefficient was also analysed to assess whether there is a significant relationship between the predicted foetal biometrics and the neonatal measurements recorded at delivery time (provided in Additional file 3: Table S3).

The development of new foetal weight prediction models based on combinations of maternal and estimated foetal biometric characteristics

Bernoulli distribution with the event probability (p) of 70% was used to randomly divide our data into two sets: model development (training) data ($n = 89$) and model efficacy assessment (testing) data ($n = 38$).

Based on the training data set, simple and multivariate linear regressions were used to develop our proposed models. The best subset selection methodology together with correlation coefficient (r), coefficient of determination (R^2), standard deviation (S), Mallows C_p, and variance inflation factor (VIF) were deployed to identify the most suitable subset of predictors. Analysis of variance (ANOVA) together with t-test statistics was used to simultaneously and partially confirm the significance of predictors' contribution in the regression models. Diagnostic tests of residuals were used to confirm the validity of the regression models.

Since our aim is to investigate whether a combination of maternal and foetal factors could improve foetal weight prediction accuracy, we have utilised the most commonly recommended formulas of ultrasonic foetal measurement standards (based on GA) to predict the measurements of foetal biometrics in our local population. This prediction is one way to fill in the foetal database gaps during pregnancy in the absence of ultrasound. The estimates of these two most significant characteristics of foetal biometry, such as HC and AC were then combined with maternal FH to develop the prediction models. The idea of this combination was to evaluate whether it could improve the prediction accuracy of foetal weight.

Our delivery date in our data ranged from 32 to 41 weeks. The ultrasonic formulas were deployed to estimate foetal HC and foetal AC at the given GA for each individual patient and used to estimate the delivery weight. Therefore, the mean time between the last measurements of FH and GA as well as the last estimates of foetal HC and foetal AC and birth was assumed to be 0 days.

The efficacy assessment of the proposed models

The testing data set was used to validate and assess the efficacy of the proposed models. The potential bias due to growth between the last measurements and birth of the developed models for estimating foetal weight was assessed by calculating the mean prediction error [the average of the differences between the ith actual values of birth weight (ABW_i) and the ith predicted values of foetal weight based on the proposed models (EFW_{p_i})] $= \sum_{i=1}^{n} \frac{(ABW_i - EFW_{p_i})}{n}$. The mean absolute percentage prediction error or $MAPE = \sum_{i=1}^{n} \frac{|(\frac{ABW_i - EFW_{p_i}}{ABW_i} \times 100)|}{n}$ was also calculated to represent the dispersion of the errors [42]. In addition, the median absolute percentage prediction error or $MEDAPE = Median\,|(\frac{ABW_i - EFW_{p_i}}{ABW_i} \times 100)|$ was measured and used for assessing the efficacy of the models. The later measurement is more resistant to outlier distortion (due to the presence of extreme deviations) than the mean; therefore, deploying *MEDAPE* would eliminate the false interpretation of forecast accuracy [43].

The efficacy of the proposed models was also assessed by the number of estimates within 10% of ABW. A two independent sample t-test was used to decide if there is a significant difference between the observed or actual values of birth weight (ABW), EFW_r, and estimated foetal weights based on the proposed models (EFW_p). Multiple comparisons were carried out between our proposed models, eleven existing clinical models, and six existing ultrasonic models to select the most effective models for estimating foetal weights at a given GA.

Results

Out of 146 women who received ANC services and gave birth in the selected primary health care centre, 127 (87%) women met the study criteria (Fig. 2). These women delivered live singletons with normal delivery weights between 32 and 41 weeks of GA. We excluded 19 (13%) women due to incomplete information on the required characteristics listed in Fig. 2, such as no records of GA, FH, and FS ($n = 3$), GA > 41 weeks ($n = 2$), been referred to hospitals due to pregnancy complications ($n = 6$), and abnormal birth weight babies ($n = 8$).

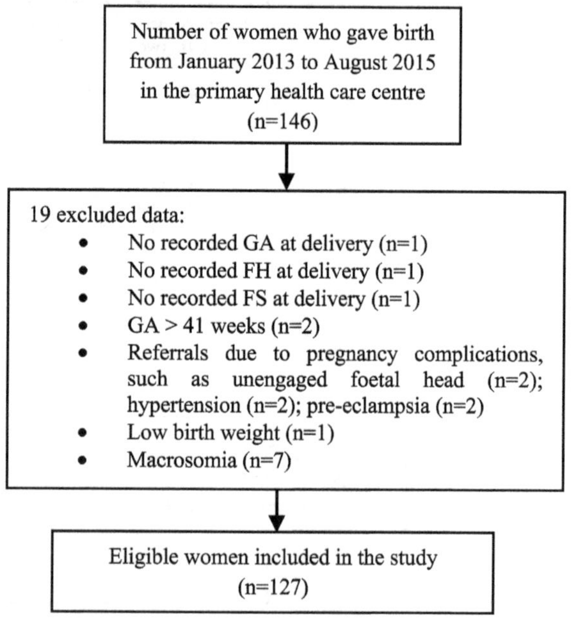

Fig. 2 Flowchart of recruitment of participants through the study

General information on the study population

Descriptive statistics on baseline characteristics of mother and new-born of the study population ($n = 127$) are presented in Table 1. Overall, the pregnant women were well-nourished (arm circumference = 25.5 cm) and had normal haemoglobin level (11.6 g/dl) and body mass index (24.4 kg/m^2). The median age, height, weight, and FH for women were 28 years (range 16–44 years), 156 cm (range 148–176 cm), 60 kg (range 44–83 kg), and 32 cm (range 27–36 cm), respectively. The outcomes of pregnancy were in a normal average of GA (38 weeks), delivery weight (3252.8 g), birth length (50.2 cm), neonatal HC (33.5 cm), and neonatal AC (34.5 cm).

The reliability assessment of existing ultrasonic formulas in estimating foetal biometrics

This section presents the results of reliability analysis among three existing ultrasonic formulas [30–32] listed in Additional file 1: Table S1 in predicting foetal biometrics when ultrasound facilities are not accessible.

The intraclass and interclass correlation coefficient analyses are presented in Additional files 2 and 3: Table S2 and S3, respectively. The results presented in Additional file 2: Table S2 indicate that all three formulas have excellent reliability/consistency in predicting foetal HC and foetal AC at a given GA (the obtained ICC values are 0.957 and 0.996, respectively). Therefore, either of the existing formulas can be deployed in our study population.

Additional file 3: Table S3 shows that the estimated ultrasonic HC has a significant relationship with the neonatal HC (p-value < 0.0005) based on the existing models although the relationship was weak ($0.191 < r < 0.212$). Meanwhile, there is no significant correlation between the estimated ultrasonic AC and the neonatal AC ($0.076 < r < 0.078$, p-value > 0.05). However, since the Australian standard formulas produced slightly higher interclass correlation coefficients (between the estimates of foetal biometrics and the neonatal measurements) and more estimates falling within 10% of the neonatal measurements; therefore, the ultrasonic formulas based

Table 1 Maternal and neonatal baseline characteristics of study population ($n = 127$)

Characteristics	Missing data	Mean	Standard deviation	Median	Minimum	Maximum
Maternal age (years)	–	27.6	4.9	28	16	44
Maternal height (cm)	3	156.5	5.0	156	148	176
Maternal weight (kg)	–	59.9	7.5	60	44	83
Maternal body mass index (kg/m^2)	3	24.4	3.1	24.3	16.5	34.2
Maternal arm circumference (cm)	1	25.5	1.7	25	22	31
Maternal haemoglobin level (g/dl)	–	11.6	0.7	11.4	9	13.2
Maternal fundal height (FH) at delivery time (cm)	–	32.2	2.4	32	27	36
Gestational age (GA) at delivery time (weeks)	–	38.6	1.5	39	32	41
Actual birth weight (ABW) (g)	–	3252.8	340.8	3300	2600	4000
Neonatal birth length (cm)	–	50.2	2	50	40	56
Neonatal head circumference (HC) (cm)	–	33.5	1.3	33	29	37
Neonatal abdominal circumference (AC) (cm)	–	34.5	1.9	35	28	37

on the Australian population will be deployed to fill the foetal database gaps and assist the development of our proposed models.

Correlation analysis

Prior to developing models, correlations between the potential predictors of foetal weight estimation based on 127 data were investigated. The correlation analysis is presented in Additional file 4: Table S4.

Additional file 4: Table S4 shows that maternal FH has a significant correlation with the EFW_r and the ABW ($r = 0.952$, p-value < 0.0005 and $r = 0.795$, p-value < 0.0005, respectively). Unlike FH, GA has no significant correlation with the EFW_r and ABW.

Optimal models based on the best subset selection algorithm

Deploying the best subset selection algorithm, we have summarised the models developed based on the EFW_r (provided in Additional file 5: Table S5). These models were based on one, two, and three independent variables. The table also lists their corresponding R^2, Mallows Cp, S, and VIF statistics.

Additional file 5: Table S5 shows that the first model incorporated only one predictor: FH. The second, third, and fourth models incorporated two predictors: FH and GA, FH and estimated foetal HC, and FH and estimated foetal AC, respectively. The last model was developed based on three predictors: FH, estimated foetal HC, and estimated foetal AC.

Overall, the developed models had equal capability in predicting foetal weight estimation (coefficient of determination between 88.3 and 88.8%). However, using Mallows Cp index and S, we concluded that Models (3) and (4) were the best fit models with the least predicting errors. Models based only on estimated foetal HC or estimated foetal AC was excluded from the analysis due to the insignificant R^2. Model (5) was excluded due to the presence of severe multicollinearity ($VIF > 193$) (provided in Additional file 5: Table S5).

Table 2 presents the coefficients of the predictors for the chosen models together with the corresponding p-values of ANOVA, t-test statistics, and diagnostics of residuals.

Table 2 shows that for each individual model, the p-value corresponding to independent predictors is significant. Since our sample size is large, statistically significant non-normality of residuals was accepted. However, the authors have deployed robust regression to find the best fit models. Unfortunately, the best fit models proposed by robust regression had slightly larger prediction errors than those selected through the best subset models. Therefore, our further analysis is carried out using the OLS regression models presented in Table 2.

The accuracy comparison of the proposed and existing models

The two most commonly used models in Indonesia for estimating delivery weight are the Johnson-Toshach and the Risanto models. Both models estimate foetal weight based on FH. However, the Johnson-Toshach formula, which is nationally well-recognised, requires additional information on the status of the FS [44].

As listed in Table 2, the first model recommended through the best selection algorithm was Model (1) which is also developed based on FH only. Therefore, the authors carried out further comparisons between the proposed Model (1) and the widely used the Johnson-Toshach [14, 15] and the Risanto models [22, 23] as well as other existing models for estimating foetal weight based only on FH (the Niswander, the modified Niswander, the Mhaskar, the Gayatri-Afiyanti, the Buchmann-Tlale, the Santjaka-Handayani, the Mongelli-Gardosi, and the Yiheyis [16–18, 22–25, 45]). We also compared Models (2), (3), and (4) with the existing models based on ultrasonic measurements of foetal

Table 2 Predictor analysis of the proposed models

Model	Parameters	Estimated coefficients	Simultaneous p-value (ANOVA)	Partial p-value (t-test)	VIF	Residuals
(1)	β_0 (Intercept)	− 1538.3	< 0.0005***	2.66e-12***	–	Non-normal (p-value < 0.005)
	β_1 (FH)	150. 3		< 2e-16***	–	
(2)	β_0 (Intercept)	− 959	< 0.0005***	0.011*		Non-normal (p-value < 0.005)
	β_1 (GA)	−15.8		0.071*	1.01	
	β_2 (FH)	151.2		< 0.0005***	1.01	
(3)	β_0 (Intercept)	− 634.3	< 0.0005***	0.2304	–	Non-normal (p-value < 0.005)
	β_1 (FH)	151.2		< 2e-16***	1.01	
	β_2 (estimated HC)	−2.8		0.0682*	1.01	
(4)	β_0 (Intercept)	−996.8	< 0.0005***	0.00548**	–	Non-normal (p-value < 0.005)
	β_1 (FH)	151.2		< 2e-16***	1.01	
	β_2 (estimated AC)	−1.6		0.07066*	1.01	

***Significant at p-value < 0.0005
**Significant at p-value < 0.05
*Significant at alpha p-value < 0.1

biometrics, such as foetal HC and foetal AC (the Jordaan, the Weiner, the Hadlock 1984, and the Stirnemann [10, 42, 46, 47]). Details for the proposed and existing models are presented in Additional file 6: Table S6.

The prediction accuracy of the proposed (Models (1), (2), (3), and (4) in Table 2) and the existing models were assessed using the testing data set. The predicting errors were calculated as the mean prediction error (the average of the differences between ABW_i and EFW_{p_i}), the *MAPE*, and the *MEDAPE*. The results are presented in Table 3.

Table 3 shows that the mean prediction errors recorded for the proposed models are significantly smaller (between − 0.2 and 2.4 g) than those recorded for other existing models. Similarly, the MAPEs and MEDAPEs recorded for the proposed models are significantly smaller (between 5.0 and 5.1% and between 4.1 and 4.2%, respectively) than those recorded for other existing models. Therefore, we concluded that our four proposed models were capable to predict estimated foetal weight with less errors compare with the existing models between 35 and 41 weeks of pregnancy. The visualisation of these multiple comparisons can be seen in Fig. 3.

Furthermore, a two independent sample t-test (provided in Additional file 7: Table S7) was also used to investigate if there is a significant difference between the observed and estimated foetal weights based on the proposed models. The results show that there is no significant difference between the observed and estimated foetal weights based on the proposed models (p-value > 0.05).

Assessing the prediction accuracy based on proportion falling between 10% of actual values

Table 3 presents the prediction ability of the proposed models, 11 existing clinical models (based on FH only), and 6 existing ultrasonic models (based on ultrasonic measurements of foetal HC and foetal AC as well as based on GA only). The table provides the total number of predictions falling within 10% of ABW.

Table 3 shows that 92% of the predicted values produced by our proposed Model (1) fall within the 10% of ABW compared with 89% for the Johnson-Toshach model and 84% of the Risanto models. However, Model (1) only uses FH to predict foetal weight, while the Johnson-Toshach model requires information on FH as well as FS. Therefore, we recommend that Model (1) be used instead of the Johnson-Toshach model.

Model (1) (based on FH only) is equally capable to estimate foetal weight as Models (2) and (4). These results imply that the inclusion of GA (which is not a biometric measurement of foetus) and estimated foetal AC do not have an impact on estimated foetal weight accuracy. Our results are in agreement with the previous study conducted by Huber (2014) [48].

Comparing the accuracy of Model (3) (based on FH and estimated foetal HC) and Model (4) (based on FH and estimated foetal AC) with the Hadlock 1984 model (based on ultrasonic measurements of foetal HC and foetal AC) [10], we concluded that both proposed Models (3) and (4) were significantly more capable in predicting foetal weight than the Hadlock model. Table 3 shows that the proportion of predicted birth weights falling within the 10% of ABW for Models (3) and (4) are more than double the proportion based on the Hadlock model.

Discussion

Our study highlights that the use of combined maternal and estimated foetal biometric characteristics can provide a reliable estimate of delivery weights

Table 3 Accuracy comparisons between the proposed and existing models

Sample size $n = 38$					
(ABW - EFW_p)	Mean prediction error (g)	MAPE (%)	MEDAPE (%)	Error distribution	Number of estimates within 10% of ABW (%)
Our recommended models					
Model (1)	2.42	5.01	4.10	Normal (p-value > 0.05)	92
Model (2)	−0.20	5.10	4.16		92
Model (3)	−1.62	5.10	4.22		89
Model (4)	−0.29	5.10	4.16		92
Existing clinical models					
Johnson (1957) [15]	31.18	5.28	4.73	Normal (p-value > 0.05)	89
Risanto I (1995) [22]	149.56	5.95	5.37		84
Risanto II (2014) [23]	152.37	6.00	5.45		84
Niswander (1970) [16]	400.95	12.24	12.07		37
Mod Niswander (1999) [17]	457.68	13.70	14.16		29
Mhaskar (2003) cited in [65]	405.26	12.59	12.86		32
Gayatri (2006) [24]	471.05	14.02	15.15		26
Buchmann-Tlale (2009) [18, 66]	571.05	17.12	18.18		11
Santjaka (2011) [25]	− 2411.95	75.33	72.24		0
Mongelli-Gardosi (2004) [19]	1348.35	41.93	42.40		0
Yiheyis (2016) [45]	363.95	11.12	11.05		45
Existing ultrasonic models					
Jordaan (1983) [46]	− 277.09	14.64	14.43	Normal (p-value > 0.05)	39
Weiner II (1985) cited in [60]	486.29	15.90	12.86		32
Hadlock 1984 [10]	−96.83	12.67	12.64		45
Hadlock 1991 [67]	− 42.75	11.74	9.88		50
Stirnemann 2016 [42]	−31.46	12.20	10.88		39
Sotiriadis 2017 [68]	230.72	10.88	9.43		50

between 35 and 41 weeks of GA. This result confirms the previous study that shows a significant association between birth weight and characteristics of mother and foetus [1, 26].

Both clinical and estimates of ultrasonic predictors are used in our proposed models. Maternal FH measurement was selected as one of the clinical predictors as it is one of the most recommended and accessible predictors to estimate foetal weight and monitor foetal growth during pregnancy [3, 23, 49, 50]. Although the clinical approach using FH screening had reportedly low sensitivity for detecting intergrowth and birth weight abnormalities (ranged 16–45%) [51, 52], it is a simple and inexpensive clinical activity [29, 53], especially true in rural areas where ultrasound machines and skilled personnel are not always available. The utility of FH remains an important first level screening tool, widely used during routine ANC in both high and low income settings [29] even though it had high false-negative rates for small for GA [53].

In ultrasonic settings, foetal biometric characteristics monitored during pregnancy include HC, biparietal diameter (BPD), occipitofrontal diameter (OFD), AC, and femur length (FL). These characteristics are routinely measured by ultrasound every 5 weeks after the first initial dating scan (between 8 and 14 weeks' gestation). The standard ranges for ultrasonic measurements are (14–18), (19–23), (24–28), (29–33), (34–38), and (39–42) weeks [54] or at least once every trimester of pregnancy, i.e. between weeks 10–14 (first trimester), 20–24 (second trimester), and 30–32 (third trimester) [55].

Assessment of foetal biometric characteristics during ANC is vital to ensuring normal foetal size and safe delivery. In the absence of ultrasound facility, particularly in low-resource primary health care settings, the measurements of these characteristics are not always accessible. Therefore, a reliable prediction of these characteristics during pregnancy would be a proxy of foetal biometrics and vitally improve the quality of

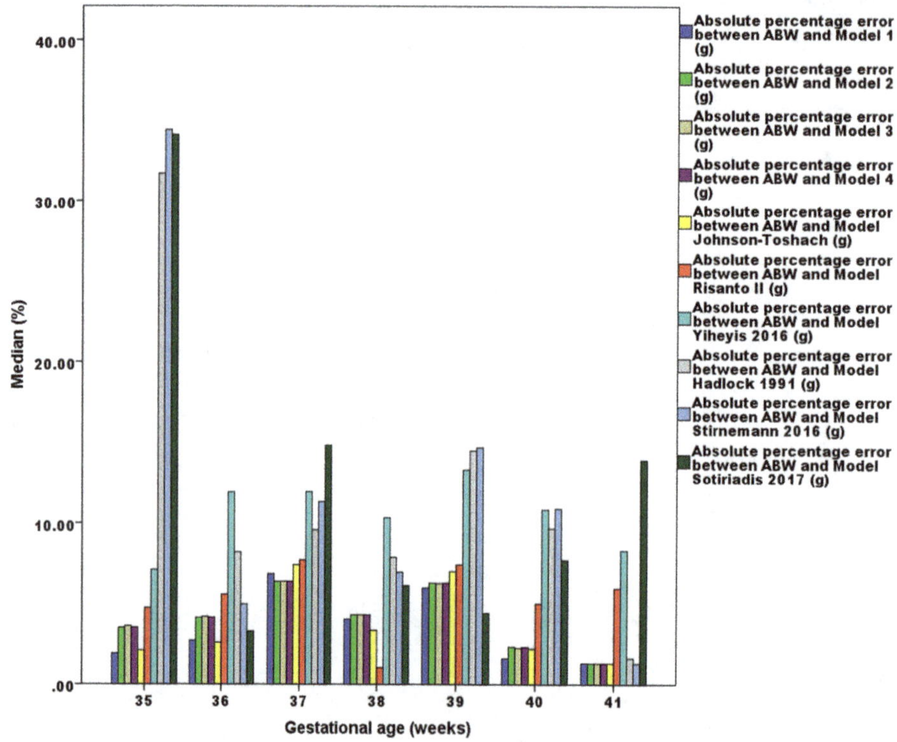

Fig. 3 MEDAPEs comparison between the proposed and commonly used models ordered by GA

ANC services in monitoring foetal inter growth assessment which currently remain low due to the database gaps [56–59].

Several ultrasonic formulas to estimate the foetal characteristics at different GA have been developed [30–32]. The foetal HC and foetal AC are widely recognised as the most influential predictors for predicting foetal weight [10, 11, 46, 60, 61]. Our results show that the best fit formulas to estimate these foetal characteristics at a given GA in our population were based on the Australian population [30].

To the best of our knowledge, in the majority of Indonesian primary health care centres where ultrasound facility is not accessible, none of the existing ultrasonic formulas were adopted to estimate foetal HC and foetal AC. Therefore, the formulas potentially can be deployed to fill in the database gaps on the inter growth process of foetus during pregnancy. Consequently, early informed intervention could be initiated to prevent abnormal growth and delivery weights.

Several techniques have been available to reduce collinearity, such as centering, multiplying variables by various constants (scaling), the use of orthogonal polynomials, and other transformations [62]. Currently, the use of automated machine learning, such as Genetic Algorithm rather than a conventional fractional polynomial approach has also been applied to model multiple biometric variables of foetus that are highly correlated [54].

In this paper, we used the best subset selection algorithm to prevent the inclusion of highly correlated variables and select the best subset of predictors to be included in the models. It has been emphasized that a formula for estimating foetal weight should be simple and straightforward to be used by doctors and midwives and be easily understood by patients [63]. This would improve the quality of communication, information, and education as part of routine ANC service in low-resource primary health care centres.

Based on our comparison analysis, the proposed Models (1), (2), (3), and (4) produced the least mean prediction errors (between − 0.2 and − 2.4 g), the MAPEs (between 5.01 and 5.10%), and the MEDAPEs (between 4.10 and 4.22%). The mean percentage prediction error (MPE) steadily tended towards zero as the time interval between the last scan and birth decreased [42]. Our MPEs were ranged between − 0.1 and − 0.3% in those born within 0 day ($n = 38$) which are lower than the previous research [42] reported by − 0.8% in those born within 1 day ($n = 198$).

Our proposed models were unbiased for predicting weight between 35 and 41 weeks of GA. In the group born within 0 day of the last measurements, the MAPEs were ranged between 5.0 and 5.10% with 89–92% of predicted weights falling within 10% of the true birth weights which are smaller than those reported in previous study [42]. This was particularly for Model (1) which was simply developed based on FH only.

The comparison between the proposed Model (1) and the widely used Johnson-Toshach model shows that Model (1) (developed based on the Indonesian data) was more accurate in predicting the estimated foetal weight than the Johnson-Toshach model (developed based on the United States data). Furthermore, the Johnson-Toshach model requires the knowledge of FS. The results presented in Table 3 also shows that the inclusion of FS in the model has not reduced the prediction errors in foetal weight estimations yet raise a subjectivity issue unless there is a standard protocol to determine FS with less error [20]. Therefore, we recommend the proposed Model (1) be deployed in Indonesia and other countries with similar health systems and challenges for weight prediction.

Our comparison study confirms that the proposed Models (3) (based on FH and estimates of foetal HC) and (4) (based on FH and estimates of foetal AC) perform better than the ultrasonic models: the Jordaan, the Weiner II, the Hadlocks, the Stirnemann, and the Sotiriadis models. The incorporation of estimated foetal HC or estimated foetal AC has increased R^2 slightly (provided in Additional file 5: Table S5), but it did not improve the predicting accuracy (Table 3). However, access to these values will enable the practitioners to monitor foetal growth during pregnancy where advanced equipment, such as ultrasound, is not always available. Consequently, detecting foetal growth abnormality, such as small for GA, prematurity, intrauterine growth retardation, and LBW during pregnancy will be possible.

Strengths and limitations

Our retrospective study has investigated the utilisation of some commonly used foetal weight prediction models in Indonesia. Particularly, the combination between maternal and estimated foetal biometric characteristics was proposed. The aim of this combination was whether it could improve the prediction accuracy of foetal weight at any given GA in the absence of ultrasound machines and trained ultra-sonographers.

The retrospective cohort study was undertaken to provide baseline data on the selected primary health care centre. It is possible that women have used different health services than that reviewed in this study. Although this may result in underestimation in data records, it is unlikely to impact on the validity of the analyses. This study also encountered limitations associated with the accuracy of the information recorded on the manual pregnancy register or inaccurate data transfer to the electronic database. However, monitoring and controlling the process of data transfer was conducted to reduce potential error. Further study should be conducted to assess the efficacy of the proposed models using prospective data [64].

The proposed prediction models are linear regressions. However, the authors have investigated non-linear models. The non-linear models did not improve the estimation accuracy. Therefore, complex models do not guarantee significant improvement in the prediction accuracy. Furthermore, due to the fact that the objective of the study is to provide simple yet reliable foetal weight estimating models for low-resource areas, we are recommending the proposed models. We believe that the findings can be applied in other low-resource settings to improve ANC services.

Conclusion

This research has developed models to predict the estimated foetal weight at varying gestational age where ultrasound facilities do not exist. Since birth weight is one of the most important indicators of neonatal survival, a reliable estimate of foetal weight at different stages of pregnancy would facilitate the intervention plan for medical practitioners to prevent the risk of abnormal delivery weights. Further, the models will lead to the development of foetal inter growth charts, which are currently unavailable in the Indonesian primary health care systems.

Additional files

Additional file 1: Table S1. Existing ultrasonic formulas to estimate foetal HC and AC based on GA. Table S1 consists of the existing ultrasonic formulas to estimate foetal head circumference (HC) and foetal abdominal circumference (AC) which were developed based on the Australian foetal biometry data (measured between 11 and 41 weeks), the UK foetal biometry data (measured between 13 and 42 weeks), and the international foetal biometry data (measured between 14 and 42 weeks or until birth) [29–31].

Additional file 2: Table S2. Intraclass correlation coefficient analysis of the existing ultrasonic formulas in predicting foetal biometrics. Table S2 shows a reliability analysis using intraclass correlation coefficient (ICC) to assess the consistency of the ultrasonic formulas for Indonesian population. The obtained ICC values were computed by single-rating, consistency, and two-way random effects models for the foetal biometrics with three raters (different ultrasonic formulas) across 127 subjects (pregnant women).

Additional file 3: Table S3. Interclass correlation coefficient analysis for predicting foetal biometrics. Table S3 describes interclass (Pearson) correlation coefficient to assess whether there is a significant relationship between the predicted foetal biometrics and the neonatal measurements recorded at delivery time.

Additional file 4: Table S4. Correlation coefficient of the potentially clinical predictors of foetal weight estimation. Table S4 presents the investigation of correlations between the potential predictors of foetal weight estimation based on 127 data.

Additional file 5: Table S5. Models recommended by the best subset selection algorithm together with corresponding analysis of variance information. Table S5 summarises the models developed based on the recorded estimated foetal weight (EFW,) using the best subset selection algorithm. These models were based on one, two, and three independent variables. The table also lists their corresponding R^2, Mallows C_p, *S*, and *VIF* statistics.

Additional file 6: Table S6. List of the proposed and existing models based on clinical and ultrasonic variables. Table S6 lists the proposed models and the existing clinical and ultrasonic models for estimating foetal weight.

Additional file 7: Table S7. Two independent sample t-tests between ABW, EFW_r, and EFW_p. Table S7 provides a two independent sample t-test to investigate if there is a significant difference between the observed or actual values of birth weight (ABW), recorded foetal weight estimation (EFW_r), and estimated foetal weights based on the proposed model (EFW_p).

Abbreviations

ABW: Actual birth weight; ABW_i: The ith actual values of birth weight; AC: Abdominal circumference; ANC: Antenatal care; ANOVA: Analysis of variance; BPD: Biparietal diameter; CIE: Communication, information, and education; EFW_p: Estimated foetal weight based on the proposed model; EFW_r: Recorded foetal weight estimation; EFW_{pi}: The ith predicted values of foetal weight based on the proposed models; FH: Fundal height; FL: Femur length; FS: Foetal head engagement/foetal station; GA: Gestational age; HC: Head circumference; ICC: Intraclass correlation coefficient; LBW: Low birth weight; MAPE: Mean absolute percentage prediction error; MEDAPE: Median absolute percentage prediction error; MPE: Mean percentage prediction error; OFD: Occipitofrontal diameter; OLS: Ordinary least square; *r*: Correlation coefficient; R^2: Coefficient of determination; S: Standard deviation; *VIF*: Variance inflation factor

Acknowledgements

We are grateful to the Australian Agency for International Development (AusAID) for funding DA's PhD scholarship in Mathematical Sciences at the School of Science, RMIT University, Melbourne, Australia.
The authors would like to thank Feri Anita Wijayanti, M.Mid, Bd. for the provision of antenatal care references in the Indonesian context. We would also thank the dedicated midwives for their roles in supervising the data measuring and recording task in the primary health care centre.
The authors are greatly indebted to the Higher Degree Research (HDR) Language and Learning Advisor of RMIT University, Dr. Ken Manson, for his roles in providing language help and proofreading the article.

Funding

Not applicable. This research did not receive any specific grant from funding agencies in the public, commercial, or not-for-profit sectors. However, the Australian Agency for International Development (AusAID) has granted DA's PhD scholarship in Mathematical Sciences at the School of Science, RMIT University, Melbourne, Australia. This analysis is part of DA's thesis.

Authors' contributions

DA and MA contributed in the conception and design of the study. DA provided the literature review and information summary on relevant research articles and policies in Indonesia. DA performed data collection, pre-processing data, analysis, and interpretation. DA prepared the manuscript. MA and KM provided data analysis, advice, proofreading, and critical revision of the manuscript. All of the authors read and approved the final manuscript.

Authors' information

DA: PhD candidate in the Mathematical Sciences (Applied Statistics), School of Science (Mathematical and Geospatial Sciences), College of Science, Engineering, and Health, RMIT University, Melbourne, Australia and Junior Lecturer at Study Program of Statistics, Faculty of Mathematics and Natural Sciences, University of Lambung Mangkurat (ULM), South Kalimantan, Indonesia.
MA: Senior Lecturer of Statistical Quality Control and its applications in: manufacturing industry, air pollution control, software quality, univariate and multivariate processes, health industry, and the banking system, School of Science (Mathematical and Geospatial Sciences), College of Science, Engineering, and Health, RMIT University, Melbourne, Australia.
KM: Senior Lecturer of Applied Statistics and Mathematics, Market Research, and Numerical Analysis in aerospace engineering, clinical sciences, geomatic engineering, and oncology and carcinogenesis, College of Science, Engineering, and Health, RMIT University, Melbourne, Australia.

Ethics approval and consent to participate

This study is a part of doctoral degree research and has obtained two ethics clearances:

1. The Ethical Committees of Medical Research, Medical Faculty, University of Lambung Mangkurat (ULM), Banjarmasin, South Kalimantan (Indonesia), on March 10th, 2016, with registration number: 018/KEPK-FK UNLAM/EC/III/2016. Permission to access unidentified secondary data in the preganancy register available at the selected primary health care was also granted under this ethical consideration.

2. The Science, Engineering, and Health College Human Ethics Advisory Network (CHEAN) of Royal Melbourne Institute of Technology (RMIT) University, Melbourne, Victoria (Australia), on March 16th, 2016, with registration number: ASEHAPP 19-16/RM No: 19974.

Research permissions were obtained from the Indonesian national, provincial, and local governments.

Competing interests

The authors declare that they have no competing interests.

References

1. Njim T, Atashili J, Mbu R, Choukem S-P. Low birth weight in a sub-urban area of Cameroon: an analysis of the clinical cut-off, incidence, predictors and complications. BMC Pregnancy Childbirth. 2015;15(1):288.
2. Gibson KS, Waters TP, Gunzler DD, Catalano PM. A retrospective cohort study of factors relating to the longitudinal change in birth weight. BMC Pregnancy Childbirth. 2015;15(1):1.
3. Parvin Z, Shafiuddin S, Uddin MA, Begum F. Symphysio fundal height (SFH) measurement as a predictor of birth weight. Faridpur Med Coll J. 2013;7(2): 54–8.
4. Lalys L, Pineau J-C, Guihard-Costa A-M. Small and large foetuses: identification and estimation of foetal weight at delivery from third-trimester ultrasound data. Early Hum Dev. 2010;86(12):753–7.
5. Sharma SR, Giri S, Timalsina U, Bhandari SS, Basyal B, Wagle K, Shrestha L. Low birth weight at term and its determinants in a tertiary hospital of Nepal: a case-control study. PLoS One. 2015;10(4):e0123962.
6. Willocks J, Donald I, Duggan T, Day N. Foetal cephalometry by ultrasound. BJOG Int J Obstet Gynaecol. 1964;71(1):11–20.
7. Robson SC, Gallivan S, Walkinshaw SA, Vaughan J, Rodeck CH. Ultrasonic estimation of fetal weight: use of targeted formulas in small for gestational age fetuses. Obstet Gynecol. 1993;82(3):359–64.
8. Spinnato JA, Allen RD, Mendenhall HW. Birth weight prediction from remote ultrasound examination. Obstet Gynecol. 1988;71(6):893–8.
9. Shepard M, Richards V, Berkowitz R, Warsof S, Hobbins J. An evaluation of two equations for predicting fetal weight by ultrasound. Am J Obstet Gynecol. 1982;142(1):47–54.
10. Hadlock F, Harrist R, Carpenter R, Deter R, Park S. Sonographic estimation of fetal weight. The value of femur length in addition to head and abdomen measurements. Radiology. 1984;150(2):535–40.
11. Hadlock FP, Harrist R, Sharman RS, Deter RL, Park SK. Estimation of fetal weight with the use of head, body, and femur measurements—a prospective study. Am J Obstet Gynecol. 1985;151(3):333–7.

12. Campbell S, Wilkin D. Ultrasonic measurement of fetal abdomen circumference in the estimation of fetal weight. BJOG Int J Obstet Gynaecol. 1975;82(9):689–97.
13. Combs CA, Jaekle RK, Rosenn B, Pope M, Miodovnik M, Siddiqi TA. Sonographic estimation of fetal weight based on a model of fetal volume. Obstet Gynecol. 1993;82(3):365–70.
14. Johnson R, Toshach C. Estimation of fetal weight using longitudinal mensuration. Am J Obstet Gynecol. 1954;68(3):891–6.
15. Johnson RW. Calculations in estimating fetal weight. Am J Obstet Gynecol. 1957;74(4):929.
16. Niswander KR, Capraro VJ, Van Coevering RJ. Estimation of birth weight by quantified external uterine measurements. Obstet Gynecol. 1970;36(2):294–8.
17. Farid SW. Child weight prediction based on the modification of the Niswander formula (Taksasi berat badan anak berdasarkan modifikasi rumus Niswander). Majalah Obstetri dan Ginekologi Indonesia. 1999;23(4):188–93.
18. Buchmann E, Tlale K. A simple clinical formula for predicting fetal weight in labour at term: derivation and validation. SAMJ. 2009;99(6):457–60.
19. Mongelli M, Gardosi J. Estimation of fetal weight by symphysis–fundus height measurement. Int J Gynecol Obstet. 2004;85(1):50–1.
20. Bothner B, Gulmezoglu A, Hofmeyr G. Symphysis fundus height measurements during labour: a prospective, descriptive study. Afr J Reprod Health. 2000;4(1):48–55.
21. Dare F, Ademowore A, Ifaturoti O, Nganwuchu A. The value of symphysio-fundal height/abdominal girth measurements in predicting fetal weight. Int J Gynecol Obstet. 1990;31(3):243–8.
22. Siswosudarmo H. Detection of low birth weight babies at term pregnancy with fundal height measurements (Deteksi bayi berat lahir rendah pada kehamilan aterm dengan pengukuran tinggi fundus). Berkala Epidemiologi Klinik Biostatika Indonesia. 1995;1(20):78–84.
23. Siswosudarmo R, Titisari I. Developing a new formula for estimating birth weight at term pregnancy. Jurnal Kesehatan Reproduksi. 2014;1(2):145–149.
24. Gayatri D, Afiyanti Y. Validation of fetal weight estimation formula (TBJ) for prediction of birth weight based on uterine fundal height of pregnant women (Validasi rumus taksiran berat janin (TBJ) untuk prediksi berat badan lahir berdasarkan tinggi fundus uterus ibu hamil). Jurnal Keperawatan Indonesia. 2006;10(1):24–9.
25. Santjaka HI, Handayani R. Study of the accuracy of fetal weight estimates based on statistics and fundal height (Studi ketepatan taksiran berat janin berdasarkan statistik dan tinggi fundus uteri). Jurnal Bidan Prada. 2011;2(01):21–34.
26. Kiserud T, Piaggio G, Carroli G, Widmer M, Carvalho J, Jensen LN, Giordano D, Cecatti JG, Aleem HA, Talegawkar SA. The World Health Organization fetal growth charts: a multinational longitudinal study of ultrasound biometric measurements and estimated fetal weight. PLoS Med. 2017;14(1):e1002220.
27. Anggraini D, Abdollahian M, Marion K. Review of low birth weight prediction models in Indonesia. Int J Adv Sci Eng Technol. 2015;3(4):105–11.
28. Abdollahian M, Ahmad S, Huda S, Nuryani S, Anggraini D. Investigating the relationship between neonatal mortality rate and mother's characteristics. In: Proceedings of the International Conference on Information and Knowledge Engineering (IKE); The Steering Committee of the World Congress in Computer Science, Computer Engineering, and Applied Computing (WorldComp); CSREA Press; 2012. p. 1.
29. Papageorghiou AT, Ohuma EO, Gravett MG, Hirst J, da Silveira MF, Lambert A, Carvalho M, Jaffer YA, Altman DG, Noble JA. International standards for symphysis-fundal height based on serial measurements from the fetal growth longitudinal study of the INTERGROWTH-21st project: prospective cohort study in eight countries. BMJ. 2016;355:i5662.
30. Westerway SC, Davison A, Cowell S. Ultrasonic fetal measurements: new Australian standards for the new millennium. Aust N Z J Obstet Gynaecol. 2000;40(3):297–302.
31. Loughna P, Chitty L, Evans T, Chudleigh T. Fetal size and dating: charts recommended for clinical obstetric practice. Ultrasound. 2009;17(3):160–6.
32. Papageorghiou AT, Ohuma EO, Altman DG, Todros T, Ismail LC, Lambert A, Jaffer YA, Bertino E, Gravett MG, Purwar M. International standards for fetal growth based on serial ultrasound measurements: the fetal growth longitudinal study of the INTERGROWTH-21 st project. Lancet. 2014; 384(9946):869–79.
33. Achadi E, Jones G. Health sector review: maternal, neonatal, and child health. In: Jakarta: Ministry of National Development Planning/Bappenas, Republic of Indonesia; 2014.
34. UNICEF-Indonesia. Issues briefs: maternal and child health. In: UNICEF Indonesia; 2012. p. 1–6.
35. MoH. Indonesia health profile (Profil kesehatan Indonesia) 2012. In: Jakarta: Ministry of Health, Republic of Indonesia; 2013.
36. Bellio R, Ventura L. An introduction to robust estimation with R functions. Proceedings of 1st International Work; 2005. p. 1–57.
37. Fox J, Weisberg S. An R companion to applied regression: Sage; 2010.
38. Renaud O, Victoria-Feser M-P. A robust coefficient of determination for regression. J Statist Plann Inference. 2010;140(7):1852–62.
39. Faraway JJ. Practical regression and ANOVA using R. In: University of Bath; 2002.
40. Landers R. Computing Intraclass Correlations (ICC) as estimates of interrater reliability in SPSS. The Winnower 2: e143518. 81744; 2015. https://doi.org/10.15200/winn.143518.81744.
41. Koo TK, Li MY. A guideline of selecting and reporting intraclass correlation coefficients for reliability research. J Chiropr Med. 2016;15(2):155–63.
42. Stirnemann J, Villar J, Salomon L, Ohuma E, Ruyan P, Altman D, Nosten F, Craik R, Munim S, Cheikh Ismail L. International estimated fetal weight standards of the INTERGROWTH-21st project. Ultrasound Obstet Gynecol. 2017;49(4):478–86.
43. Levenbach H. Training EDC: The Myth of the MAPE and how to avoid it. 2015.
44. Anggraini D, Abdollahian M, Marion K. Accuracy assessment on prediction models for fetal weight based on maternal fundal height. In: Information technology: new generations. Cham: Springer; 2016. p. 859–68.
45. Yiheyis A, Alemseged F, Segni H. Johnson's formula for predicting birth weight in pregnant mothers at Jimma University Teaching Hospital, South West Ethiopia. Med J Obstet Gynecol. 2016;4(3):1087–93.
46. Jordaan HV. Estimation of fetal weight by ultrasound. J Clin Ultrasound. 1983;11(2):59–66.
47. Weiner Z, Ben-Shlomo I, Beck-Fruchter R, Goldberg Y, Shalev E. Clinical and ultrasonographic weight estimation in large for gestational age fetus. Eur J Obstet Gynecol Reprod Biol. 2002;105(1):20–4.
48. Huber C, Zdanowicz JA, Mueller M, Surbek D. Factors influencing the accuracy of fetal weight estimation with a focus on preterm birth at the limit of viability: a systematic literature review. Fetal Diagn Ther. 2014;36(1):1–8.
49. Morse K, Williams A, Gardosi J. Fetal growth screening by fundal height measurement. Best Pract Res Clin Obstet Gynaecol. 2009;23(6):809–18.
50. Titisari HI, Siswosudarmo R. Risanto's formulas is more accurate in determining estimated fetal weight based on maternal fundal height. Indones J Obstet Gynecol. 2013;1(3):149–51.
51. Sparks TN, Cheng YW, McLaughlin B, Esakoff TF, Caughey AB. Fundal height: a useful screening tool for fetal growth? J Matern Fetal Neonatal Med. 2011; 24(5):708–12.
52. Curti A, Zanello M, De Maggio I, Moro E, Simonazzi G, Rizzo N, Farina A. Multivariable evaluation of term birth weight: a comparison between ultrasound biometry and symphysis-fundal height. J Matern Fetal Neonatal Med. 2014;27(13):1328–32.
53. Pay ASD, Wiik J, Backe B, Jacobsson B, Strandell A, Klovning A. Symphysis-fundus height measurement to predict small-for-gestational-age status at birth: a systematic review. BMC Pregnancy Childbirth. 2015;15(1):22.
54. Papageorghiou AT, Kemp B, Stones W, Ohuma EO, Kennedy SH, Purwar M, Salomon LJ, Altman DG, Noble JA, Bertino E. Ultrasound-based gestational-age estimation in late pregnancy. Ultrasound Obstet Gynecol. 2016;48(6): 719–26.
55. Postoev VA, Grjibovski AM, Nieboer E, Odland JØ. Changes in detection of birth defects and perinatal mortality after introduction of prenatal ultrasound screening in the Kola Peninsula (North-West Russia): combination of two birth registries. BMC Pregnancy Childbirth. 2015;15(1):1.
56. Gardosi J. Fetal growth standards: individual and global perspectives. Lancet. 2011;377(9780):1812–4.
57. Gardosi J. Customised assessment of fetal growth potential: implications for perinatal care. Arch Dis Child Fetal Neonatal Ed. 2012. https://doi.org/10.1136/fetalneonatal-2012-301708.
58. Moxon SG, Ruysen H, Kerber KJ, Amouzou A, Fournier S, Grove J, Moran AC, Vaz LM, Blencowe H, Conroy N. Count every newborn: a measurement improvement roadmap for coverage data. BMC Pregnancy Childbirth. 2015;15(2):S8.
59. Kerber KJ, Mathai M, Lewis G, Flenady V, Erwich JJH, Segun T, Aliganyira P, Abdelmegeid A, Allanson E, Roos N. Counting every stillbirth and neonatal death through mortality audit to improve quality of care for every pregnant woman and her baby. BMC Pregnancy Childbirth. 2015;15(2):S9.
60. Abele H, Hoopmann M, Wagner N, Hahn M, Wallwiener D, Kagan KO. Accuracy of sonographic fetal weight estimation of fetuses with a birth weight of 1500g or less. Eur J Obstet Gynecol Reprod Biol. 2010;153(2):131–7.

61. Dudley N. A systematic review of the ultrasound estimation of fetal weight. Ultrasound Obstet Gynecol. 2005;25(1):80–9.
62. Kleinbaum D, Kupper L, Nizam A, Rosenberg E. Applied regression analysis and other multivariable methods: Nelson Education; 2013.
63. Salomon LJ, Bernard JP, Ville Y. Estimation of fetal weight: reference range at 20–36 weeks' gestation and comparison with actual birth-weight reference range. Ultrasound Obstet Gynecol. 2007;29(5):550–5.
64. Asiki G, Baisley K, Newton R, Marions L, Seeley J, Kamali A, Smedman L. Adverse pregnancy outcomes in rural Uganda (1996–2013): trends and associated factors from serial cross sectional surveys. BMC Pregnancy Childbirth. 2015;15(1):1.
65. Gayatri D, Afiyanti Y. Comparison of some formulas for predicting birth weight based on height measurement of fundus uteri (Perbandingan beberapa rumus untuk memprediksi berat badan lahir berdasrkan pengukuran tinggi fundus uteri). Jurnal Keperawatan Indonesia. 2004;8(1):18–22.
66. Rusdy RS, Yasmin FA, Putri LA, Oktrian O, Pusponegoro A. Comparison of Johnson-Tohsach formula with South Africa formula in determining fetal weight estimation at Puskesmas Kecamatan Pasar Rebo, East Jakarta (Perbandingan rumus Johnson-Tohsach dengan rumus South Africa dalam menentukan taksiran berat janin di Puskesmas Kecamatan Pasar Rebo, Jakarta Timur). eJurnal Kedokteran Indonesia. 2014;2(1):33–6.
67. Hadlock FP, Harrist RB, Martinez-Poyer J. In utero analysis of fetal growth: a sonographic weight standard. Radiology. 1991;181(1):129–33.
68. Sotiriadis A, Eleftheriades M, Papadopoulos V, Sarafidis K, Pervanidou P, Assimakopoulos E. Divergence of estimated fetal weight and birth weight in singleton fetuses. J Matern Fetal Neonatal Med. 2018;31(6):761–9.

12

The impact of postpartum psychosis on partners

Nia Holford[1], Sue Channon[2*], Jessica Heron[3] and Ian Jones[4]

Abstract

Background: Postpartum Psychosis is a severe mental health condition following childbirth, with a psychosis and associated mood disturbance. Research to date has primarily focused on mothers' experiences, and on identifying risk factors, aetiology, and intervention efficacy. Within both research and clinical communities, there has been little acknowledgement of partners' experiences of Postpartum Psychosis, nor the important support role that partners can provide. The aim of this study was to consider the lived experiences of partners of women who have had Postpartum Psychosis, and the impact that it has had on their lives and relationships.

Methods: Participants ($N = 8$) were partners recruited through the charity Action on Postpartum Psychosis. Partners completed an in-depth, semi-structured interview regarding their experiences of Postpartum Psychosis. Interpretative Phenomenological Analysis was used to analyse the interview transcripts.

Results: Seven superordinate themes emerged from the interview data: loss; powerlessness; united vs. individual coping; hypothesising and hindsight; barriers to accessing care and unmet needs; managing multiple roles; and positive changes from Postpartum Psychosis.

Conclusions: These findings provide a rich illustration of the experiences of partners, including some previously unidentified findings relating to partner hypervigilance to signs of relapse and positive changes in their attitudes and relationships. Areas where support could be provided for partners are also highlighted.

Keywords: Postpartum Psychosis, Partners, Experience, Loss, Support, Relationship

Background

Postpartum Psychosis (PP) is a severe mental health condition, with a psychotic element and associated mood disturbance following childbirth, and is often described as a 'psychiatric emergency' [1, 2]. Postpartum Psychosis occurs in 1 to 2 per 1000 births, with a peak window of onset within the first two weeks after birth [3]. The onset of PP is typically sudden, unexpected and severe [4, 5]. As an emerging field of research, studies have primarily focused on identifying incidence rates, aetiology, exploring genetic susceptibility and risk factors [6–10]. Risk factors that have been identified include having a pre-existing mental health problem (such as Bipolar Disorder), primiparity, marital conflict, lack of social support, and the presence of stressful life events.

The London School of Economics report an 8.1 billion pound spend to cover the direct and indirect costs of perinatal mental health for each annual birth cohort within the United Kingdom [11]. Current National Institute for Health and Care Excellence (NICE) guidance on antenatal and postnatal mental healthcare, recommend that healthcare professionals be alert to any possible symptoms of PP within the first two weeks after childbirth [12]. However, only half of women have access to specialist perinatal mental health services, and both personal and service level barriers to receiving appropriate care have been outlined [11]. Other NICE recommendations include for mental healthcare providers to: establish a co-ordinated care plan; provide medical and therapeutic interventions; and consider the support role of the partner, and the potential effect of the perinatal episode on the couple relationship.

Pregnancy and childbirth are times of considerable change, placing increased demands on a couple. The

* Correspondence: channons2@cardiff.ac.uk
[2]Centre for Trials Research, Cardiff University, Cardiff, UK

relationship that a couple have with each other, and the relationship that they build with their infant during the postnatal window, helps to provide a foundation for infant development and secure attachment [13–15]. Establishing this foundation can be difficult in the best of circumstances, but perinatal mental health problems cause an additional challenge. The treatment of, and the course of recovery from, PP has been described as 'a long and difficult process', often involving a psychiatric admission of the mother to a general psychiatric ward, or admission of the mother and infant to a Mother and Baby Unit (MBU) ([1], p.155). Whilst the understanding of the impact of perinatal mental health problems for the mother might be improving, the literature provides little information on the impact of such difficulties on partners, or on their relationships with their new infant and the mother.

From the limited research that has been conducted to date, partners typically described the support they felt that the mother required, or lacked, and neglected to mention their own needs; instead, they identified that they struggled to ask for help and felt isolated and overwhelmed [16]. Partners were provided with little support or information regarding PP, and wanted greater support and information for themselves [17]. Although Engqvist and Nilsson [18] sought views from both the mothers and their partners on the recovery process from PP, only four out of twenty-four quotes within this article were from partners, and regarded their interpretation of the mother's needs at different stages, or their needs as a couple, rather than their own individual needs. Partners were included in the work by Wyatt et al. [19] but this study examined the impact of PP on the relationship and used dyadic interviews. Only one published study was identified to date that focused solely on partners' experiences of PP [20], drawing on interviews with men during their partners admission to an MBU for first episode PP.

The relevance and importance of pursuing further research into PP can be drawn from considering other neighbouring, but distinct, fields of research, namely that relating to Postnatal Depression (PND). Research by Reid and Taylor [21] into PND has already stressed the protective nature of a supportive couple relationship in the development of postnatal mental health difficulties. Moreover, common themes faced by couples experiencing PND have been identified as including a perceived fracturing of the family unit, a sense of loss, and maternal absence [22, 23].

The aim of the current study was to consider the lived experiences of partners of women who have had Postpartum Psychosis, and the impact that it has had on their lives and relationships.

Methods

Interpretative Phenomenological Analysis (IPA) was utilised in this study as it is a form of qualitative analysis that allows for the exploration of individuals' lived experiences with the aim of capturing the insider's perspective, both unique and collective experiences. Through the process of analysis, data is gained from each individual participant and overarching themes emerge as to what it can be like for someone to go through such an event. This study utilised IPA to explore the lived experiences of partners of women who had been diagnosed with PP as it is an analytic process which allows for both the meaning that partners have made of their experiences to be identified, but also allows for reflection on their affective responses.

The study aim was addressed through semi-structured interviews with partners. In addition, a short online questionnaire was devised and completed at the recruitment stage in order to identify socio-demographic details. Interpretative Phenomenological Analysis (IPA) was applied to the interview transcripts to try to develop an in-depth exploration of partners' experiences of PP [24]. The use of IPA allows for the identification of some experiences, which may be shared among partners, but also those uniquely expressed. Previous research exploring the impact of Postnatal Depression (PND) on partners has used a similar IPA approach [22].

Recruitment

The study was given ethical approval from Cardiff University (EC.14.11.11.3914R2A). Participants were recruited through the UK based charity Action on Postpartum Psychosis (APP www.app-network.org). Permission to recruit through APP was obtained from the charity's director and leadership team. An advertisement for the current research, featuring a brief description of the study and call for participants, was posted on the APP forum website, Facebook page, and Twitter feed. The advertisement included a link to more information regarding the study, a consent form, and access to an online questionnaire for partners to complete and to register if they wished to be contacted with more information regarding an interview. To be eligible for the interview the episode of PP was to have occurred more than 6 months ago but less than 10 years ago, to try and limit emotional distress and for recollection purposes. A further consent form was completed in writing immediately prior to an interview about their experiences of PP.

Sample

A sample size between 4 to10 is deemed adequate for the completion of IPA [24]. A total of nine partners completed the online questionnaire and agreed to be contacted for an interview, of which eight completed the interview. The ninth partner opted to withdraw from the research prior to an interview being arranged due to their other commitments. The questionnaire data from the ninth participant was subsequently excluded from analysis. All partners who volunteered were male, although the study was open to all couples. The most common age bracket for partners was between 30- to 34-years-old ($n = 4$), although ages ranged from 30- to 49-years-old. Most partners were married ($n = 7$), and all noted they were still with the mother ($N = 8$). The partners' highest level of educational attainment varied, but the majority had either a master's degree qualification (n = 4), or an undergraduate degree ($n = 3$), with only one partner noting no qualifications. All partners were in full-time work (N = 8). In terms of the episode of PP experienced, most involved the admission of the mother to either a psychiatric ward or a MBU ($n = 5$). The onset of each episode was typically within the first 2 weeks of childbirth ($n = 7$), with partners reporting the duration of the episode varying between 1 and 3 months to over 1 year.

Data collection

All of the interviews were completed by the first author (NH) between April and June 2015. Partners were interviewed in their homes ($n = 1$), via SKYPE ($n = 3$), or on the telephone ($n = 4$), based on the participant's preference. Only one of the eight partners interviewed opted for a face-to-face interview, with most noting that it was easier, and felt more private, for them to complete an interview via a video link or on the telephone. A semi-structured interview design was adopted (Additional file 1). At the start of each interview, the partner was invited to describe their experiences of PP. The subsequent interview schedule was led by the participant, but covered topics relating to partner relationships with the mother and infant, role, decision regarding future pregnancies, and coping and support.

All interviews were audio recorded and subsequently transcribed with all potential identifiers removed. Audio recordings of completed interviews were destroyed once transcription was completed. All data associated with the interviews was stored using awarded pseudonyms.

Data analysis

All interviews were transcribed by NH to help full immersion in the data. A step-by-step procedure for completing IPA outlined by Smith et al. [21] on the lined, numbered interview transcripts was followed (see Table 1).

Respecting the ethos of IPA, analysis of the interview data focused on developing an understanding of the meaning that each partner made of their experience of PP. Both Yardley's [25] and Elliott, Fischer, and Rennie's [26] criteria for assessing quality in qualitative research were considered throughout to ensure IPA was completed to a high standard. Yardley's criteria included exploring: sensitivity to the context, commitment and rigour, transparency and coherence, and the impact and

Table 1 Smith et al.'s [21] stages of IPA

Stage	Description of Stage
1	Reading a transcript
2	Initial notation of a transcript
3	Development of emergent subordinate themes
4	Connections across emergent subordinate themes
5	Moving to the next transcript and repeating stages 1–4
6	Looking across transcripts
7	Testing coherence and plausibility of theme structure
8	Developing a narrative of results and a personal reflection

importance of the research. Similarly Elliott et al.'s criteria involved: considering one's own perspective, situating the sample, providing credibility checks, establishing coherence, accomplishing general and specific research tasks, and ensuring the research resonates with readers. Due to the subjective nature of interpretation, the researcher held an awareness of the different hermeneutic levels involved. The researcher kept a reflexive diary of their experiences at each stage of the research, and any personal or prior experiences that they felt were relevant to reflect upon and bracket during the research process. During the analysis stage the researcher separately noted and bracketed any personal thoughts in order to concentrate on the partner's own interpretation. After all transcripts had been separately analysed, similarities or differences in themes communicated across partners were identified. The researcher formed an overarching summary depicting a list of superordinate themes across partners. To test coherence and plausibility of the emergent theme structure, the researcher arranged separate meetings with the other research team members, and the charity APP, to discuss the identified themes.

Results

Seven superordinate themes and 20 subordinate themes were identified across the eight interview transcripts depicting partners' experiences of PP (see Table 2):

Loss

Loss was strongly communicated by partners: from a loss of what was expected in having a child to loss of the couple relationship; physical loss or separation due to hospital admissions; and a feeling that life stops.

> You would think that the first time after having a baby you go round obviously showing her off to everybody, and we couldn't do that purely because [the mother] wasn't there. *(James)*

Table 2 Theme structure

Superordinate Themes	Subordinate Themes
Loss	Expectation and Loss
	Loss within Couple Relationship
	Trauma
	Life Stops
Powerlessness	Control and Exclusion
	Overwhelming Uncertainty and Unexpectedness
United vs. Individual Coping	Coping Strategies
	Questioning Own Limits
	Couple Unity
	Support and Recovery
Hypothesising and Hindsight	Theorising and Meaning Making
	Guilt and Regret
Barriers to Accessing Care and Unmet Needs	Unrecognised and Unmet Care Needs
	Lack Continuity in Care
	Partner Unmet Support Needs
	Calls for Change
Managing Multiple Roles	Role Alteration
	Neglecting Own Needs
Positive Changes from Postpartum Psychosis	Positives Noted
	Relationship Changes

> At a lot of times, we would go up to [MBU] in the car and I'd go "who is she"[the mother], and I suppose those were the most difficult times. (Mark)

> Essentially, I had gained a child on one day and lost my partner on the next day. (Henry)

> ...during it all there was no husband and wife relationship, which we had been having you know a week or so before [infant] was born. (Peter)

Partners used quite visceral language to refer to their experience of loss, which emphasised the physical and emotional pain felt due to being separated from the mother and infant.

> You can't get a cuddle, that sort of closeness is ripped apart...I felt I had lost not only my wife but my little one, he was in the MBU. (Ben)

A subordinate theme of trauma emerged due to the perceived threatened loss of the mother through PP. Partners described PP as a traumatic experience, stressing their feelings of loss for both the mother and infant. The grief and sense of abandonment experienced by partners is manifest by the frequent use of the word 'lost' across the interviews.

> I didn't recognise her at all... it just wasn't her, but it was almost like she was kind of possessed. I was just terrified really that she... that I had lost her really. (David)

> There were times there where we felt, I felt, that we had lost all of our family, that I wasn't going to have [the mother]. (Ben)

Powerlessness

Partners noted a sense of powerlessness, encompassing a general lack of control and uncertainty stemming from the birth and ongoing throughout the mother's PP episode. There was a sense of partners not knowing what was wrong, or how to help the mother, or whether the mother would get better.

> But I had no control on the situation, no input into it. I was just holding the sick bowl. (Henry)

> I didn't quite know what was going to happen next really. I think even with my mum and dad, because we just didn't know what was going on. We didn't know how to treat it. (Ben)

The language that partners used to describe their experiences highlighted their feelings of being overwhelmed, excluded, and the perceived gravity and enormity of their experience.

> I don't think I could have coped much longer... I honestly don't think I could have survived much longer [without MBU]. (Ben)

> Well it was pretty terrifying really. (David)

Most partners described the unexpected and sudden onset of PP, with the mother having had positive pregnancy experiences up until that point. The language used by partners stressed the severity and swift escalation of PP.

> ...very rapidly. I mean, thinking back at it, it happened within an hour, or hour and half, of [son] being born. (Stuart)

> So, it was all a bit... exploding all of a sudden. (John)

Partners also emphasised their sense of exclusion and not being heard by healthcare professionals, further contributing to their feelings of powerlessness....as a

> partner, I wasn't allowed to know what was happening...(Henry)

United vs. individual coping

Different coping styles were adopted; some partners clearly communicated a unified approach to coping as a couple, whereas for others, coping occurred as a separate and dividing process between the partner and the mother.

> ...we thought something was wrong but we didn't know what. (John)

> [To the mother] "Look, you have to snap out of things, and if you don't I'm out of here because I can't cope with this". (Henry)

A variety of individualised coping strategies were identified by partners. Some partners focused on practicalities (such as care routines), or pursuing normality, or taking an approach of planning one day at a time. Others had to learn to talk about their emotions, to speak as a couple; and some found dry humour to be helpful. Some partners reported needing their own space (so took the dog for a walk), or found it useful to vent to friends. For others, partners needed to seek out other people who had experienced PP, or search for information on PP. Utilising familiar work-stress management strategies were adopted by some, as was attributing blame (for example, believing that the mother's birth plan choices resulted in the episode). All partners questioned their ability to cope and sought support, even if that was anonymised support through an online forum. Partners noted it was 'impossible' (David) to comprehend how they would have coped without familial support.

> The thought of being a father was going to be tough and then you have that on top of it. Your world comes crashing down all around you. Looking back now you kind of think I don't know how I got through that. (Mark)

Coping often involved partners having to become a 'specialist' (Mark) in PP in order to understand what was happening to the mother, and answer questions that healthcare professionals had failed to address. The word 'specialist' demonstrated the need to self-educate about the nature and development of PP, to become expert in order for partners to better cope and understand the experience. Furthermore, it implied a lack of communication and information from healthcare professionals, which motivated partners to commence a process of information seeking and assimilation, in order to generate answers to partners' outstanding queries regarding PP. Partners often referred to needing to research PP but the language that Mark used captured the extent to which partners can adopt information gathering as a means to better cope with their experience.

> I'm now a specialist in postpartum psychosis medication involved, because I am one of those people who will research in terms of Google and APP networks and what not. I guess that had been my idea of finding out what is actually going on. (Mark)

Issues that partners highlighted encountering when trying to cope included: having to compromise their values; having no opportunity to vent their emotions and to prioritise the mother's needs; and continuing to question the mother's behaviour (including her humour or signs of energy) after recovery for fear the mother was becoming unwell again.

> She had to stop breastfeeding which she didn't want to do... (Ben)

> ...I analyse our conversations more than I should really. (James)

Partners although praising the support provided by families, also reported the difficulties in setting boundaries for extended family involvement in providing care.

> I think it strained... because the in-laws came and lived over at the house for a bit and helped out quite a bit. Which was good but hard to tell them to back off. (John)

Partners noted that generally they were not offered any support from healthcare professionals, and when it was offered struggled to understand the nature of the support and failed to believe any reassurances given.

> I didn't know what sort of support I needed. In fact I would say they didn't help... I was completely lost as to what a social worker does and what benefit it was to me. (Henry)

> ...I thought she [nurse] was trying to comfort me rather than it actually being true...it was pretty hard, impossible to believe really at the time. (David)

Hypothesising and hindsight

Partners typically developed a specific theory about what they felt may have triggered the mother's episode of PP. These hypothesised triggers differed across partners and included postnatal difficulties such as poor sleep, exhaustion, pressures or problems breastfeeding, and pressures relating to feeling unable to following a child rearing book. Other hypothesised triggers related to the birthing experience, such as, experiencing a difficult labour, unexpected changes to the birth plan, and or developing a sense of loss of control during the birthing process. Physiological changes due to labour were also considered by partners to be potential triggers, such as hormonal changes and anaemia.

Finally, delays in appropriate treatment were considered as significant in the further development of symptoms, for example, delayed access to appropriate perinatal mental health services and mothers being prescribed antidepressant medication which appeared to worsen symptoms. The benefit of reflection was remarked upon, especially as a couple, in making sense of their experiences. James reflected upon their infant as 'this little person,' highlighting the sense of reality, responsibility and vulnerability faced by partners in trying to adequately meet their infants' care needs in the context of also trying to care for the mother.

> ...we feel that the sleeplessness was very much a big thing... we have actually got this little person to look after.... *(James)*

Partners also communicated feelings of guilt and regret, often commenting on things they felt they 'should have' done.

> ...there is a huge amount of guilt I felt that I had pushed her into going out and things like that... because I'd been told to. But actually that didn't help her at all and I felt masses amount of guilt. (Ben)

> I suppose just feeling negative... that I let [the mother] down, when I should have been...[partner paused]. (Stuart)

> ...I probably felt if anything guilty that I wasn't there in the Unit. (David)

A final regret reported by partners was that of not being provided with information to make an informed decision as to whether to have a second child, and thus opting not to.

> ...it would have changed my mind, having read other stories, evidence and stuff, I think we would have been in a better position to do that [decision to not have a second child]. (Ben)

Barriers to accessing care and unmet needs

Partners identified barriers to accessing care for the mother. These included healthcare professionals failing to accurately identify what was wrong with the mother due to poor understanding, the lack of empathy from primary care services, and the lack of consistency in care and communication between healthcare professionals.

> ...[GP] just told [the mother] to go and have a bath, try and chill out for a bit, and take some natural sleeping remedies and you'll be fine...that's another day or two down the line and we tried that and she just got worse and worse and worse. (James)

> ...people in the healthcare profession, they could have helped more, and got to get us support sooner, that is at the centre of everything. (Stuart)

> ...the locum at the end was "you'll have to try harder than that to kill yourself", and I could have disappeared I was so angry. (Ben)

Partners described not being heard, either individually or as a couple, by healthcare professionals, and if they were listened to then it was only after the mother had reached crisis point. For most partners, no enquiry was made by healthcare professionals to the partner's own needs and no support offered.

> ...when the medical teams would be coming around and I would be talking to them, and thinking back, ignoring every single word I said...From the typical bloke perspective it was just kind of assumed by everyone that everything would be okay. There was never much discussion, even from family, but certainly not from any of the medical services, as to how I was, what concerns did I have. I was very much left to feel that you have got to cope... [this interview] ...is probably the first time I actually had the opportunity to express it because going right back to day one no one ever really asks. (Peter)

Partners advocated that some changes need to happen, for instance: increasing the number of local MBUs, having noted them to be a 'lifesaver' (Mark); raising awareness of PP among primary care staff; educating partners about PP and increasing the support offered to them; and helping couples to be aware of PP and feel prepared for it, as this had helped some partners following later pregnancies.

> The whole MBU staff was fantastic because they know it, and I think, at that point that was the first thing I'd heard of postpartum psychosis. (Ben)

> ...those places [MBU] are a lifesaver, because if you are not in that specialism no one else can really understand. (Mark)

Managing multiple roles

Partners commented on the conflict between their many new roles and meeting the care needs of their family, particularly in the context of trying to maintain a job. In order to manage, partners would typically prioritise the mother's, or infant's, needs above their own, and would often then have to prioritise whether to care for the mother or their infant.

> ...I still had to work, there was no one who could cover my job, and look after a newborn, not getting much sleep, my wife is potentially on suicide watch, and being watched 24/7...There wasn't really time to stop and think how am I feeling because there was no choice but to deal with everything. (Peter)

> ...I felt I struggled to sleep, because I wanted to make sure that she was sleeping and that put me on edge and I felt very agitated myself. (James)

Partners noted a shift in their couple relationship. David's quote signified a shift in the partner's role within the couple relationship, from one of mutual supporter to that of protector and carer. The perceived vulnerability of the mothers by partners altered the relationship dynamic, and for some resulted in adopting a modified, non-egalitarian and paternalistic communication style.

> ...it was almost like speaking to a child I guess in a way... (David)

Positive changes from postpartum psychosis

The majority of partners detailed a number of personal positive changes that had occurred due to PP, including increasing partners' own empathy and understanding towards mental health issues in general.

> ...it gave us an empathy, not even with PP... people going through depression... I was probably being a bloke's bloke beforehand in terms of thinking about people with depression. "Just snap out of it" type, sort of thing. (Ben)

> I think I am far more aware of how [the mother], or how I perceive [the mother] to be feeling, so even without her saying anything I will find myself second-guessing how I think she is feeling... (Peter)

Furthermore, there was recognition for MBUs assistance in establishing a care routine for their infant.

> ...If there was any silver lining to be had out of this whole story, it was that the Mother and Baby Unit taught you how to look after a little one. (Ben)

Positive changes to the couple relationship were also noted by some partners. Following the episode of PP, some couple relationships had reportedly strengthened and became more supportive. Moreover, partners had experienced more time to bond with their infant, and had concentrated on redressing their work-life priorities.

> I've always said that it has got better. It's got stronger, that sounds really odd... I always say that we are actually stronger for it. These things make you feel stronger, I guess...My focus used to be very different. I used to be quite career driven... whereas now I'm like it's just get through the day, get home. I use to work 90% of this time. Whereas now I'm out the door at one minute past five. (Mark)

> ...we are both very supportive of each other in life... when one seems exhausted and drained then we give each other a break, but then we kind of more sympathetic than before. (David)

Discussion

The aim of the study was to develop an understanding of the lived experiences of partners of woman with Postpartum Psychosis (PP). Seven themes were identified: loss; powerlessness; united vs. individual coping; hypothesising and hindsight; barriers to accessing care and unmet needs; managing multiple roles; and positive changes arising from PP.

Several of the themes were comparable to those found in perinatal mental health research. The sense of loss communicated across many dimensions including loss of the expected future echoed the findings with mothers who had experienced PP [1] and reflects the work on expectation-loss theory of what might, or what could, have been [27]. Themes identified in studies exploring partners' experience of PND [22, 23] also centred on loss including loss of control, intimacy, expectation and routine, alongside feelings of helplessness in caring for their family and the "fracturing" ([22], p717) of the family unit.

The powerful individual narratives and the themes that have emerged underline the impact of PP on the partners and further evidence the need for implementation of the NICE recommendations for mental health providers to consider the needs of the partner and the effect of PP on the couple relationship [12]. Women who have experienced PP recognise that their partners need access to psychological support [1]. However, partners in this study neglected their own needs (similar to previous findings [16]), so without the healthcare professionals being alert to this it will be difficult to reduce the known risk to partners mental health when a woman has postnatal mental health problems [28–30]. This is an important consideration for the well-being of all members of the family unit including the infant; the partners in this study took on a greater caregiving role for the infant than they had planned and research suggests that partners take on a buffering role in the development of attachment in their infant, in the context of postnatal mental health problems [31, 32]. Interestingly the positive changes described by some partners as a result of PP often related to this shift in role, having more time to bond with their infant and changing priorities away from work to prioritising time with their family.

Partners described a range of coping strategies. Alongside well recognised strategies previously identified in this context [28] such of seeking normality, and trying to source information, there were other strategies which required couples to compromise on their values in order to cope, for example, making the decision for the mother not to breastfeed in order to receive medication. This type of compromise appears common when there are postnatal mental health problems; unfulfilled dreams or wishes was a theme extracted from narratives of women who had experienced PP [33]. In order to try and make sense of their experience many partners developed their own theory about the trigger for the PP. Some included those postulated within the existing research literature, for example, sleep loss, or antidepressant medication resulting in mania [9, 34] but others were quite specific and particular to their family circumstances.

The benefit of familial support was clearly communicated by partners, noting that it would have been 'impossible' to comprehend coping without such support, echoing the views of women who experienced PP [1]. However, some partners identified the need to establish boundaries around familial support, and at times felt the need for families to step back. This has not previously been noted within the research literature, but may link to the sense of powerlessness that partners report during the episode of PP, and their need to feel in some way in control of the situation.

Significant expectation was placed on partners, by both family members and healthcare professionals, to provide support. However, they felt that their concerns were unheard and they were largely excluded from the mother's care and treatment which exacerbated the sense of powerlessness and uncertainty. The lack of clear consistent communication from the healthcare professionals had several consequences. The importance of reassurance by healthcare professionals has previously been identified from research with mothers [35] but the partners in this study reported that they struggled to believe any of the reassurances, due to previous inaccurate information about the mother's condition. Similarly they found it difficult to trust the recovery process as they continued 'second guessing' whether the mother would become unwell again, misinterpreting humour, or energy, as a sign of mania or psychosis returning. This finding has not previously been identified within the PP research literature, but links with the change in the relationship dynamic and a potential shift in the partner's frame of reference by which they interpret and understand the mother's actions which may endure after the mother is considered recovered.

Partners identified a number of barriers to care and unmet needs, many of which indicated a failure of services to adhere to the gold standard described in the NICE guidelines [12], and reflected the lack of access in the UK to perinatal mental healthcare services [11]. The requirement for improvements in perinatal mental health service provision was recognised in the Chief Medical Officer's annual report in England, and the Together for Mental Health Delivery Plan 2016–2019 in Wales [36, 37] so services may have improved in response. However, based on these findings, the implications for practice broadly fall into three domains: types of service provision, improved knowledge and communication both between healthcare professionals and between the professionals and family. Those who had access to an MBU clearly valued the service so broader availability of this type of service is a priority. There needs to be improvements in knowledge about PP and its management in primary and secondary care in order to improve the quality and accuracy of communication. Continuity of care would be improved by an assigned care co-ordinator acting as a point of reference for partners and other healthcare professionals. Partners play such a significant role in PP that any education package for healthcare professionals must underline the need to involve them, listen to them but also to be alert to their mental health needs as well. Campaigns targeted at parents-to-be to inform them of signs of perinatal mental health difficulties and how to seek help could also help to raise awareness in the population.

There is a growing literature on partners' experiences in the context of perinatal mental health but this exploration of partners' own experiences of PP is largely unique at this time. The qualitative design of the current study is a strength as it attempts to maintain the voice and personal experiences of partners. It has led to findings which fit with the existing research in areas such as PND but also advances our understanding of the experience of PP and therefore offers information to inform improvements in practice.

One potential limitation with regards to data analysis is that all initial coding was completed one researcher, however, criteria for assessing quality in qualitative research was considered throughout to try to ensure that IPA was completed to a high standard. The approach to sampling was appropriate to the method but as the partners were all recruited through a charity other potential participants would have been missed and it might also be the case that allowing for an upper time-frame of 10 years could have had an impact on recall. The fact that all couples were still together could potentially have biased the reporting of changes in the couple relationship as it is known that there are high rates of separation and divorce following postnatal mental health problems [38]. Some of the themes extracted that relate to partner experiences could be argued to represent the experiences of new fathers, without the context of PP; qualitative research with first time fathers [39] suggests there is some overlap, for example, in the theme of helplessness mirroring to some degree the theme of powerlessness, but many of the other themes appear to denote more about the practical demands placed on new fathers, such as the theme of trial and error parenting.

Conclusions

We believe the current study will help develop a more thorough understanding of PP and the impact that it can have on partners and the couple relationship. In order to support partners, services need to be aware of and responsive to their experiences which may include loss and trauma, emotional responses (such as feelings of guilt, regret and self-blame), the multiple roles they are managing, and the impact on the couple relationship. The study has also helped to identify current barriers to care and unmet needs, from a lack of awareness of PP and delays in accessing appropriate treatment, to a lack of support for, or consideration of, partners. Overall, the impact of PP on partners is broad and substantial and requires consideration by healthcare professionals in order to secure the best clinical outcomes for all members of the new family unit.

Abbreviations

APP: Action on Postpartum Psychosis; IPA: Interpretative Phenomenological Analysis; MBU: Mother and Baby Unit; PND: Postnatal Depression; PP: Postpartum Psychosis

Acknowledgements

We wish to thank the partners who openly shared their experiences in this study, and Action for Postpartum Psychosis for their assistance in the development of the research, the recruitment process and providing feedback on the results. This work was completed as part of work presented for a Doctorate thesis by NH.

Funding

No funding has been provided to complete this research.

Authors' contributions

NH lead the study design, conducted all the interviews and lead the data analysis. NH also took the lead in drafting the article for publication. SC contributed to the study design and data analysis. IJ and JH contributed to the study design and data analysis. All authors read and approved the final manuscript.

Ethics approval and consent to participate

The study was given ethical approval from Cardiff University. Two written consent forms were provided to participants along with information sheets. The first consent form was completed prior to brief online questionnaire collecting largely sociodeomographic information. A further consent form was completed immediately prior to an interview about their experiences of PP. All information gathered as part of the study was obtained with the participant's consent and agreement for that information to be used anonymously when writing up the research for publication.

Consent for publication

Not applicable.

Competing interests

The authors declare that they have no competing interests.

Author details

[1]South Wales Clinical Psychology Doctorate Programme, Cardiff University, Cardiff, UK. [2]Centre for Trials Research, Cardiff University, Cardiff, UK. [3]Action on Postpartum Psychosis, Department of Psychiatry, The Barberry National Centre for Mental Health, University of Birmingham, Birmingham, UK. [4]National Centre for Mental Health, Division of Psychological Medicine and Clinical Neurosciences, MRC Centre for Neuropsychiatric Genetics and Genomics, Cardiff University, Cardiff, UK.

References

1. Heron J, Gilbert N, Dolman C, Shah S, Beare I, Dearden S, et al. Information and support needs during recovery from postpartum psychosis. Arch Womens Ment Health. 2012;15:155–65.
2. Jones I, Chandra PS, Dazzan P, Howard LM. Bipolar disorder, affective psychosis, and schizophrenia in pregnancy and the post-partum period. Lancet. 2014;384(9956):1789–99.
3. Mishra S, Kar S, Reddy P, Swain S. Postpartum Psychosis: Review. The Orissa. J Psychiatry. 2011;2:5–9.
4. Appleby L, Mortensen PB, Faragher EB. Suicide and other causes of mortality after post-partum psychiatric admission. Br J Psychiatry. 1998;173: 209–11.
5. Heron J, McGuinness M, Robertson Blackmore E, Craddock N, Jones I. Early postpartum symptoms in puerperal psychosis. Br J Obstet Gynaecol. 2008; 115:348–53.

6. Di Florio A, Jones L, Forty L, Gordon-Smith K, Robertson Blackmore E, Heron J, et al. Mood disorders and parity – a clue to the aetiology of the postpartum trigger. J Affect Disord. 2014;152:334–9.
7. Jones I, Craddock N. Familiarity of the puerperal trigger in bipolar disorder: results of a family study. Am J Psychiatr. 2001;158:913–7.
8. Jones I, Craddock N. Bipolar disorder and childbirth: the importance of recognising risk. Br J Psychiatry. 2005;186:453–4.
9. Lawson A, Murphy K, Sloan E, Uleryk E, Dalfen A. The relationship between sleep and postpartum mental disorders: a systematic review. J Affect Disord. 2015;176:65–77.
10. Stewart DE, Klompenhouwer JL, Kendall RE, Van Hulst AM. Prophylactic lithium in puerperal psychosis: the experience of three centres. Br J Psychiatry. 1991;158:393–7.
11. Baucer A, Parsonage M, Knapp M, Lemmi V, Adelaja B. The costs of perinatal mental health problems: London School of Economics; 2014. http://eprints.lse.ac.uk/59885/1/__lse.ac.uk_storage_LIBRARY_Secondary_libfile_shared_repository_Content_Bauer%2C%20M_Bauer_Costs_perinatal_%20mental_2014_Bauer_Costs_perinatal_mental_2014_author.pdf Accessed 11 May 2017
12. National Institute for Health and Care Excellence. Antenatal and postnatal mental health: clinical management and service guidance. NICE 2014. www.nice.org.uk/guidance/cg192 Accessed 2 Jan 2016.
13. Ainsworth M. The development of infant-mother attachment. In: Cardwell B, Ricciuti H, editors. Review of child development research. Chicago: University of Chicago Press; 1973. p. 1–94.
14. Bowlby J. Attachment and loss. Vol. 1: Attachment. New York: Basic Books; 1969.
15. Bowlby J. Attachment and loss, Vol.2: separation. New York: Basic Books; 1973.
16. Doucet S, Letourneau N, Robertson Blackmore E. Support needs of mothers who experience postpartum psychosis and their partners. J Obstet Gynecol Neonatal Nurs. 2012;41:236–45.
17. Action on Post-partum Psychosis. Postpartum psychosis: A guide for partners. https://www.app-network.org/wp-content/uploads/2011/10/2018-Insider-Guide_Partners.pdf. Accessed 3rd October 2018.
18. Engqvist I, Nilsson K. The recovery process of postpartum psychosis from both the women's and next of kin's perspective – an interview study in Sweden. Open Nurs J. 2014;8:8–16.
19. Wyatt C, Murray C, Davies J, Jomeen J. Postpartum psychosis and relationships: their mutual influence from the perspective of women and significant others. J Reprod Infant Psychol. 2015;33(4):426–42. https://doi.org/10.1080/02646838.2015.1027181.
20. Boddy R, Gordon C, MacCallum F, McGuinness M. Men's experiences of having a partner who requires mother and baby unit admission for first episode postpartum psychosis. J Adv Nurs. 2017;73(2):399–409.
21. Reid KM, Taylor MG. Social support, stress, and maternal postpartum depression: a comparison of supportive relationships. Soc Sci Res. 2015;54: 246–62.
22. Beestin L, Hugh-Jones S, Gough B. The impact of maternal postnatal depression on men and their ways of fathering: an interpretative phenomenological analysis. Psychol Health. 2014;29:717–35.
23. Meighan M, Davis M, Thomas S. Living with postpartum depression: the father's experience. Am J Matern Child Nurs. 1999;24(4):202–8.
24. Smith JA, Flowers P, Larkin M. Interpretative phenomenological analysis: theory, method, and research. London: SAGE Publications; 2009.
25. Yardley L. Dilemmas in qualitative health research. Psychol Health. 2000;15: 215–28.
26. Elliott R, Fischer CT, Rennie DL. Evolving guidelines for publication of qualitative researcher studies in psychology and related fields. Br J Clin Psychol. 1999;38:215–29.
27. Luterman D. Counseling persons with communication disorders and their families. 5th ed. Austin: ProEd; 2008.
28. Marrs J, Cossar J, Wroblewska A. Keeping the family together and bonding: a father's role in a perinatal mental health unit. J Reprod Infant Psychol. 2014;32(4):340–54.
29. Blackmore E, Rubinow D, O'Connor T, Liu X, Tang W, Craddock N, et al. Reproductive outcomes and risk of subsequent illness in women diagnosed with postpartum psychosis. Bipolar Disord. 2013;15:394–404.
30. Lovestone S, Kumar R. Postnatal psychiatric illness: the impact on partners. Br J Psychiatry. 1993;163:201–16.
31. Albertsson-Karlgren U, Graff M, Nettelbladt P. Mental disease postpartum and parent-infant interaction – evaluation of videotaped sessions. Child Abuse Rev. 2001;10:5–17.
32. Edhborg M, Lundh W, Seimyr L, Widstrom A. The parent-child relationship in the context of maternal depressive mood. Arch Womens Ment Health. 2003;6:211–6.
33. Engqvist I, Ferszt G, Ahlin A, Nilsson K. Psychiatric nurses' descriptions of women with postpartum psychosis and nurses' responses – an exploratory study in Sweden. Issues Ment Health Nurs. 2012;30:23–30.
34. Burt VK, Rasgon N. Special considerations in treating bipolar disorder in women. Bipolar Disord. 2004;6:2–13.
35. McGrath L, Peters S, Wieck A, Wittkowski A. The process of recovery in women who experienced psychosis following childbirth. BioMed Central Psychiatry. 2013;13:341.
36. Department of Health. Annual report of the Chief Medical Officer, 2014, The health of the 51%: women. Department of Health. 2015. www.gov.uk/government/uploads/system/uploads/attachment_data/file/484383/cmo-report-2014.pdf Accessed 2 Jan 2016.
37. Welsh Government Consultation Document. Together for Mental Health Delivery Plan: 2016-2017 (Number: WG27588). Welsh Government 2016. https://gov.wales/topics/health/nhswales/plans/mental-health/?lang=en. Accessed 2 Jan 2016.
38. Milgrom J, McCloud P. Parenting stress and postnatal depression. Stress Med. 1996;12:177–86.
39. Kowlessar O, Fox JR, Wittkowki A. First-time fathers' experiences of parenting during the first year. J Reprod Infant Psychol. 2015;33:4–14.

13

Multilevel analysis of factors associated with assistance during delivery in rural Nigeria: implications for reducing rural-urban inequity in skilled care at delivery

Bola Lukman Solanke* and Semiu Adebayo Rahman

Abstract

Background: Studies have observed rural-urban inequity in the use of skilled delivery in Nigeria. A number of studies have explicitly examined associated factors of assistance during delivery in rural areas. However, the studies so far conducted in rural Nigeria have investigated mainly individual-level characteristics with near exclusion of community-level characteristics. Also, most of the studies that have investigated community-level influence on use of maternal healthcare services in Nigeria did not isolate rural areas for specific research attention. The objective of this study was to investigate the individual-level and community-level characteristics associated with assistance during delivery in rural Nigeria.

Methods: The study analysed women data of 2013 Nigeria Demographic and Health Survey. A weighted sample size of 12,665 rural women was analysed. The outcome variable was assistance during delivery, dichotomised into 'skilled assistance' and 'unskilled assistance'. The explanatory variables are selected individual-level characteristics (maternal education, parity, age at first birth, religion, healthcare decision, employment status, access to mass media, and means of transportation); and selected community-level characteristics (community literacy level, community childcare burden, proportion of women employed outside agriculture, proportion of women who perceived distance to facility as a big problem, community poverty level, and geographical region). The mixed-effects logistic regression was applied.

Results: During the most recent deliveries, 23.0% of rural women utilised skilled assistance compared with 77.0% who utilised unskilled assistance. Maternal education, parity, religion, healthcare decision, access to mass media, and means of transportation were the individual-level characteristics that revealed significant effects on the likelihood of utilising skilled assistance during delivery, while community literacy level, community poverty level, community perception of distance to health facility, and geographic region were the community-level characteristics that revealed significant effects on the odds of using skilled assistance during delivery. Results of Intra-Class Correlation (ICC) supported significant community-level effects on the likelihood of using skilled assistance during delivery.

Conclusions: Assistance during delivery is influenced by individual-level and community-level characteristics. Health policies and programmes seeking to reduce rural-urban inequity in skilled delivery should endeavour to identify and address important factors at both the individual and community levels of the social environment.

Keywords: Skilled assistance, Individual-level, Community-level, Delivery, Rural women, Nigeria

* Correspondence: modebolasolanke@gmail.com; bsolanke@oauife.edu.ng
Department of Demography and Social Statistics, Faculty of Social Sciences, Obafemi Awolowo University, Ile-Ife, Nigeria

Background

Rural areas in Nigeria have 51% population compared with 49% urban population [1], the rural areas also have higher incidences of pregnancies, child deliveries, and preventable maternal and child morbidities and mortality compared with the urban areas [2]. This makes the provision of maternal healthcare services across the continuum of maternal health care more compelling in the rural areas. However, evidence abounds that infrastructure for healthcare delivery particularly infrastructure for skilled care at delivery is markedly different between rural and urban areas, with the rural areas suffering infrastructural neglect in the country [3]. The existing rural health facilities in Nigeria are often bereft of adequate equipment, competent health personnel, and are largely inaccessible due to distance and poor road networks [2]. This situation which also exists in several sub-Saharan Africa countries often culminates not only in disparity in where rural and urban women deliver their babies [4], but also in disparity in the competency of persons providing assistance during delivery [5–7].

Assistance during delivery refers to the person attending child delivery. The person may be a 'skilled attendant' such as a doctor, nurse and midwife or an 'unskilled attendant' such as a traditional birth attendant, community extension worker, and friend/relative. The skills and competency of the person attending child delivery determine to a large extent whether complications during delivery are promptly identified and well-managed, as well as ensuring that hygienic practices are upheld during delivery [2]. While percentage of birth delivered by a skilled attendant in the urban areas of Nigeria increased from 65.4% in 2008 to 67.0% in 2013, the proportion in the rural areas of Nigeria, declined from 27.7% in 2008 to 22.7% in 2013 [8, 9]. This not only depict inequity in skilled care at delivery within Nigeria, it may continue to adversely affect birth outcome [10], exert negative impact on use of skilled delivery services by rural women [11], and may be a contributory factor to current poor maternal and newborn health in the country [2]. In addition, the situation of skilled delivery in Nigeria is a far cry from global expectation that all pregnant women irrespective of location be assisted by skilled attendants during delivery [12].

Health interventions in Nigeria such as the Midwives Service Scheme (MSS), which was established to improve human resources for health often, fail to reduce rural-urban disparity in skilled care at delivery due to challenges such as difficulty in retaining health personnel for rural health practice [13, 14]. The situation is aggravated by the unwillingness of many students undergoing medical training to take up future appointments in the rural and remote areas of the country [15]. Though, the World Health Organization (WHO) has made useful suggestions for recruiting and retaining rural health workforce [16], but achieving current and future human resource needs for sexual and reproductive health including maternal and child health in sub-Saharan Africa countries remains a huge challenge [17]. Thus, amid rural neglect and poor health delivery system, understanding the wide spectrum of factors affecting assistance during delivery remains relevant in reproductive health research in Nigeria.

Numerous studies across the world have confirmed that use of maternal healthcare services including assistance during delivery is mainly affected by a mixture of individual characteristics such as gender inequality [18, 19], maternal education [20], socio-economic inequality [21], spousal violence [22, 23], birth order and pregnancy wantedness [24], and community characteristics such as type of residence [25, 26], prevalence of larger family size [27], community education, community perception of distance to health facility, and community media saturation [28, 29]. Though, a number of studies have explicitly examined associated factors of assistance during delivery in rural areas [30–36], the studies so far conducted in rural Nigeria have investigated mainly individual-level characteristics with near exclusion of the community-level characteristics associated with assistance during delivery in rural areas [37–41]. Also, most of the studies that have investigated community-level influence on use of maternal healthcare services in Nigeria [28, 42–44] did not isolate rural areas for specific research attention.

This may undermine understanding the role of community-level characteristics (the characteristics of the social groups' individual belong) in influencing utilisation of skilled care at delivery, and how community-level characteristics may contribute to developing effective community-based responses that could address existing inequity in utilisation of skilled care at delivery in the country. Community-level characteristics represent a unique social context that not only affect how individuals perceived and respond to health or other issues in the social environment, but also exert independent effects on the health outcomes of individuals in the community. Such independent effects made it possible for two women with identical socio-demographic and health characteristics to have different likelihood of using or not using skilled care at delivery. Thus, community-level characteristics may affect assistance during delivery by moderating how individuals in the community perceive the relevance and quality of assistance during child delivery. Increasing numbers of studies have provided research evidence that such social context is crucial for improving health behaviour [45–49].

The objective of the study was therefore, to examine the individual-level and community-level characteristics associated with assistance during delivery in rural Nigeria. This was with the view to providing additional policy-relevant information for addressing current rural-urban inequity in skilled care at delivery, and promoting equity in utilisation of skilled care at delivery in the country. The study was guided by the research question: to what extent are individual-level and community-level characteristics associated with assistance during delivery in rural Nigeria? The socio-ecological theory of health behaviour provides the theoretical underpinning of the study. The theory asserts that human health behaviour such as the use of maternal healthcare service is influenced at multiple levels within the social and physical environment such as the individual, household, community, societal and policy environment levels [50].

Methods

Study context

The study location is Nigeria, the most populous country in Africa [1]. Nigeria has a weak health delivery system that contributes to adverse maternal and child health outcomes [10, 51]. Also, the health delivery system in the country is inadequately funded [52]. Average national indices of maternal and child health, particularly utilisation of crucial maternal healthcare services such as skilled care delivery in the country is among the poorest in sub-Saharan Africa [2]. In the 5 years preceding the 2013 Nigeria Demographic and Health Survey (NDHS), among women who had a live birth, 61% received antenatal care from a skilled health provider; a lower proportion (51%) reported the recommended four or more antenatal care visits; 36% had facility-delivery, and 38% of deliveries were attended by a skilled health provider [9]. These show that utilisation of maternal healthcare services in the country need improvement. The Integrated Maternal, Newborn and Child Health (IMNCH) Strategy currently being implemented in the country seeks to boost utilisation of essential maternal care services across the continuum of maternal healthcare [2]. For instance, some of the IMNCH priority actions include increasing the coverage and quality of the Focused Antenatal Care; increasing demand for facility-based deliveries with skilled birth attendance; and ensuring that all mothers and newborns receive prompt postnatal check within 2 days. Nevertheless, the coverage of the IMNCH interventions is still very low particularly in rural and remote areas of the country [53]. The Federal Government has also made efforts to boost the funding of maternal and child health delivery in the country through The Subsidy Reinvestment and Empowerment Programme [51]. The programme has however recorded only marginal improvement in the situation of maternal, newborn and child health in the country, as drop out from the continuum of maternity care remain high in the country [54] with substantial rural-urban differentials in the use of maternal healthcare services [55].

Some health practitioners have commenced advocacy for free maternal and child health in the country to further boost utilisation of maternal healthcare services [56]. Some other health professionals have also advocated for the implementation of Conditional Cash Transfer (CCT) Scheme in the country, as another means of encouraging maternal healthcare use, particularly among socially disadvantaged women [57]. In spite of this efforts, negative perception of public health facilities may have continue to hinder improved utilisation among women in the country [58]. The Community-based health insurance programme, another initiative designed to enhance access to healthcare in the country is yet to successfully commence in many communities in the country [59]. These have provided compelling need for further investigation of associated factors of maternal healthcare use in the country.

Data source and sample

This study was based on data collected from women of reproductive age in the 2013 NDHS. The 2013 NDHS is part of the series of cross-sectional Demographic and Health Survey (DHS) conducted across developing countries to provide reliable and internationally comparable information on the current state of fertility, childhood and adult mortality, family planning, and other sexual and reproductive health issues in developing countries. Relevant information about the design and implementation of the survey has been published [9]. In this study, only rural women were analysed. The study however, excluded women who were not currently married, and women who had no live birth in the 5 years preceding the survey. A weighted sample of 12,665 women were analysed in the study. A formal request to analyse the dataset was made to MEASURE DHS (the custodian of the DHS data) through online platform. Authorisation was granted.

Outcome variable

The outcome variable in the study was assistance during delivery. This was a dichotomous variable with 'skilled assistance' and 'unskilled assistance' as categories. Skilled assistance in the study refers to delivery assistance provided by a doctor, nurse, midwife, or auxiliary nurse/midwife. This was based on the classification of skilled and unskilled health provider adopted in the 2013 NDHS [9]. But in some other countries, auxiliary nurse/midwife may not be classified as a skilled health provider [60]. Unskilled assistance in the study refers to delivery assistance provided by community extension worker, traditional birth attendants, friends/relatives, and no one. The category of interest in the study was the skilled assistance category.

Explanatory and control variables

The explanatory variables in the study are individual-level and community-level characteristics. The individual-level characteristics analysed are maternal education, healthcare decision, parity, age at first birth, religion, employment status, access to mass media, and means of transportation. These characteristics were selected for analysis because previous studies have established their associations with utilisation of maternal healthcare services particularly in developing countries [20, 21, 23–26, 61–65]. Some of the variables were re-coded to suit the analytic framework of the study. Healthcare decision was based on whether women were involved in making decision about their own healthcare. Women who solely or jointly with male partner had final say on their healthcare decision were grouped as 'participation', while other women who had no say in the decision were grouped as 'no participation'. Women's access to the mass media was based on the frequency of listening to radio, watching television, or reading newspaper weekly. Women who did not listen to radio, watch television, or read newspaper during the week were grouped as 'no access', while those who listened to radio, watched television, or read newspaper at least once weekly were grouped as 'moderate' access. Women who listened to radio, watched television, or read newspaper more than once weekly were grouped as 'high' access. Women's parity was divided into primiparity (one child ever born), multiparity (two to four children ever born), and grand multiparity (five or more children ever born).

Six community-level characteristics were analysed in the study. These are community childcare burden (proportion of women who had five or more children), community literacy level (proportion of women who cannot read and write at all), community poverty level (proportion of women in the poorest household quintile), proportion of women employed outside agricultural sector, community perception of distance to health facility (proportion of women who perceived distance to health facility as a big problem), and geographic region. The community-level characteristics were derived by aggregating the selected characteristic at the cluster level and then dividing into suitable categories. This was done because the variables are not directly available in the DHS data. Most studies that have analysed community-level variables using DHS data adopted the method [28, 29, 48]. In addition, to the selected individual-level and community-level variables, three variables were selected for statistical control. These are household wealth quintile, number of antenatal care visits, and timing of first antenatal care visits. The selection of these variables was guided by literature [24–27, 66].

Data analysis

Three levels of statistical analyses were employed. The univariate analysis describes assistance during delivery using the pie chart, while respondents' characteristics were presented using frequency distributions and percentages. At the bivariate level of analysis, cross tabulation of the research variables were carried out to show percentage of skilled assistance as changes in the categories of the explanatory variable occurs. This analytic level also describes the relationship between the variables using unadjusted binary logistic regression coefficient to reveal whether the relationships are positive or negative. Before the multivariate analysis was carried out, a Variance Inflation Factor (VIF) was calculated to detect extent of multi-collinearity of the independent variables using the mean VIF score. This was needed to determine the suitability of the selected variables for multivariate analysis. As a rule of thumb in regression analysis, a mean VIF score of less than 5 is tolerated, while a mean VIF score of 5–10 suggests that the regression coefficients might be inadequately estimated [67, 68]. At the multivariate level, the mixed-effects logistic regression was used to determine extent of variation in the use of skilled assistance attributable to individual-level and community-level characteristics. The mixed-effects logistic regression model consists of two parts, namely, the fixed effect and the random effect [43]. The model was specified as:

$$\log\left(\frac{\pi_{ij}}{1-\pi_{ij}}\right) = \beta_0 + \beta_1 x_{ij} + \beta_2 x_{2ij} + \ldots + \beta_8 x_{8ij} + \beta_9 z_{1j} + \beta_{10} z_{2j} + \ldots \beta_{14} z_{6j} + \mu_{0j}$$

Where:

π_{ij} is the log of odds of skilled assistance.

$(1 - \pi_{ij})$ is the log of unskilled assistance.

x and z are the explanatory variables for the likelihood of skilled assistance.

x_1 to x_8 are the individual-level characteristics.

z_1 to z_6 are the community-level characteristics.

$\beta_0$is the overall intercept.

$\beta_1 \ldots \beta_{14}$ are the regression coefficients for the explanatory variables x_1 to x_8, and z_1 to z_6.

u_{0j} is the community-level random effect (assumed to be normally distributed with mean equal to 0 and variance equal to $\sigma_{\mu 0^2}$).

The fixed effects were estimated using odds ratio of adjusted binary logistic regression, while the random effects were estimated using the Intra-Class Correlation (ICC) calculated as: $\frac{\tau}{\tau+\left[\frac{\pi^2}{3}\right]}$ where τ is the estimated community-level variance [43]. The ICC ranges from 0 to 1, with ICC of 1 indicating that women in the community have identical use of skilled assistance during delivery, and with ICC of 0 indicating that women in the community do not have identical use of skilled assistance in the community. Four models were fitted in the study. Model 1 included only individual-level characteristics, while Model 2 was based solely on community-level characteristics. Model 3 included both individual-level and community-level characteristics. Model 4 was the full model that included the explanatory and control variables. The models were fitted using the *xtmelogit* command of Stata version 12 [69]. Model adequacy was examined using the Wald chi-square which assesses the statistical significance of the model. The 5% alpha level was considered statistically significant. Analyses were performed using Stata version 12.

Results

Univariate results

Figure 1 presents distribution of respondents by assistance during delivery. As shown in the figure, during their most recent deliveries, slightly less than a quarter of respondents (23.0%) utilised 'skilled assistance' while the majority of respondents (77.0%) utilised 'unskilled assistance'. Table 1 presents respondents' socio-demographic profile. Nearly two-thirds of the respondents' had no formal education. However, among respondents with educational attainments, primary education was dominant. The majority of respondents were either multiparous (42.7%) or grand multiparous (41.7%) women. Reproductive age interval of 15–19 years was the dominant age interval at first birth among the respondents. The proportion of the respondents who had first birth at age twenty-five or older ages was less than one-tenth of the respondents. The majority of the respondents were employed during the survey. However, slightly more than one-third of the respondents were unemployed during the survey. Muslim women compared with women practicing Christianity or other religions were dominant among respondents.

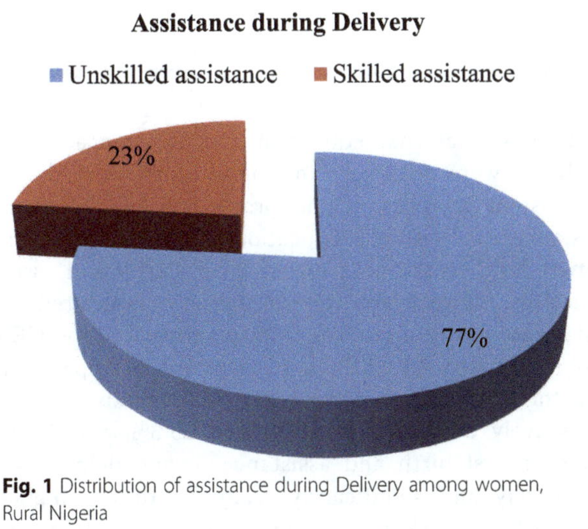

Fig. 1 Distribution of assistance during Delivery among women, Rural Nigeria

More than two-thirds of the respondents did not participate in their healthcare decision. Slightly more than two-fifths of respondents had no access to the mass media. However, nearly one-third of the women had 'high' access to the mass media. More than two-fifths of respondents either had no modern means of transportation or had animal-drawn cart as means of transportation. Motorcycle/scooter was the dominant modern means of transportation available to the respondents who reported a modern means of transportation. Higher proportions of the respondents were in the poorest (34.7%) and poorer (31.1%) wealth quintiles compared with the respondents in other wealth categories. Nearly half of the respondents (49.5%) had no antenatal care visits prior to their most recent deliveries, while nearly half of respondents reported some numbers of antenatal care visits. However, more than one-third of the respondents (37.6%) reported the recommended four or more antenatal care visits prior to their most recent deliveries. Distribution of respondents by timing of first antenatal care visits however revealed that nearly half of the respondents had their first antenatal care visit in the third trimester of pregnancy, while slightly more than one-third of respondents (35.6%) had their first antenatal care visit in the second trimester of pregnancy.

More than one-third of the respondents live either in communities with low (36.3%) or moderate (39.0%) childcare burden that is communities with low or medium proportion of high parous women but nearly one-quarter of the respondents live in communities with high childcare burden. In contrast, more than one-third of the respondents live in communities with either medium or high proportions of women who cannot read or write at all. Likewise, the distribution of respondents by community poverty level showed that the proportions of women who live in communities with either medium or high poverty level were more than one-third of respondents. The proportions of respondents employed outside agriculture were similar in the communities, though with slightly higher proportion of respondents living in communities with high proportion of women employed outside agriculture. More respondents live in communities where more than half of the women perceived distance to health facility as a big problem. Women from the northern region of the country were dominant among the respondents.

Bivariate results

Table 2 presents proportions of skilled assistance and the bivariate relationships between the research

Table 1 Respondents socio-demographic characteristics, rural Nigeria, 2013

Characteristic	Number of women (n = 12,665)	Percentage
Maternal Education		
None	8100	64.0
Primary	2294	18.1
Secondary	1992	15.7
Higher	278	2.2
Parity		
Primiparity	1.979	15.6
Multiparity	5411	42.7
Grandmultiparity	5275	41.7
Age at first birth (years)		
14 or less	1248	9.8
15–19	7405	58.5
20–24	2999	23.7
25 or older	1013	8.0
Employment status		
Unemployed	4361	34.4
Employed	8304	65.6
Religion		
Christianity	3608	28.5
Islam	8816	69.6
Others	241	1.9
Healthcare decision		
No Participation	9139	72.2
Participate	3526	27.8
Access to mass media		
No access	5654	44.6
Moderate access	2860	22.6
High access	4151	32.8
Means of Transportation		
None/animal cart	5108	40.3
Boat/canoe	210	1.7
Bicycle	1710	13.5
Motorcycle/scooter	5064	40.0
Car/truck	573	4.5
Household wealth quintile		
Poorest	4400	34.7
Poorer	3937	31.1
Middle	2560	20.2
Richer	1306	10.3
Richest	462	3.7

Table 1 Respondents socio-demographic characteristics, rural Nigeria, 2013 *(Continued)*

Characteristic	Number of women (n = 12,665)	Percentage
Number of antenatal care visit		
No Visit	6279	49.5
1–3 Visits	1629	12.9
4 or more visits	4756	37.6
Timing of first antenatal visit		
1st Trimester	1831	14.5
2nd Trimester	4508	35.6
3rd Trimester	6326	49.9
Community childcare burden		
Low	4602	36.3
Medium	4934	39.0
High	3129	24.7
Community literacy level		
Low	3552	28.0
Medium	4522	35.7
High	4591	36.3
Community poverty level		
Low	3761	29.7
Medium	4237	33.4
High	4667	36.9
Proportion employed outside agriculture		
Low	4120	32.5
Medium	4156	32.8
High	4389	34.7
Proportion who perceived distance as a big problem		
Low	6556	51.8
High	6109	48.2
Geographic Region		
Northern region	10,303	81.4
Southern region	2362	18.6

Source: Author's analysis based on 2013 Nigeria Demographic and Health Survey

variables. Maternal education and assistance during delivery were positively and significantly related with consistent increase in the proportion of skilled assistance as maternal education improves from one lower level to the next higher level. Parity and assistance during delivery were negatively associated. As maternal parity increased from primiparity (one-CEB) to multiparity (4-CEB), and to grand multiparity (5 or more CEB), proportion of skilled assistance respectively decreased from 29.9 to 25.3%, and 18.9%. Age at first birth and assistance during delivery are positively and significantly related with the highest proportion of skilled assistance among women who

Table 2 Proportion of skilled assistance and unadjusted binary logistic regression coefficients showing bivariate relationships, Rural Nigeria, 2013

Characteristic	% of Skilled assistance	Coeff.	95% CI
Maternal education			
None[RC]	9.1	–	–
Primary	35.0	1.684*	1.476–1.891
Secondary	58.8	2.658*	2.450–2.866
Higher	87.0	4.205*	3.728–4.683
Parity			
Primiparity[RC]	29.9	–	–
Multiparity	25.3	−0.230**	−0.370, −0.091
Grandmultiparity	18.9	−0.604*	−0.746, −0.462
Age at first birth (years)			
14 or less[RC]	14.6	–	–
15–19	17.7	0.232**	0.036–0.428
20–24	33.5	1.080*	0.865–1.294
25 +	45.0	1.566*	1.278–1.855
Employment status			
Unemployed[RC]	16.8	–	–
Employed	26.7	0.591*	0.411–0.770
Religion			
Christianity[RC]	51.3	–	–
Islam	11.9	−2.053*	−2.280, −1.825
Others	20.8	−1.388*	−2.002, −0.774
Healthcare decision			
No participation[RC]	16.3	–	–
Participation	41.4	1.287*	1.124–1.451
Access to mass media			
No access[RC]	12.9	–	–
Moderate access	20.5	0.556*	0.341–0.770
High access	39.5	1.487*	1.298–1.676
Means of transportation			
None/animal cart[RC]	21.6	–	–
Boat/canoe	15.2	−0.430	−0.955, 0.094
Bicycle	15.3	−0.423**	−0.682, – 0.164
Motorcycle/scooter	25.4	0.211**	0.030–0.391
Car/truck	47.0	1.167*	0.887–1.447
Household wealth quintile			
Poorest	4.8	–	–
Poorer	16.1	1.333*	1.081–1.586
Middle	38.4	2.509*	2.235–2.782
Richer	58.3	3.317*	3.011–3.622
Richest	78.2	4.258*	3.834–4.682
Number of antenatal care visits			
No visit	5.6	–	–
1–3 visits	22.4	1.583*	1.352–1.814
4 or more visits	47.1	2.711*	2.496–2.925
Timing of first antenatal care visit			
1st trimester	51.9	–	–
2nd trimester	37.7	−0.576*	−0.745, −0.408
3rd trimester	4.8	−3.066*	−3.297, −2.835
Community childcare burden			
Low	36.1	–	–
Medium	16.5	−1.051*	−1.398, −0.704
High	15.2	−1.150*	−1.524, −0.776
Community Literacy Level			
Low	56.5	–	–
Medium	17.0	−1.850*	−2.128, – 1.573
High	3.9	−3.462*	−3.772, – 3.153
Community Poverty Level			
Low	52.9	–	–
Medium	18.4	−1.606*	– 1.903, – 1.309
High	3.9	−3.315*	−3.627, – 3.004
Proportion employed outside agriculture			
Low	22.0	–	–
Medium	23.3	0.074	−0.286, 0.434
High	24.7	0.152	−0.216, 0.520
Proportion who perceived distance as a big problem			
Low	13.1	–	–
High	34.3	1.244*	0.936–1.552
Geographic region			
Northern region	14.8	–	–
Southern region	60.6	2.180*	1.891–2.470

Notes: Coeff. (Coefficient), RC (Reference Category), $*p < 0.01$, $**p < 0.05$

had their first birth at age 25 years or older ages (45.0%). Likewise, employment status was positively and significantly associated with assistance during delivery ($\beta = 0.591$; CI: 0.411–0.770). Employed women had higher skilled assistance compared with unemployed women (26.7% vs. 16.8%).

Religion was negatively associated with assistance during delivery. Christian women compared with Muslim and other women had higher prevalence of skilled assistance. The relationship between healthcare decision and assistance during delivery was significantly positive ($\beta =$ 1.287; CI: 1.124–1.451) with higher prevalence of skilled assistance among women who participated in the decision compared with women who did not participate in the decision (41.4% vs. 16.3%). Access to mass media and assistance during delivery were significantly positively related. As access to mass media improve from 'none' to 'moderate' and 'high', the proportion of skilled delivery increased from 12.9 to 20.5%, and 39.5% respectively. Means of transportation had mixed relationship with assistance during delivery. The relationship was negative among women whose means of transportation were boat/canoe or bicycle but positive among women whose means of transportation were motorcycle/scooter or car/truck. However, the proportion of skilled assistance was highest among women whose means of transportation were car or truck (47.0%).

Household wealth quintile had significant positive relationship with assistance during delivery. As wealth quintile improved from one lower wealth group to another higher wealth group, the proportion of skilled assistance progressively improved. For instance, proportion of skilled assistance improved from 38.4% among women in 'middle' wealth group to 58.3% among women in 'richer' wealth group. Antenatal care visits relates positively with assistance during delivery. The proportion of skilled assistance was 5.6% among women who had no antenatal care visit but increased to 22.4% among women who had 1–3 antenatal care visits. It further increased to 47.1% among women who had the recommended four or more antenatal care visits. Timing of first antenatal care visit was negatively associated with assistance during delivery with lowest proportion of skilled assistance (4.8%) among women whose first antenatal care visits took place in the third trimester of pregnancy compared with 51.9% of skilled assistance among women whose first antenatal care visit took place within the first trimester of pregnancy.

Community childcare burden was negatively associated with assistance during delivery with reduction in the proportions of skilled assistance as childcare burden increases in the communities. The relationship between community literacy level and assistance during delivery was also negative with lowest proportion of skilled assistance (3.9%) among women in communities with high proportion of women who cannot read or write at all. Community poverty level was negatively associated with assistance during delivery. The proportion of skilled assistance was highest among women who live in communities with low proportion of women in the poorest wealth group. Proportion of women employed outside agricultural sector relates positively with assistance during delivery. The proportion of skilled assistance increased as the proportion of women employed outside agriculture improved. For instance, the proportion of skilled assistance was higher among women who live in communities with high proportion of women employed outside agricultural sector compared with women in communities with low proportion of women employed outside agriculture (24.7% vs. 22.0%). Community perception of distance to health facility was positively associated with assistance during delivery with lower proportion of skilled assistance (13.1%) among women who live in communities with low perception of distance to health facility as a big problem to accessing healthcare. Likewise, geographic region and assistance during delivery were significantly positively related ($\beta = 2.180$; CI: 1.891–2.470). Southern women compared with their northern counterpart had higher use of skilled assistance (60.6% vs. 14.8%).

Multivariate results

Prior to fitting the multivariate models, the VIF computed revealed a mean VIF score of 3.36. This not only confirms that the explanatory variables were not significantly multi-collinear, it also suggest that the variables were sufficient for adequate estimation of the regression coefficients. The variables were then included in the mixed-effects analyses. Table 3 presents the fixed-effects on the likelihood of skilled assistance during delivery. The Wald chi-square confirm that all the fitted models were statistically significant ($p < 0.01$). In Model 1 (Wald $\chi^2 = 288.3$; $p < 0.01$), six individual-level characteristics, namely, maternal education, parity, religion, healthcare decision, access to mass media, and means of transportation had significant effects on the likelihood of skilled assistance. For instance, grand multiparous women were 48.2% less likely to utilise skilled assistance compared with primiparous women (OR = 0.518: CI: 0.420–0.640). In contrast, women who participated in healthcare decision were 43.5% more likely to utilise skilled assistance compared with women who did not participate in healthcare decision (OR = 1.435; CI: 1.215–1.693).

In Model 2 (Wald $\chi^2 = 333.4$; $p < 0.01$), four community-level characteristics, namely, community literacy level, community poverty level, community perception of distance to health facility, and geographic region revealed significant independent effects on the likelihood of skilled assistance. For instance, women in communities with high proportion of women who cannot read or write at all were less likely to utilise skilled assistance compared with women in communities with low proportion of women who cannot read or write at all (OR = 0.072; CI: 0.040–0.128). Likewise, women in communities with high proportion of women in poorest wealth group were less likely to utilise skilled assistance compared with women in communities with low proportion of women in poorest wealth group (OR = 0.159; CI: 0.090–0.282). The inclusion of both individual-level and community-level characteristics in Model 3 (Wald $\chi^2 = 367.9$; $p < 0.01$) reinforced the

Table 3 Odds ratio of adjusted binary logistic regression showing fixed effects on the likelihood of skilled assistance

Characteristic predicting skilled assistance	Model 1 (Wald $\chi^2 = 288.3$; $p < 0.001$)		Model 2 (Wald $\chi^2 = 333.4$; $p < 0.001$)		Model 3 (Wald $\chi^2 = 367.9$; $p < 0.001$)		Model 4 (Wald $\chi^2 = 474.9$; $p < 0.001$)	
	Odds Ratio	95% CI	Odds Ratio	95% CI	Odds Ratio	95% CI	Odds Ratio	95% CI
Maternal education								
None[RC]	–	–			–	–	–	–
Primary	1.994*	1.623–2.450			1.481*	1.215–1.806	1.205	0.996–1.458
Secondary	3839*	2.583–5.706			2.703*	2.120–3.447	1.840*	1.464–2.313
Higher	4.131*	3.184–5.358			13.114*	7.533–22.831	5.793*	3.474–9.660
Parity								
Primiparity[RC]	–	–			–	–	–	–
Multiparity	0.538*	0.440–0.657			0.532*	0.437–0.648	0.575*	0.476–0.695
Grand multiparity	0.518*	0.420–0.640			0.506*	0.411–0.624	0.564*	0.462–0.689
Age at first marriage (years)								
14 years or less[RC]	–	–			–	–	–	–
15–19 years	0.843	0.654–1.086			0.839	0.654–1.077	0.811	0.635–1.035
20–24 years	1.104	0.840–1.453			1.044	0.798–1.366	0.981	0.755–1.275
25 years or older	1.121	0.800–1.571			1.033	0.743–1.437	0.945	0.685–1.304
Employment Status								
Unemployed[RC]	–	–			–	–	–	–
Unemployment	1.169	0.991–1.378			1.094	0.931–1.286	1.033	0.883–1.208
Religion								
Christianity[RC]	–	–			–	–	–	–
Islam	0.317*	0.237–0.423			0.741**	0.560–0.982	0.750**	0.577–0.974
Traditional/others	0.354**	0.188–0.664			0.558	0.299–1.040	0.712	0.390–1.300
Healthcare Decision								
No Participation[RC]	–	–			–	–	–	–
Participation	1.435*	1.215–1.693			1.290**	1.100–1.513	1.213**	1.041–1.413
Access to mass media								
None[RC]	–	–			–	–	–	–
Moderate	1.138	0.932–1.388			1.039	0.856–1.260	0.934	0.774–1.127
High	1.817*	1.506–2.193			1.562*	1.304–1.871	1.255**	1.055–1.494
Means of Transportation								
None/animal cart[RC]	–	–			–	–	–	–
Boat/canoe	0.513**	0.293–0.900			0.386*	0.226–0.659	0.392*	0.234–0.659
Bicycle	0.966	0.748–1.249			1.028	0.800–1.321	1.052	0.824–1.341
Motorcycle/scooter	1.425*	1.207–1.683			1.383*	1.177–1.626	1.222**	1.046–1.429
Car/truck	2.169*	1.566–3.003			1.984*	1.447–2.719	1.438**	1.055–1.960
Community childcare burden								
Low[RC]			–	–	–	–	–	–
Medium			0.886	0.623–1.260	1.071	0.759–1.511	1.079	0.796–1.462
High			0.752	0.505–1.116	0.936	0.635–1.380	0.978	0.694–1.378
Community literacy level								
Low[RC]			–	–	–	–	–	–
Medium			0.208*	0.136–0.319	0.389*	0.256–0.591	0.489*	0.339–0.706
High			0.072*	0.040–0.128	0.170*	0.095–0.302	0.346*	0.208–0.575

Table 3 Odds ratio of adjusted binary logistic regression showing fixed effects on the likelihood of skilled assistance *(Continued)*

Characteristic predicting skilled assistance	Model 1 (Wald $\chi^2 = 288.3$; $p < 0.001$)		Model 2 (Wald $\chi^2 = 333.4$; $p < 0.001$)		Model 3 (Wald $\chi^2 = 367.9$; $p < 0.001$)		Model 4 (Wald $\chi^2 = 474.9$; $p < 0.001$)	
	Odds Ratio	95% CI	Odds Ratio	95% CI	Odds Ratio	95% CI	Odds Ratio	95% CI
Community poverty level								
Low[RC]			–	–	–	–	–	–
Medium			0.382*	0.252–0.579	0.447*	0.299–0.670	0.602**	0.421–0.860
High			0.159*	0.090–0.282	0.213*	0.122–0.370	0.402*	0.241–0.670
Proportion employed outside agriculture								
Low[RC]			–	–	–	–	–	–
Medium			1.065	0.747–1.518	1.064	0.749–1.511	0.932	0.683–1.274
High			1.416	0.982–2.043	1.331	0.923–1.919	1.084	0.783–1.502
Proportion who perceived distance as big problem								
Low[RC]			–	–	–	–	–	–
High			2.774*	1.999–3.850	2.433*	1.770–3.345	1.815*	1.374–2.397
Geographic region								
Northern[RC]			–	–	–	–	–	–
Southern			2.103*	1.399–3.162	1.750**	1.163–2.634	1.818**	1.265–2.611
Household wealth quintile								
Poorest[RC]							–	–
Poorer							1.261	0.990–1.606
Middle							1.630**	1.227–2.166
Richer							1.819**	1.296–2.552
Richest							2.834*	1.761–4.560
Number of antenatal care visits								
None[RC]							–	–
1–3							1.430	0.991–2.064
4+							2.602*	1.803–3.756
Timing of first antenatal visit								
1st trimester[RC]							–	–
2nd trimester							0.802**	0.680–0.946
3rd trimester							0.252*	0.173–0.369

Notes: *$p < 0.001$, **$p < 0.05$

statistical significance of the individual-level and community-level characteristics which showed significant effects in the earlier models.

In the full model (Wald $\chi^2 = 474.9$; $p < 0.01$), the inclusion of the three control variables did not result in any substantial change in the pattern of the fixed effects on assistance during delivery. In the model, the likelihood of utilising skilled assistance increased significantly as maternal education improved. For instance, women who attained higher education were nearly six times more likely to use skilled assistance compared with uneducated women (OR = 5.793: CI: 3.474–9.660). Likewise, multiparous women (OR = 0.575; CI: 0.476–0.695) and grand multiparous women (OR = 0.564; CI: 0.462–0.689) were less likely to utilise skilled assistance compared with primiparous women. Also, Muslim women were 25% less likely to utilise skilled assistance compared with Christian women (OR = 0.750; CI: 0.577–0.974). Women who participated in healthcare decision were 21.3% more likely to utilise skilled assistance compared with women who did not participate in healthcare decision (OR = 1.213; CI: 1.041–1.413). Access to mass media revealed significant effect on the odds of skilled assistance. Women who had high access to the mass media were 25.5% more likely to utilise skilled assistance compared with women in the reference category (OR = 1.255; CI: 1.055–1.494). Similarly, women who had car/truck were 43.8% more likely to use skilled assistance compared with women who had no means of transportation (OR = 1.438; CI: 1.055–1.960).

Community literacy level exerted significant influence on the likelihood of using skilled assistance. Women who live in communities with high proportion of women who cannot read or write at all were 65.4% less likely to utilise skilled assistance compared with women in communities with low proportion of women who cannot read or write at all (OR = 0.346; CI: 0.208–0.575). Also, community poverty level revealed significant influence on the odds of skilled assistance. Women in communities with high proportion of women in poorest wealth group were 59.8% less likely to use skilled assistance during delivery compared with women in communities with low proportion of women in poorest wealth group (OR = 0.402; CI: 0.241–0.670). Women in communities where high proportion of women perceived distance to health facility as a big problem were more likely to use skilled assistance during delivery compared with women in the reference category (OR = 1.815; CI: 1.374–2.397). Women in southern region of Nigeria were almost twice more likely to use skilled assistance compared with women in northern region of the country (OR = 1.818; CI: 1.265–2.611). The three selected control variables showed significant influence on the likelihood of using skilled assistance during delivery. The odds of using skilled assistance during delivery increased progressively as household wealth group improved. Women who had four or more antenatal care visits were almost three times more likely to utilise skilled assistance during delivery compared with women who had no antenatal care visits (OR = 2.602; CI: 1.803–3.756). Women whose first antenatal visit took place either in the second or third trimester were less likely to use skilled assistance during delivery compared with women whose first antenatal visit took place in the first trimester of pregnancy.

Table 4 presents the random effects of the mixed-effects models. As shown in the table and using the significance of the LR test, all the models fitted showed a good fit. In the absence of individual-level and community-level characteristics, the result of the ICC in the empty model reveal that the use of skilled assistance was highly identical among women in the community (ICC = 0.705). When only individual variables were included in Model 1, the ICC reduced to 0.515 to indicate that higher proportion of variation in the use of skilled assistance was attributable to community-level characteristics (ICC = 0.515). This proportion further reduces to 0.381 in Model 2. With the combination of individual-level and community-level characteristics in Model 3, the variation in the use of skilled assistance attributable to community-level characteristics remained substantial (ICC = 0.359) indicating that more than one-third of the women in the communities had identical use of skilled assistance during delivery. In the full model, more than a quarter of variation in the use of skilled assistance during delivery were attributable to community-level characteristics (ICC = 0.286).

Discussion

This study examined individual-level and community-level characteristics associated with assistance during delivery in rural Nigeria. It improves research attention on skilled delivery in the rural areas which in spite of poor health infrastructure is usually the area with higher incidences of pregnancies and child deliveries in Nigeria [2, 8, 9]. The study not only compliment existing studies that have explicitly examined associated factors of assistance during delivery in rural areas [30–33], it also analysed community-level influence on the use of assistance during delivery in rural areas of Nigeria compared with previous rural studies that investigated mainly individual-level characteristics [34–38]. The study provided additional support for the socio-ecological model [50] by confirming the significance of factors operating at both individual and community levels, and thus consistent with previous studies that stressed the importance of community factors in initiatives to improve human health behaviour particularly health-seeking behaviour [45–49]. Based on this finding, it is plausible to assert that factors affecting utilisation of skilled assistance during delivery in rural areas of Nigeria operates at multiple levels, which require that initiatives seeking to boost utilisation of skilled assistance during delivery should endeavour to identify and address the important factors at each distinct level of the social environment.

The study found that utilisation of skilled assistance at delivery is very poor in the rural areas of Nigeria. Though, the 23.0% prevalence of skilled assistance found in the study was higher than the 13.0% reported in an earlier study in Nigeria [53], it corroborates prevalence reported in both the 2008 and 2013 NDHS [8, 9]. There are two possible reasons for poor utilisation of skilled

Table 4 Random Effects showing influence of community characteristics on use of skilled assistance during delivery

Parameter	Empty Model	Model 1	Model 2	Model 3	Model 4
Community level variance (SE)	7.850 (0.925)	3.488(0.449)	2.023 (0.258)	1.840 (0.243)	1.320 (0.177)
Log likelihood	− 5028	− 4698.3	− 4761.8	− 4550.8	− 4229.6
LR test	$\chi^2 = 4192.2$; $p < 0.001$	$\chi^2 = 1231.1$; $p < 0.001$	$\chi^2 = 1024.3$; $p < 0.001$	$\chi^2 = 781.2$; $p < 0.001$	$\chi^2 = 571.9$; $p < 0.001$
ICC	0.705	0.515	0.381	0.359	0.286

assistance at delivery in rural Nigeria. The first reason may relate to poor health infrastructure in rural areas of the country which made unskilled health providers more accessible to rural women [2]. In many rural and remote areas of the country, there are no Primary Health Care (PHC) centres, and where the PHCs are available, many of the health personnel including skilled birth attendants are usually unwilling to reside in the rural communities [13]. The implementation of the MSS was expected to improve maternity care in the rural areas of Nigeria, but it is yet to yield significant positive results due to challenges such as retention of health personnel in rural areas, availability and training of midwives, and lack of political will by States and Local government in the country [14]. Also, where PHCs are available, several adjoining communities may have to depend on its services. This usually creates distance barrier to some of the communities and may affect utilisation. This implies that utilisation of skilled delivery may likely improve in the rural areas if more health centres are provided with qualified health personnel. As evident in the study, though a high proportion of the women perceived distance to health facility as a big problem, but they reported a higher use of skilled assistance than the proportion who perceived distance to health facility as not a big problem which indicates that distance to health facility may not be as important as the availability of health facilities and accessibility to desired services. It is therefore important that government at all tiers of the Nigerian federation should improve public investment on the provision of more health facilities for rural dwellers. In the interim, the staff strength at existing rural health facilities could be expanded by the recruitment of more qualified health personnel especially those already trained in delivery care.

The second reason that may account for poor use of skilled assistance among rural women is the socio-demographic condition of the women. As found in the study, educational attainment was poor among the women, the majority of them were multiparous, had no autonomy on their healthcare, and belong to poorest household wealth group. Such social conditions have been found in earlier studies [2, 51, 53] to promote non-use of maternal healthcare services. Beyond the provision of healthcare centres in rural areas, it is imperative that more concerted efforts be made to improve the socio-economic conditions of rural women. This could be achieved through more rural development efforts such as the creation of more roads to enhance economic activities of rural women, and strengthening existing rural empowerment programmes. The advocacy for free Maternal and Child Health (MCH) services [56] should be given fresh impetus in the country to encourage more States of the federation to implement free MCH services particularly for rural families. This will reduce the economic burden of healthcare among rural women. Where free MCH services are not feasible, rural women could be assisted to improve their use of skilled delivery through the design and implementation of more CCT programme already piloted in some States of the country [57].

Hence, individual characteristics of women cannot be ignored in interventions to improve utilisation of skilled assistance during delivery. Existing initiatives should endeavour to focus more on three specific characteristics, namely, education, autonomy on healthcare decision, and religion. Education is central to all efforts aiming to improve use of skilled delivery in the rural areas because in spite of the effectiveness of existing interventions, utilisation may remain low in the absence of widespread awareness of the dangers of unskilled delivery. Also, several socio-cultural practices such as unequal power relations between male and female partners, and lack of male involvement in maternal healthcare [19] that undermine prompt health-seeking behaviour are best confronted through the provision of accurate information, communication and education on maternal and child health issues. It is thus important that the current IMNCH strategy reposition its information and communication initiative through massive public health education messages using the mass media particularly the radio which are more widely used in the rural areas.

This should be complimented by promoting women autonomy in the communities. Men in the communities should be mobilised through public campaigns to encourage women to have sole autonomy on issues affecting their reproductive life. Also, there should be more interventions to focus on Muslim women. As evident in this study and consistent with findings in similar previous studies [63, 65], there is unequal likelihood of maternal healthcare services utilisation among Christian and Muslim women. This may indicate that the different religions have different practices that impact women's perception and use of services. This differences in religious beliefs as it relates to maternal health should not only be fully understood by health policy planners, it is also important that religion be made an important component of future maternal healthcare interventions in line with the submission of several scholars on the subject [61, 62, 64, 70].

The study further found that community-level characteristics are crucial for improvement of the use of skilled assistance at delivery in the rural areas. This necessitates more community-based maternal healthcare interventions in rural Nigeria to increase the coverage of the existing community-based programme of the IMNCH Strategy [2]. Community-based interventions are more important in the rural areas because women in the rural communities tend to have identical perception and use of accessible health services. Findings from the study provided evidence that community-level factors such as community poverty or literacy levels have important effects on use of skilled assistance during delivery. Hence, existing community-based intervention such as the community extension workers programme [2] needs to be strengthened in the country. Finally, the antenatal care programme should be appropriately perceived as a veritable means of reaching rural women about other services within the continuum of maternal and child healthcare. In many rural communities and as found in this study, high proportions of women had no antenatal care visits. Also, among those who reported antenatal care visits, more than one-third of the visits took place in the third trimester of pregnancy. Such visitations may not be as a result of seeking adequate antenatal information and counselling, but more likely to be a response to complications or health challenges. Thus, there should be renewed efforts to strengthen the antenatal care programme not only in terms of expanding its coverage to all rural communities to enhance visits in the first trimester of pregnancy, but to also ensure that women who visited health facility for antenatal care are followed up, retained in the continuum to ensure facility deliveries and use of skilled attendants during delivery, and ultimately to reduce rate of drop out from maternity care [31, 54].

This study cannot claim to have established a cause-effect relationship between the explanatory and outcome variables of the study due to the cross-sectional nature of the data analysed. The study however buttress existing observation that both individual-level and community-level characteristics have important implications for the use of maternal healthcare services among women. Likewise, the socio-ecological theory could not be applied in its original form because the data analysed did not provide sufficient information required to capture all its theoretical constructs. It is not impossible that a different pattern of relationship between the variables may be observed if all the theoretical constructs are derivable. Future studies on the subject matter may therefore consider the use of primary data to enhance availability of all needed information.

Conclusions

This study provided additional empirical evidence that utilisation of maternal healthcare services particularly skilled delivery service is influenced by individual-level characteristics such as maternal education, parity, religion, and healthcare decision, and community-level characteristics such as community poverty level, and community literacy level. The study provided evidence that to a significant extent, individual-level and community-level characteristics are associated with assistance during delivery in rural Nigeria. Initiatives seeking to reduce rural-urban inequity in skilled delivery should endeavour to identify and address the important factors at the individual and community levels of the social environment.

Abbreviations

DHS: Demographic and Health Survey; FMoH: Federal Ministry of Health; MSS: Midwives Service Scheme; NDHS: Nigeria Demographic and Health Survey; PRB: Population Reference Bureau; WHO: World Health Organization

Acknowledgements

The author expresses gratitude to the National Population Commission (NPC) [Nigeria], ICF International and MEASURE DHS Project for granting prompt authorisation to analyse the data.

Funding

Not applicable.

Authors contribution

BLS developed the concept, carried out the statistical analyses, and interpreted the results. RAY reviewed literature. Both authors discussed the results, and read through the manuscript for intellectual content. Both authors read and approved the final manuscript.

Author information

BLS has a PhD in Demography and Social Statistics from Obafemi Awolowo University, Ile-Ife, Nigeria. His research interests are fertility, contraception, and women's health issues. He is a Senior Lecturer. RAY is a postgraduate student in the Department.

Consent for publication

Not applicable.

Competing interests

The authors declares that they have no competing interests.

References

1. Population Reference Bureau. 2017 World Population Data Sheet with a special focus on Youth. https://assets.prb.org/pdf17/2017_World_Population.pdf. Accessed 27 May 2018.
2. Federal Ministry of Health. Saving newborn lives in Nigeria: Newborn health in the context of the Integrated Maternal, Newborn and Child Health Strategy. 2nd ed. Abuja: Federal Ministry of Health, Save the Children, Jhpiego; 2011.
3. Mafimisebi TE, Oguntade AE. Health Infrastructure Inequality and Rural-Urban Utilization of Orthodox and Traditional Medicines in Farming Households: A Case Study of Ekiti State, Nigeria. 2011. https://doi.org/10.5772/19798. Accessed 20 July 2017.
4. Adewuyi EO, Zhao Y, Auta A, Lamichhane R. Prevalence and factors associated with non-utilization of healthcare facility for childbirth in rural and urban Nigeria: analysis of a national population-based survey. Scand J Public Health. 2017:1–8. https://doi.org/10.1177/1403494817705562.
5. Limwattananon S, Tangcharoensathien V, Sirilak S. Trends and inequities in where women delivered their babies in 25 low-income countries: evidence from demographic and health surveys. Reprod Health Matters. 2011;19(37):75–85. https://doi.org/10.1016/S0968-8080(11)37564-7.

6. Bobo FT, Yesuf EA, Woldie M. Inequities in utilization of reproductive and maternal health services in Ethiopia. Int J Equity Health. 2017;16:105. https://doi.org/10.1186/s12939-017-0602-2.
7. Crowe S, Utley M, Costello A, Pagel C. How many births in sub-Saharan Africa and South Asia will not be attended by a skilled birth attendant between 2011 and 2015? BMC Pregnancy Childbirth. 2012;12(4). https://doi.org/10.1186/1471-2393-12-4.
8. National Population Commission (NPC) [Nigeria] & ICF International. Nigeria Demographic and Health Survey. Abuja, Nigeria, and Rockville, Maryland. USA: NPC and ICF International; 2008. p. 2009.
9. National Population Commission (NPC) [Nigeria] & ICF International. Nigeria Demographic and Health Survey. Abuja, Nigeria, and Rockville, Maryland. USA: NPC and ICF International; 2013. p. 2014.
10. Nkwo PO, Lawani LO, Ezugwu EC, Iyoke CA, Ubesie AC, Onoh RC. Correlates of poor perinatal outcomes in non-hospital births in the context of weak health system: the Nigerian experience. BMC Pregnancy Childbirth. 2014;14(341). https://doi.org/10.1186/1471-2393-14-341.
11. Koblinsky M, Matthews Z, Hussein J, Mavalankar D, Mridha MK, Anwar I, et al. Going to scale with professional skilled care. Lancet. 2006:3. https://doi.org/10.1016/S0140-6736(06)69382-3.
12. Adegoke AA, van den Broek N. Skilled birth attendance-lessons learnt. BJOG. 2009;116(Suppl. 1):33–40. https://doi.org/10.1111/j.1471-0528.2009.02336.x.
13. Ebuehi OM, Campbell PC. Attraction and retention of qualified health workers to rural areas in Nigeria: a case study of four LGAs in Ogun state. Nigeria Rural Remote Health. 2011;11:1515.
14. Abimbola S, Okoli U, Olubajo O, Abdullahi MJ, Pate MA. The midwives service scheme in Nigeria. PLoS Med. 2012;9(5):e1001211. https://doi.org/10.1371/journal.pmed.1001211.
15. Ossai EN, Azuogu BN, Uwakwe KA, Anyanwagu UC, Ibiok NC, Ekeke N. Are medical students satisfied with rural community posting? A survey among final year students in medical schools of south-East Nigeria. Rural Remote Health. 2016;16:3632.
16. Rourke JWHO. Recommendations to improve retention of rural and remote health workers - important for all countries. Rural Remote Health. 2010;10:1654.
17. Guerra Arias M, Nove A, Michel-Schuldt M, de Bernis L. Current and future availability of and need for human resources for sexual, reproductive, maternal and newborn health in 41 countries in sub-Saharan Africa. Int J Equity Health. 2017;16:69. https://doi.org/10.1186/s12939-017-0569-z.
18. Adjiwanou V, LeGrand T. Gender inequality and the use of maternal healthcare services in rural sub-Saharan Africa. Health Place 2014; 29:67–78, http://dx.doi.org/https://doi.org/10.1016/j.healthplace.2014.06.001
19. Morgan R, Tetui M, Kananura RM, Ekirapa-Kiracho E, George AS. Gender dynamics affecting maternal health and health care access and use in Uganda. Health Policy Plan. 2017;32:v13–21. https://doi.org/10.1093/heapol/czx011.
20. Ahmed S, Creanga AA, Gillespie DG, Tsui AO. Economic status, education and empowerment: implications for maternal health service utilization in developing countries. PLoS One. 2010;5(6):e11190. https://doi.org/10.1371/journal.pone.0011190.
21. Obiyan MO, Kumar A. Socioeconomic inequalities in the use of maternal health Care Services in Nigeria: trends between 1990 and 2008. SAGE Open. 2015:1–11. https://doi.org/10.1177/2158244015614070.
22. Solanke BL. Association between intimate partner violence and utilisation of maternal health services in Nigeria. Afr Popul Stud. 2014;28(2 Suppl):933–45 https://doi.org/10.11564/28-0-547.
23. Ononokpono DN, Azfredrick EC. Intimate partner violence and the utilization of maternal health Care Services in Nigeria. Health Care Women Int. 2014;35:973–89. https://doi.org/10.1080/07399332.2014.924939.
24. Worku AG, Yalew AW, Afework MF. Factors affecting utilization of skilled maternal care in Northwest Ethiopia: a multilevel analysis. BMC Int Health Hum Rights. 2013;13(20). https://doi.org/10.1186/1472-698X-13-20.
25. Singh PK, Kumar C, Rai RK, Singh L. Factors associated with maternal healthcare services utilization in nine high focus states in India: a multilevel analysis based on 14385 communities in 292 districts. Health Policy Plan. 2014;29:542–59. https://doi.org/10.1093/heapol/czt039.
26. Jat TR, Ng N, San Sebastian M. Factors affecting the use of maternal health services in Madhya Pradesh state of India: a multilevel analysis. Int J Equity Health. 2011;10:59 https://doi.org/10.1186/1475-9276-10-59.
27. Yadav A, Kesarwani R. Effect of individual and community factors on maternal health care service use in India: a multilevel approach. J Biosoc Sci. 2016;48:1–19. https://doi.org/10.1017/S0021932015000048.
28. Babalola S, Fatusi A. Determinants of use of maternal health services in Nigeria – looking beyond individual and household factors. BMC Pregnancy Childbirth. 2009;9:43. https://doi.org/10.1186/1471-2393-9-43.
29. Babalola SO. Factors associated with use of maternal health services in Haiti: a multilevel analysis. Rev Panam Salud Publica. 2014;36(1):1–9.
30. Yanagisawa S, Oum S, Wakai S. Determinants of skilled birth attendance in rural Cambodia. Tropical Med Int Health. 2006;11(2):238–51. https://doi.org/10.1111/j.1365-3156.2005.01547.x.
31. Magoma M, Requejo J, Campbell OMR, Cousens S, Filippi V. High ANC coverage and low skilled attendance in a rural Tanzanian district: a case for implementing a birth plan intervention. BMC Pregnancy Childbirth. 2010;10(13). https://doi.org/10.1186/1471-2393-10-13.
32. Crissman HP, Engmann CE, Adanu RM, Nimako D, Crespo K, Moyer CA. Shifting norms: pregnant women's perspectives on skilled birth attendance and facility–based delivery in rural Ghana. Afr J Reprod Health. 2013;17(1):15–26.
33. Adamu YM, Salihu HM. Barriers to the use of antenatal and obstetric care services in rural Kano, Nigeria. J Obstet Gynaecol. 2002;22(6):600–3. https://doi.org/10.1080/0144361021000020349.
34. Adjiwanou V, LeGrand T. Does antenatal care matter in the use of skilled birth attendance in rural Africa: a multi-country analysis. Soc Sci Med. 2013;86:26–34 https://doi.org/10.1016/j.socscimed.2013.02.047.
35. Vidler M, Ramadurg U, Charantimath U, Katageri G, Karadiguddi C, Sawchuck D, et al. Utilization of maternal health care services and their determinants in Karnataka state. India Reproductive Health. 2016;13(Suppl 1):37. https://doi.org/10.1186/s12978-016-0138-8.
36. Sakeah E, Doctor HV, McCloskey L, Bernstein J, Yeboah-Antwi K, Mills S. Using the community-based health planning and services program to promote skilled delivery in rural Ghana: socio-demographic factors that influence women utilization of skilled attendants at birth in northern Ghana. BMC Public Health. 2014;14:344. https://doi.org/10.1186/1471-2458-14-344.
37. Ejembi CL, Alti-Muazu M, Chirdan O, Ezeh HO, Sheidu S, Dahiru T. Utilisation of maternal health services by rural Hausa women in Zaria environs, northern Nigeria: has primary health care made a difference? J Comm Med Prim Health Care. 2004;16(2):47–54.
38. Osubor KM, Fatusi AO, Chiwuzie JC. Maternal health-seeking behavior and associated factors in a rural Nigerian community. Matern Child Health J. 2006;10(2):159–69. https://doi.org/10.1007/s10995-005-0037-z.
39. Ebuehi OM, Akintujoye IA. Perception and utilization of traditional birth attendants by pregnant women attending primary health care clinics in a rural local government area in Ogun state, Nigeria. Int J Womens Health 2012; 4:25–34. https://doi.org/10.2147/IJWH.S23173
40. Emelumadu OF, Ukegbu AU, Ezeama NN, Kanu OO, Ifeadike CO, Onyeonoro UU. Socio-demographic determinants of maternal health-care service utilization among rural women in Anambra state, south East Nigeria. Ann Med Health Sci Res. 2014;4:374–82. https://doi.org/10.4103/2141-9248.133463.
41. Oguntunde O, Aina O, Ibrahim MS, Umar HS, Antenatal Care PP. Skilled birth attendance in three communities in Kaduna state. Nigeria Afr J Reprod Health. 2010;14(3):89–96.
42. Ononokpono DN, Odimegwu CO, Imasiku E, Adedini S. Contextual determinants of maternal health care service utilization in Nigeria. Women Health. 2013;53(7):647–68. https://doi.org/10.1080/03630242.2013.826319.
43. Aremu O, Lawoko S, Dalal K. Neighborhood socioeconomic disadvantage, individual wealth status and patterns of delivery care utilization in Nigeria: a multilevel discrete choice analysis. Int J Womens Health. 2011; 3:167–174. https://doi.org/10.2147/IJWH.S21783
44. Ononokpono DN, Odimegwu CO. Determinants of maternal health care utilization in Nigeria: a multilevel approach. Pan Afr Med J. 2014;17(Supp 1):2. https://doi.org/10.11694/pamj.supp.2014.17.1.3596.
45. Lippman SA, Leslie HH, Neilands TB, Twine R, Grignon JS, MacPhail C, et al. Context matters: community social cohesion and health behaviors in two south African areas. HEALTH PLACE 2018; 50:98–104. https://doi.org/10.1016/j.healthplace.2017.12.009
46. Elmusharaf K, Byrne E, O'Donovan D. Strategies to increase demand for maternal health services in resource-limited settings: challenges to be addressed. BMC Public Health. 2015;15:870. https://doi.org/10.1186/s12889-015-2222-3.
47. Chikhungun LC, Madise NJ, Padmadas SS. How important are community characteristics in influencing children's nutritional status? Evidence from Malawi population-based household and community surveys. Health Place. 2014; 30:187–195. https://doi.org/10.1016/j.healthplace.2014.09.006

48. Akinyemi JO, Adedini SA, Odimegwu CO. Individual v. community-level measures of women's decision-making involvement and child survival in Nigeria. S Afr J Child Health. 2017;11(1):26–32. https://doi.org/10.7196/SAJCH.2017.v11i1.1148.
49. Ngome E, Odimegwu C. The social context of adolescent women's use of modern contraceptives in Zimbabwe: a multilevel analysis. Reprod Health. 2014;11(64). https://doi.org/10.1186/1742-4755-11-64.
50. McLeroy KR, Bibeau D, Steckler A, Glanz K. An ecological perspective on health promotion programs. Health Educ Q. 1988;15:351–77.
51. Yaya S, Bishwajit G, Uthman OA, Amouzou A. Why some women fail to give birth at health facilities: a comparative study between Ethiopia and Nigeria. PLoS One 2018; 13(5): e0196896. https://doi.org/10.1371/journal.pone.0196896
52. Adinma ED, Adinma JIB, Obionu CC, Asuzu MC. Effect of government-community healthcare co-financing on maternal and child healthcare in Nigeria. West Afr J Med. 2011;30(1):35–41.
53. Doctor HV, Findley SE, Ager A, Cometto G, Afenyadu GY, Adamu F, Green C. Using community-based research to shape the design and delivery of maternal health services in northern Nigeria. Reprod Health Matters. 2012;20(39):104–12. https://doi.org/10.1016/S0968-8080(12)39615-8.
54. Akinyemi JO, Afolabi RF, Awolude OA. Patterns and determinants of dropout from maternity care continuum in Nigeria. BMC Pregnancy Childbirth. 2016;16:282. https://doi.org/10.1186/s12884-016-1083-9.
55. Adewuyi EO, Auta A, Khanal V, Bamidele OD, Akuoko CP, Adefemi K, et al. Prevalence and factors associated with underutilization of antenatal care services in Nigeria: a comparative study of rural and urban residences based on the 2013 Nigeria demographic and health survey. PLoS One 2018;13(5): e0197324. https://doi.org/10.1371/journal.pone.0197324
56. Okonofua F, Lambo E, Okeibunor J, Agholor K. Advocacy for free maternal and child health care in Nigeria—results and outcomes. Health Policy. 2011;99:131–8. https://doi.org/10.1016/j.healthpol.2010.07.013.
57. Okoli U, Morris L, Oshin A, Pate MA, Aigbe C, Muhammad A. Conditional cash transfer schemes in Nigeria: potential gains for maternal and child health service uptake in a national pilot programme. BMC Pregnancy Childbirth. 2014;14(408). https://doi.org/10.1186/s12884-014-0408-9.
58. Onyeneho NG, Amazigo UV, Njepuome NA, Nwaorgu OC, Okeibunor JC. Perception and utilization of public health services in Southeast Nigeria: implication for health care in communities with different degrees of urbanization. Int J Equity Health. 2016;15:12. https://doi.org/10.1186/s12939-016-0294-z.
59. Odeyemi IAO. Community-based health insurance programmes and the national health insurance scheme of Nigeria: challenges to uptake and integration. Int J Equity Health. 2014;13:20. https://doi.org/10.1186/1475-9276-13-20.
60. Utz B, Siddiqui G, Adegoke A, vAN Den Broek N. Definitions and roles of a skilled birth attendant: a mapping exercise from four south-Asian countries. Acta Obstet Gynecol Scand. 2013;92:1063–9. https://doi.org/10.1111/aogs.12166.
61. Gitsels–van der Wal JT, Manniën J, Gitsels LA, Reinders HS, Verhoeven PS, Ghaly MM, et al. Prenatal screening for congenital anomalies: exploring midwives' perceptions of counselling clients with religious backgrounds. BMC Pregnancy Childbirth. 2014;14(237). https://doi.org/10.1186/1471-2393-14-237.
62. Aziato L, Odai PNA, Omenyo CN. Religious beliefs and practices in pregnancy and labour: an inductive qualitative study among post-partum women in Ghana. BMC Pregnancy Childbirth. 2016;16:138. https://doi.org/10.1186/s12884-016-0920-1.
63. Doku D, Neupane S, Doku PN. Factors associated with reproductive health care utilization among Ghanaian women. BMC Int Health and Hum Rights. 2012;12(29). https://doi.org/10.1186/1472-698X-12-29.
64. Ganle JK. Why Muslim women in northern Ghana do not use skilled maternal healthcare services at health facilities: a qualitative study. BMC Int Health and Hum Rights. 2015;15:10. https://doi.org/10.1186/s12914-015-0048-9.
65. Solanke BL, Oladosu OA, Akinlo A, Olanisebe SO. Religion as a social determinant of maternal health care service utilisation in Nigeria. Afr Popul Stud 2015; 29(2):1868–1881. https://doi.org/10.11564/29-2-761.
66. Rai RK, Singh PK, Singh L. Utilization of maternal health care services among married adolescent women: insights from the Nigeria demographic and health survey, 2008. Womens Health Issues. 2012;22(4):e407–14. https://doi.org/10.1016/j.whi.2012.05.001.
67. O'Brien RM. A caution regarding rules of thumb for variance inflation factors. Qual Quant. 2007;41:673–90. https://doi.org/10.1007/s11135-006-9018-6.
68. Akinwande O, Dikko HG, Samson A. Variance inflation factor: as a condition for the inclusion of suppressor variable(s) in regression analysis. Open J Statistics 2015; 5:754–767. https://doi.org/10.4236/ojs.2015.57075
69. StataCorp. Stata: Release 12. Statistical Software. College Station, TX: StataCorp LP; 2011.
70. Adanikin AI, Onwudiegwu U, Akintayo AA. Reshaping maternal services in Nigeria: any need for spiritual care? BMC Pregnancy Childbirth. 2014;14(196). https://doi.org/10.1186/1471-2393-14-196.

14

Pregnancy outcomes following nonobstetric surgery during gestation

Chia-Hung Yu[1], Shih-Feng Weng[2,3], Chung-Han Ho[3,4], Yi-Chen Chen[3], Jen-Yin Chen[1,5], Ying-Jen Chang[1], Jhi-Joung Wang[1,3], Ming-Ping Wu[6,7] and Chin-Chen Chu[1*]

Abstract

Background: Whether nonobstetric surgery during gestation is associated with a higher risk of spontaneous abortion or adverse delivery outcomes is still unclear.

Methods: We performed a retrospective case-control study using a Longitudinal Health Insurance Database (LHID 2000) containing claim-data of 1 million randomly selected beneficiaries. We compared the incidences and estimated the adjusted odds ratios (aOR) with 95% confidence interval (95% CI) for spontaneous abortion, adverse delivery outcomes, cesarean delivery, and prolonged hospital stay to determine the risk of adverse outcomes in women who had nonobstetric surgery during gestation as compared to those who did not have any surgery during gestation.

Results: After exclusion, we were left with 114,852 delivery and 3999 abortion cases in our study; and 462 (0.39%) of them had nonobstetric surgery under general or regional anesthesia during pregnancy. The leading surgeries were repair of cervical os (33.12%), appendectomy (17.32%), ovarian surgeries (13.64%), and fixation of fractured bone (8.01%).The risk of spontaneous abortion (4.23% vs. 2.43%, aOR:1.53; 95% CI: 1.01–2.31), antepartum hemorrhage (7.14% vs. 2.83%, aOR: 2.51; 95% CI: 1.74–3.61), pre-eclampsia/eclampsia (2.60% vs. 1.01%, aOR: 2.35; 95% CI: 1.30–4.23), gestational diabetes (2.38% vs. 0.69%, aOR: 3.12; 95% CI: 1.69–5.78), prematurity (9.06 vs. 4.90%, aOR: 3.31; 95% CI: 2.54–4.31), cesarean section (43.55% vs. 33.76%, aOR: 1.41; 95% CI: 1.17–1.71), and prolonged hospital stay (1.82% vs. 5.91%, aOR: 3.23; 95% CI: 2.16–4.83) were higher in those women who had nonobstetric surgery after adjusting for age and comorbidities.

Conclusions: Nonobstetric surgery during gestation were associated with a higher risk of spontaneous abortion, adverse delivery outcomes, cesarean section, and prolonged hospital stay.

Keywords: Pregnancy, Nonobstetric surgery, Abortion, Delivery outcome

Introduction

Nonobstetric surgeries, including those directly related to pregnancy (e.g., cerclage or ovarian cystectomy) and those which are un-related to pregnancy (e.g., appendectomy or surgery for bone fracture) [1], are performed in 0.75 to 2.0% of all pregnancies worldwide [2]. Surgery during pregnancy is associated with a higher incidence of postoperative adverse events, such as septicemia, pneumonia, urinary tract infection, and in-hospital mortality [3–5]. However, the American College of Obstetricians and Gynecologists' Committee still concluded that a pregnant woman should never be denied an indicated surgery [6]. Patients with specific disease such as acute appendicitis during pregnancy, managed conservatively, had a higher risk of shock, peritonitis, and venous thrombosis than those managed surgically [5].

* Correspondence: chinchen.chu@gmail.com
[1]Division of Women's and Children's Anesthesia, Department of Anesthesiology, Chi Mei Medical Center, 901 Zhonghua Road, Yongkang District, Tainan City 710, Taiwan

Most of the available scientific literature about this topic mainly focus on diagnosis, surgical management, and immediate maternal complications [3, 7–11]. Only few studies have reported information about abortion [12], fetal outcomes [13–15], and obstetric outcomes [13, 16] in women having nonobstetric surgery during pregnancy. Recently, a large scale British study analyzed the association of adverse obstetric outcomes in such patients [16]. However, some important adverse obstetric outcomes such as antepartum hemorrhage, premature rupture of membrane, pre-eclampsia/eclampsia, and fetal distress have still not been reported.

Besides, no similar studies are available on this topic in the Asian population. Different ethnic races may have different epidemiological profiles and perhaps different outcomes. Studies using big data from ethnicities other than Caucasian are warranted. Therefore, we aimed to assess the risk of miscarriage and adverse pregnancy outcomes following nonobstetric surgery during gestation by using a nationwide population-based database in Taiwan.

Methods

Ethical review

The present study was granted an exemption from a full ethical review by Chi Mei Hospital Institutional Review Board (Tainan, Taiwan, Chairperson Prof., Chung HsiHsing, Ethical Committee No. 10402-E04) on 12 February 2015. Since the study had a retrospective design and all types of personal identification in the database were encrypted to secure patient privacy, the committee also waived the need for obtaining informed patient consent.

Database

Taiwan launched a single-payer National Health Insurance (NHI) program on March 1, 1995. The NHI offers comprehensive medical care coverage to all Taiwan residents. As of 2015, about 22.6 million (more than 99%) of Taiwan's 22.96 million legal residents (citizens and noncitizens) were enrolled in this program. The National Health Research Dataset (NHIRD) provides encrypted patient identification numbers, gender, date of birth, dates of admission and discharge, the ICD-9-CM (International Classification of Diseases, Ninth Revision, Clinical Modification) codes of diagnoses and procedures, details of prescriptions, and costs covered and paid for by the NHI.

For longitudinal follow up of the pregnancy outcomes after nonobstetric surgery, we used the Longitudinal Health Insurance Database 2000 (LHID 2000), a sub-dataset of the NHIRD, which contains all claim data (from 1997 to 2013) of 1 million beneficiaries who were randomly selected from the system in 2000. All the registration and claim data of the sampled people constituted this longitudinal database, and their healthcare data is updated annually. There was no significant difference in age, gender, or average insured payroll-related premiums between the sample group and all enrollees. The LHID 2000 database was thus considered to have representative power of the national population [17].

Study sample

We identified delivery event using the Diagnosis Related Groups code (DRG code 0373A, 0373C, 0371A or 0373B) and abortion by the International Classification of Diseases, 9th Revision, Clinical Modification (ICD-9 CM code 634-637). They were traced back whether having a nonobstetric surgery during pregnancy (Fig. 1a and b).

Nonobstetric surgery was defined as any surgery performed during pregnancy except, (i) fetal surgery, (ii) dilatation and curettage, (iii) surgery on gestational uterus body, and (iv) cesarean delivery. Surgery on adnexa or uterine cervix was still included as nonobstetric surgery, as classified in a previous research [7].

Nonobstetric surgeries were further subclassified into four main categories: (i) digestive system (ICD-9 procedure code: 42-54), including appendectomy, biliary surgery, and hemorrhoidectomy etc., (ii) female genital system (ICD-9 procedure code: 60-64), for example, repair of cervical os and ovarian surgery etc., (iii) musculoskeletal system (ICD-9 procedure code: 76-84), e.g., open reduction and internal fixation, and (iv) other systems. Anesthesia types were identified by payment code: general (96020C~96022C) or neuraxial anesthesia (96005C~96008C). Operations performed under local or no anesthesia were excluded from the study. In addition, patients who were ever exposed to known teratogenic factors, such as chemotherapy or radiotherapy, during gestation were also excluded from the study.

Further, we determined the trimester of pregnancy by the records of the prenatal visits (sequence code v41~50). Pregnant women who had no prenatal visits or with aberrant records were excluded from the study because of the difficulty in confirming the gestational age at which the nonobstetric surgery was performed. Delivery modes were identified based on diagnosis-related groups (DRG) and surgery codes from the NHI hospital discharge data and were categorized into vaginal delivery (DRG 0373A or 0373C) and cesarean section (DRG 0371Aor 0373B).

Outcomes

We set the study outcomes as (i) abortion (ICD-9 code, 634~637), but induced abortion (635~636) was excluded, (ii) premature labor (ICD-9 code, 644), (iii) premature rupture of membrane (ICD-9 code, 658.1), (iv): Fetal distress (ICD-9 code, 656.3~4768.4), (v): antepartum hemorrhage (ICD-9 code, 641,762.0~1),(vi) pre-eclampsia/eclampsia (ICD-9 code, 642.4~642.7), (vii) gestational diabetes (ICD-9

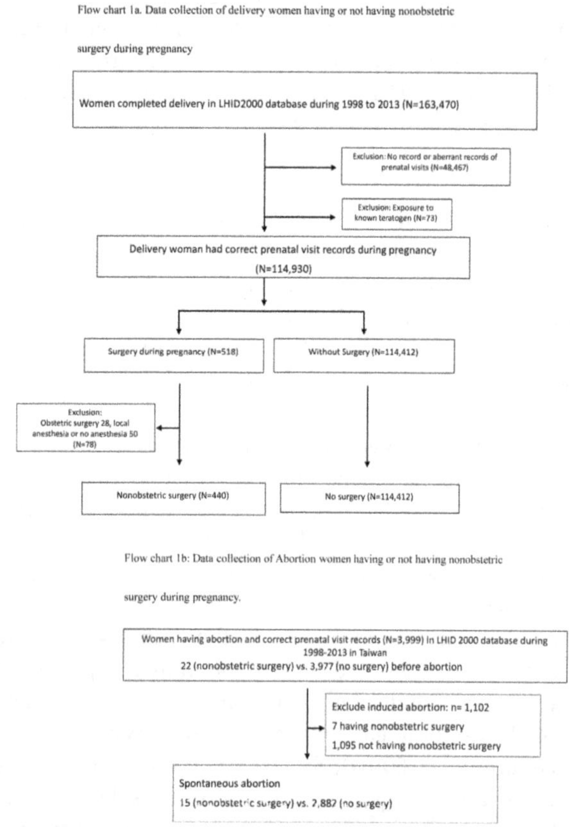

Fig. 1 Flow charts of the creation of the study sample. **a** Delivery women having or not having nonobstetric surgery during pregnancy. **b** Abortion women having or not having nonobstetric surgery during pregnancy

code, 648.8), (viii) maternal death (ICD-9 code, 761.6, 798) during delivery admission, (ix) Cesarean section (diagnosis-related group code, 0371A or 0373B), and (x) Prolonged hospital stay, defined as upper quartile of length of stay plus 1.5 times the interquartile range.

Statistical analysis

SAS 9.3.1 for Windows (SAS Institute, Inc., Cary, North Carolina, USA) was used for analysis. Continuous variables were presented as mean (SD) or median (inter-quartile range), and categorical variables were presented as number (percentile). The differences in baseline characteristics and comorbid variables between the two cohorts were evaluated using Student's t test for continuous variables and Pearson $\chi 2$or Fisher's exact tests for categorical variables. Significance was set at $p < 0.01$.

Logistic regression analyses were performed to assess the adjusted odds ratio with 95% confidence interval (CI) of adverse pregnancy outcomes between the two cohorts.

Results

Between 1997 and 2013 in LHID 2000 dataset, we identified a total of 163,470 events of delivery. After exclusion of 48,467 events without any or with aberrant prenatal visit records and 73 events having teratogenic exposures, we were left with 114,930 deliveries. After exclusion of 78 cases which underwent obstetric-related surgeries under local or no anesthesia, there were 440 deliveries which underwent nonobstetric surgeries, and 114,412 deliveries which did not undergo any surgery during pregnancy (Fig. 1a). Moreover, we identified 3999 events of abortion, and 22 of them had nonobstetric surgery during pregnancy (Fig. 1b). Totally, there were 462 (0.39%) cases having nonobstetric surgery during gestation (Table 1).

Maternal characteristics of the study groups are shown in Table 1. The proportions of patients younger than 20 years and older than 30 years were higher in the surgical group as compared to that in the non-surgical group ($p < 0.001$). Moreover, the number of pregnant mothers with incidence of multi-fetal gestation was significantly higher in the surgical group as compared to that in the non-surgical group (4.33 vs. 1.25%, $p < 0.001$). Incidence of hypertension was also significantly higher in the surgical group than that in the non-surgical group (0.87 vs. 0.17%, $p = 0.008$).

Table 1 Demographic characteristics of pregnant women in the study populations as per LHID2000[a] dataset from 1997 to 2013 in Taiwan

Characteristics	Nonobstetric surgery during pregnancy		*P*-value[b]
	No (*N* = 118,389)	Yes (*N* = 462)	
Delivery	114,412	440	
Abortion	3.977	22	
Age (Mean ± SD)	29.16 ± 4.89	29.86 ± 5.48	0.007
< 20	2810 (2.37)	16 (3.46)	< 0.001
20–29	59,426 (50.20)	189 (40.91)	
30–39	53,977 (45.59)	240 (51.95)	
≧ 40	2176 (1.84)	17 (3.68)	
Gestation			< 0.001
Singleton	116,904 (98.75)	442 (95.67)	
Multifetal	1485 (1.25)	20 (4.33)	
Comorbidities			
Diabetes mellitus	189 (0.16)	0 (0.00)	1.000
Hypertension	199 (0.17)	4 (0.87)	0.008
Ischemic heart disease	40 (0.03)	2 (0.65)	0.012
Renal disease	56 (0.05)	0 (0.00)	1.000

[a]*LHID2000* Longitudinal Health Insurance Database 2000, a sub-dataset contains all claim data of 1 million beneficiaries who were randomly selected from the system in year 2000

[b]Chi-square test or Fisher's exact test when the expected counts were fewer than 5

Data are mean ± S.D. or *n* (%). Significant different if *p*-value < 0.01

Out of the 462 cases in which non-obstetric surgeries were performed, 50.22% of surgeries were performed during 2nd trimester, whereas 36.15 and 13.64% of the surgeries were performed in the 1st and 3rd trimesters, respectively. About 76.19% of the nonobstetric surgeries were non-emergency surgeries under the Taiwan NHI definition: waiting time less than 4 h from emergency room visit to operation. Moreover, surgeries were more frequently performed under regional anesthesia in contrast to that under general anesthesia (59.74 vs. 40.26%, $p < 0.001$). The leading nonobstetric surgery was repair of cervical os (33.12%), followed by appendectomy (17.32%), ovarian surgeries (13.64%), and bone fracture surgeries (8.01%) (Table 2).

Among the 462 pregnancies with nonobstetric surgery during gestation, 440 pregnancies resulted in delivery while seven underwent induced abortion and 15 had a spontaneous abortion. The spontaneous abortion rate was higher in patients who underwent nonobstetric surgery in contrast to that in those without surgery (4.23 vs. 2.43%, $p = 0.002$). Incidence of adverse delivery events, such as premature rupture of membrane (5.63 vs. 4.33%, $p = 0.17$), fetal distress (2.16 vs. 2.64%, $p = 0.523$) and maternal death (0.23 vs. 0.06%, $p = 0.244$), were similar in these two groups (Table 3). However, patients who underwent nonobstetric surgery had a higher incidence of antepartum hemorrhage (7.14 vs. 2.83%, $p < 0.001$), pre-eclampsia/eclampsia (2.60 vs. 1.01%, $p = 0.003$), gestational diabetes (2.38 vs. 0.69%, $p < 0.001$), prematurity (9.06 vs. 4.90%, $p = 0.001$), and cesarean section (43.55 vs. 33.76%, $p < 0.001$) as compared with that in patients without any surgery. In addition, length of hospital stay for delivery was also longer in those who underwent nonobstetric surgery. (4.72 ± 4.21 vs. 3.78 ± 3.09 days, $p = 0.004$) (Table 3).

Table 2 The trimester in which the nonobstetric surgery was performed during pregnancy, as per LHID2000[a] dataset, 1997–2013, in Taiwan

Classification	*N* (%)
Surgeries	462 (100)
Trimester	
1st	167 (36.15%)
2nd	232 (50.22%)
3rd	63 (13.64%)
Emergency surgery	
Yes	110 (23.81)
No	352 (76.19)
Anesthesia	
GA	186 (40.26)
RA	276 (59.74)
Surgery	
Digestive system	115 (24.90)
Appendectomy	80 (17.32)
Hemorrhoidectomy	12 (2.60)
Biliary surgery	7 (1.52)
Others	16 (3.47)
Genital system	258 (55.85)
Repair of cervical os	153 (33.12)
Ovarian surgeries	63 (13.64)
Fallopian tube surgery	14 (3.03)
Others	28 (6.06)
Musculoskeletal system	40 (8.66)
Open reduction & internal fixation	37(8.01)
Others	3 (0.65)
Other systems	49 (10.61)

[a]*LHID2000* Longitudinal Health Insurance Database 2000, a sub-dataset containing all claims data of 1 million beneficiaries who were randomly selected from the system in year 2000

Women had nonobstetric surgery during pregnancy were associated with higher crude odds ratio of adverse outcomes, except PROM, fetal distress and maternal death during delivery. Moreover, after adjusting for age and comorbidities, pregnancies with nonobstetric surgery were still associated with a significantly higher risk of premature labor (aOR, 3.31; 95% CI, 2.54–4.31), antepartum hemorrhage (aOR, 2.51; 95% CI, 1.74–3.61), pre-eclampsia/eclampsia (aOR, 2.35; 95% CI, 1.30–4.23), gestational diabetes (aOR, 3.12; 95% CI, 1.69~5.78), cesarean section delivery (aOR, 1.41; 95% CI, 1.17–1.71), prolonged hospital stay (aOR, 3.23; 95% CI, 2.16~4.83) as compared to that in pregnancies without any surgical intervention.

The risk factors for premature labor in cases who underwent nonobstetric surgery during pregnancy were further analyzed (Table 4). Deliveries with nonobstetric surgery in the 3rd trimester had a 3.79-fold (95% CI, 1.20–11.96) odds as compared to that with surgery in the 1st trimester. Among the specific category of nonobstetric surgeries, only musculoskeletal surgery was associated with a higher risk of prematurity. Moreover, emergency cases and general anesthesia were not associated with a significantly higher risk of premature labor in contrast to non-emergency cases (aOR, 1.32; 95% CI, 0.65–2.69) or regional anesthesia (aOR, 1.78; 95% CI, 0.89–3.57).

Discussion

Using the database of 1 million randomly selected beneficiaries in Taiwan from 1997 to 2013, we noted a higher incidence and risk of spontaneous abortion, premature labor, antepartum hemorrhage, pre-eclampsia/eclampsia, gestational diabetes, and cesarean section in pregnancies with a nonobstetric surgery during their gestation in contrast to that with pregnancies without any surgery, after adjusting for age and any pre-existing comorbidities.

Table 3 The incidence, crude and adjusted odds ratio of abortion and adverse delivery outcomes in study population as per LIHD2000 dataset in Taiwan, 1997–2013

Outcome	Nonobstetric surgery during pregnancy		*P*-value	Crude OR (95% CI)[a]	Adjusted OR (95% CI)[b]
Total	No (*N* = 118,389)	Yes (*N* = 462)			
Abortion	3997 (3.36%)	22 (4.76)	0.002		
Spontaneous	2882 (2.43)	15 (4.23)		1.57 (1.04–2.36)	1.53 (1.01~2.31)
Induced	1095 (0.92)	7 (2.28)			
Delivery	114,412 (96.64)	440 (95.24)			
PROM[c]	5122 (4.33)	26 (5.63)	0.170	1.37 (0.92–2.04)	1.36 (0.91–2.02)
Fetal distress	3127 (2.64)	10 (2.16)	0.5234	0.84 (0.45–1.58)	0.83 (0.44–1.56)
Antepartum hemorrhage	3355 (2.83)	33 (7.14)	< 0.001	2.63 (1.83–3.77)	2.51 (1.74–3.61)
Pre-eclampsia/Eclampsia	1197 (1.01)	12 (2.60)	0.003	2.67 (1.50–4.74)	2.35 (1.30–4.23)
Gestational diabetes	811 (0.69)	11(2.38)	< 0.001	3.61 (1.97–6.59)	3.12 (1.69–5.78)
Prematurity	5064 (4.90)	36 (9.06)	0.001	3.43 (2.63–4.46)	3.31 (2.54–4.31)
Cesarean section	38,624 (33.76)	125 (43.55)	< 0.001	1.48 (1.22–1.79)	1.41 (1.17–1.71)
Maternal death	72 (0.06)	1(0.23)	0.244	3.62 (0.50–26.09)	3.14 (0.42–23.19)
[d]Prolonged hospital stays	2078 (1.82)	26 (5.91)	< 0.001	3.40 (2.28–5.06)	3.23 (2.16–4.83)
Hospital stay (days)					
Mean ± SD	3.78 ± 3.09	4.72 ± 4.21	< 0.001		
Median (Q1–Q4)	3 (2–5)	4 (3–5)			

Data are number (%), except hospital stay (days)
[a]*OR* odds ratio, [b]*Adjusted OR* adjusted by age and comorbidities
[c]*PROM* premature rupture of membrane, [d]Prolonged hospital stay was defined as the upper quartile of length of stay plus 1.5 times the interquartile range

Table 4 The odds ratio of premature labor in pregnant women having nonobstetric surgery as per LHID2000[a] dataset, 1997–2013, Taiwan

	Prematurity		Crude OR[b] (95% CI)	Adjusted OR[c] (95% CI)
	No = 374	Yes = 66		
Age[d] (Mean ± SD)	29.65 ± 5.61	30.86 ± 4.88	1.48 (0.93–2.35)	1.25 (0.70–2.23)
Trimester				
1st	143 (38.24)	12 (18.18)	1.00	1.00
2nd	185 (49.47)	40 (60.61)	2.58 (1.30–5.09)	2.04 (0.93–4.50)
3rd	46 (12.30)	14 (21.21)	3.63 (1.57–8.40)	4.10 (1.62–10.39)
Emergency surgery				
No	285 (76.20)	50 (75.76)	1.00	1.00
Yes	89 (23.80)	16 (24.24)	1.02 (0.56–1.89)	1.32 (0.65–2.69)
Anesthesia				
GA	159 (42.51)	15 (22.73)	1.00	1.00
RA	215 (57.49)	51 (77.27)	2.51 (1.36–4.63)	1.78 (0.89–3.57)
Surgical procedure				
Genital organ	196 (52.41)	49 (74.24)	9.00 (1.20–67.27)	5.70 (0.75–43.56)
GI	97 (25.94)	14 (21.21)	5.20 (0.66–40.95)	4.39 (0.55–34.98)
Musculoskeletal	36 (9.63)	1 (1.52)	1.00	1.00
Others	45 (12.03)	2 (3.03)	1.60 (0.14–18.36)	1.23 (0.10–14.58)

[a]*LHID 2000* Longitudinal Health Insurance Database 2000 contains claims data of 1 million beneficiaries who were randomly selected from the system in year 2000
[b]*OR* odds ratio
[c]Adjusted by age, comorbidities, and all obstetric conditions
[d]Per 10-year increase

This study is the first Asian population-based study to evaluate the pregnancy outcomes of women undergoing nonobstetric surgeries during gestation, and some of the findings are novel i.e. increased risk of antepartum hemorrhage, pre-eclampsia/eclampsia, and gestation diabetes in pregnant women who have undergone nonobstetric surgery during pregnancy.

Our analysis was based on a 17-year large-scale longitudinal database, a case control study design, and multivariable adjustments. Most previous studies were either small scale [8, 18, 19] or performed decades ago [13, 14, 19]. Although, recently, a large-scale British study [16] has been published on this topic, no similar study has been done in the Asian population; ethnic disparity may have different epidemiological profiles and diverse outcomes.

The incidence of nonobstetric surgery during pregnancy was reported to be between 0.75 and 2.0% [2]. In our study, the incidence (0.39%) is lower than 2%, which is lower as compared to that in other large-scale retrospective studies from Sweden (0.75%,1973–1981) [13] and Britain (0.73%, 2002–2012) [16]. We speculate that the racial disparity, life-style, and social-economic factors may all have contributed to this difference.

Our results revealed that the leading types of nonobstetric surgeries during pregnancy were repair of cervical os (33.1%), followed by appendectomy (17.3%), ovarian surgeries (13.6%), and repair of fractured bone (8.0%) in Asian women. Some studies excluded all surgeries on gravid uterus and fetus from nonobstetric surgeries [16]; however, some excluded only surgeries on the fetus during pregnancy from nonobstetric surgeries [7]. We followed the latter definition.

A meta-analysis of 54 studies reported that the abortion rate was 5.76% in pregnancies with nonobstetric surgeries during gestation; however, this number is difficult to interpret since matched controls were not available in that study [7]. In the recent large-scale British study, although only miscarriage during hospitalization was included, it revealed a higher spontaneous abortion rate (6.6 vs. 5.8%) in patients having nonobstetric surgery. Similarly, we also found a higher rate and risks of spontaneous abortion (4.23 vs. 2.43%, aOR 1.53, 95% CI: 1.01~2.31) in Asian women who underwent nonobstetric surgery during gestation. In contrast to the British study, we counted all abortions (both in- and out-patient services) after the nonobstetric surgery. Besides, we observed that the abortion rate was lower in Asians as compared to that in Caucasians in both groups of pregnant women i.e. those who underwent or those who did not require any nonobstetric surgery.

In previous studies, the incidence of prematurity after nonobstetric surgery was estimated to be around 3.5~8.2% [7]. In our study, risk factors associated with prematurity were analyzed further, including maternal age, trimester when the surgery was performed, emergency or elective surgery, type of surgical procedure and the choice of anesthesia. In the present study, it was observed that surgeries performed in the third trimester were associated with an increased risk of premature labor further as compared to those performed in the first and second trimester. The result is compatible with what had been observed in the study in 2001 [20].

Asides from abortion and preterm delivery, we also found increased risks of cesarean section and long hospital stays. These were similar to previous reports [16, 21, 22]. Taken together, increased abortion, preterm delivery, cesarean section rate and longer in-patient stay are the common and most reliable findings in the existing literature.

With the improvement in anesthetic techniques, perioperative care and surgical techniques, maternal death has decreased to around 0.004~0.025% [7, 11, 16, 23]. In our study, we found a relatively higher mortality rate (0.064%, 72 vs. 1 in the non-surgical and surgical group, respectively) than previous reports. Especially, the mortality in nonobstetric surgery patients yields a high mortality rate (0.23%), however, the wide range of 95% CI (0.42~23.19) indicated that our nonobstetric surgical group is not large enough to analyze the rare event of mortality. We suspected the large number of patients without prenatal visits (46,467) excluded from our study might distort the current observed results. However, the large-scale British study demonstrated a 4.67-fold increase in mortality risk (95% CI, 1.79–8.93) in the pregnant women with surgical procedure during gestation [16].

The mechanisms of our novel findings of increased risk of antepartum hemorrhage, pre-eclampsia/eclampsia and gestational diabetes were not determined, because this is a retrospective database study. However, there were some possible explanations. Firstly, the inflammatory reaction or scar formation after nonobstetric surgery may further increase the complexity of anatomy of abdominal organs and pregnancy physiology [24]. Secondly, these adverse delivery outcomes may be delayed sequelae of nonobstetric surgery, which were reportedly associated with increased risks of in-hospital pneumonia, septicemia, and postoperative bleeding [3]. Thirdly, some of the nonobstetric surgical diseases persist as long term systemic disease even after surgical treatment, e.g. patients with Crohn disease [25].

Limitations

Our findings need to be interpreted in the context of some inherent limitations of a claim database. Firstly, identifying these cases, associated comorbid disorders, and adverse outcomes was dependent upon the accuracy of the ICD-9-CM coding. Although, these codes were reviewed and validated by auditors of medical records for the insurance system to ensure the accuracy of the claims, incorrect coding might still exist. Secondly, due to lack of reporting about fetal gestational age, we had to estimate the trimester of pregnancy using the records of prenatal visits. Therefore, we had to exclude 48,467 (29.65%) pregnant women who did not have any or with aberrant prenatal visit records from our study. This might result in an equally distribution of adverse outcomes in the two groups of patients, and caused an under- or over-estimate of association of some adverse outcomes. Thirdly, some important individual data about lifestyle behaviors, such as smoking and alcohol drinking habits, body mass index, and the severity of comorbid conditions were not available in the NHIRD. Thus, we could not adjust for these variables as contributing factors. Fourthly, fetal information was lacking in the database; therefore, we could not analyze the fetal outcome, any congenital anomaly, still birth, or fetal death. This also restricted further discussion about the teratogenic effect associated with the surgeries or anesthesia. Lastly, repeat procedures in duplicate patients were excluded. This reduced the total case number to be analyzed; however, these patients might have different outcomes.

Conclusions

Nonobstetric surgery during pregnancy was associated with an increased risk of miscarriage, premature labor, and higher cesarean section rate. Further large-scale prospective studies with detailed fetal information may help to clarify the effects of nonobstetric surgery on parturient women and the newborns.

Abbreviations

95% CI: 95% confidence interval; aOR: adjusted odds ratio; ICD-9-CM: International Classification of Diseases, Ninth Revision, Clinical Modification; LHID 2000: Longitudinal Health Insurance Database 2000; NHI: National Health Insurance; OR: Odds ratio

Acknowledgements

This study is based on data from the National Health Insurance Research Database provided by the Taiwan Bureau of National Health Insurance, Department of Health, and managed by the National Health Research Institutes. The interpretation and conclusions contained herein do not represent those of the Bureau of National Health Insurance, the Department of Health, or the National Health Research.

Funding

No founding.

Authors' contributions

CHY reviewed the literature, designed the study, and drafted the manuscript. SFW, and YCC helped design the study and did the statistical analyses. JYC, YJC and MPW reviewed the literature and interpreted the results. CHH helped do the statistical analyses, and revised the manuscript. JJW revised the manuscript and provided administrative and technical support. CCC conceived and helped design the study, coordinated and interpreted the results, and revised the manuscript. All authors have read and approved the final version of this manuscript.

Authors' information

Chin-Chen Chu (M.D., Ph.D.) is a senior anesthesiologist at Chi Mei Medical Center. Chu is also a professor and works as the director of the division of women's and children's anesthesia.

Competing interests

The authors declare that they have no competing interests.

Author details

[1]Division of Women's and Children's Anesthesia, Department of Anesthesiology, Chi Mei Medical Center, 901 Zhonghua Road, Yongkang District, Tainan City 710, Taiwan. [2]Department of Healthcare Administration and Medical Informatics, Kaohsiung Medical University, 100, Shih-Chuan 1st Road, Kaohsiung 807, Taiwan. [3]Department of Medical Research, Chi Mei Medical Center, 901 Zhonghua Road, Yongkang District, Tainan City 710, Taiwan. [4]Department of Pharmacy, Chia Nan University of Pharmacy and Science, Chi Mei Medical Center, 60, Sec. 1, Erren Rd., Rende Dist., Tainan City 717, Taiwan. [5]Department of Senior Citizen Service Management, Chia Nan University of Pharmacy and Science, Chi Mei Medical Center, No.60, Sec. 1, Erren Rd., Rende Dist, Tainan City 717, Taiwan. [6]Division of Urogynecology and Pelvic Floor Reconstruction, Department of Obstetrics and Gynecology, Chi Mei Medical Center, 901 Zhonghua Road, Yongkang District, Tainan City 710, Taiwan. [7]Center of General Education, Chia Nan University of Pharmacy and Science, Chi Mei Medical Center, 60, Sec. 1, Erren Rd., Rende Dist.,, Tainan City 717, Taiwan.

References

1. Kuczkowski KM. Nonobstetric surgery during pregnancy: what are the risks of anesthesia? Obstet Gynecol Surv. 2004;59(1):52–6.
2. Reitman E, Flood P. Anaesthetic considerations for non-obstetric surgery during pregnancy. Br J Anaesth. 2011;107(Suppl 1):i72–8.
3. Huang SY, Lo PH, Liu WM, Cherng YG, Yeh CC, Chen TL, Liao CC. Outcomes after nonobstetric surgery in pregnant patients: A Nationwide Study. Mayo Clin Proc. 2016;91(9):1166–72.
4. Ali SA, Gupta S, Sehgal R, Vogel V. Survival outcomes in pregnancy associated breast cancer: a retrospective case control study. Breast J. 2012; 18(2):139–44.
5. Abbasi N, Patenaude V, Abenhaim HA. Management and outcomes of acute appendicitis in pregnancy-population-based study of over 7000 cases. BJOG. 2014;121(12):1509–14.
6. ACOG. Committee opinion number 284, august 2003: nonobstetric surgery in pregnancy. Obstet Gynecol. 2003;102(2):431.
7. Cohen-Kerem R, Railton C, Oren D, Lishner M, Koren G. Pregnancy outcome following non-obstetric surgical intervention. Am J Surg. 2005;190(3):467–73.
8. Erekson EA, Brousseau EC, Dick-Biascoechea MA, Ciarleglio MM, Lockwood CJ, Pettker CM. Maternal postoperative complications after nonobstetric antenatal surgery. J Matern Fetal Neonatal Med. 2012;25(12):2639–44.
9. Gilo NB, Amini D, Landy HJ. Appendicitis and cholecystitis in pregnancy. Clin Obstet Gynecol. 2009;52(4):586–96.
10. Coleman MT, Trianfo VA, Rund DA. Nonobstetric emergencies in pregnancy: trauma and surgical conditions. Am J Obstet Gynecol. 1997;177(3):497–502.
11. Moore HB, Juarez-Colunga E, Bronsert M, Hammermeister KE, Henderson WG, Moore EE, Meguid RA. Effect of pregnancy on adverse outcomes after general surgery. JAMA Surg. 2015;150(7):637–43.
12. Duncan PG, Pope WD, Cohen MM, Greer N. Fetal risk of anesthesia and surgery during pregnancy. Anesthesiology. 1986;64(6):790–4.
13. Mazze RI, Kallen B. Reproductive outcome after anesthesia and operation during pregnancy: a registry study of 5405 cases. Am J Obstet Gynecol. 1989;161(5):1178–85.
14. Jenkins TM, Mackey SF, Benzoni EM, Tolosa JE, Sciscione AC. Non-obstetric surgery during gestation: risk factors for lower birthweight. Aust N Z J Obstet Gynaecol. 2003;43(1):27–31.

15. Choi JJ, Mustafa R, Lynn ET, Divino CM. Appendectomy during pregnancy: follow-up of progeny. J Am Coll Surg. 2011;213(5):627–32.
16. Balinskaite V, Bottle A, Sodhi V, Rivers A, Bennett PR, Brett SJ, Aylin P. The risk of adverse pregnancy outcomes following nonobstetric surgery during pregnancy: estimates from a retrospective cohort study of 6.5 million pregnancies. Ann Surg. 2017;266(2):260–6.
17. Bureau of National Health Insurance D, Executive Yuan, Taiwan:, Database IttNHIR, (NHIRD). https://nhird.nhri.org.tw/en/Data_Subsets.html. Accessed 8 Nov 2018.
18. Shambe IH, Dikkol N, Ozoilo KN. Pregnancy outcome following non-obstetric abdominal surgery in Jos University teaching hospital: a 5-year retrospective study. Niger J Clin Pract. 2016;19(5):591–4.
19. Fardiazar Z, Derakhshan I, Torab R, Vahedi A, Goldust M. Maternal-neonatal outcome in pregnancies with non-obstetric laparotomy during pregnancy. Pak J Biol Sci. 2014;17(2):260–5.
20. Visser BC, Glasgow RE, Mulvihill KK, Mulvihill SJ. Safety and timing of nonobstetric abdominal surgery in pregnancy. Dig Surg. 2001;18(5):409–17.
21. Wei PL, Keller JJ, Liang HH, Lin HC. Acute appendicitis and adverse pregnancy outcomes: a nationwide population-based study. J Gastrointest Surg. 2012;16(6):1204–11.
22. Baldwin EA, Borowski KS, Brost BC, Rose CH. Antepartum nonobstetrical surgery at >/=23 weeks' gestation and risk for preterm delivery. Am J Obstet Gynecol. 2015;212(2):232.e1–5.
23. Sharp HT. Gastrointestinal surgical conditions during pregnancy. Clin Obstet Gynecol. 1994;37(2):306–15.
24. Tan EK, Tan EL. Alterations in physiology and anatomy during pregnancy. Best Pract Res Clin Obstet Gynaecol. 2013;27(6):791–802.
25. Hatch Q, Champagne BJ, Maykel JA, Davis BR, Johnson EK, Bleier JI, Francone TD, Steele SR. The impact of pregnancy on surgical Crohn disease: an analysis of the Nationwide inpatient sample. J Surg Res. 2014;190(1):41–6.

15

Three-dimensional power Doppler ultrasound evaluation of placental blood flow in normal monochorionic diamniotic twin pregnancies

Wei Sun[1], Shaowei Yin[2], Qiuju Wei[3], Ying Zhang[1], Zeyu Yang[1], Ailu Cai[1*], Yu Wang[1] and Wenjia Lei[1]

Abstract

Background: Monochorionic diamniotic (MCDA) twin pregnancies are at higher risk of adverse outcomes and complications, which are attributed to the influence of placental morphology in MCDA twins. Monitoring of placental function is an important index for clinical decisions. The aim of our study was to evaluate the placental blood flow estimated using three-dimensional power Doppler (3D-PD) ultrasound and the vascular indices distribution with gestational age (GA) in normal MCDA twin pregnancies.

Methods: One hundred four MCDA twin pregnancies and 106 singleton pregnancies (GA range, 14–32 weeks) were included in this prospective study. 3D-PD volume data of each fetus was obtained separately from the placenta at the site of umbilical cord insertion. We analyzed the volume data using sonobiopsy technique. The placental vascularization index (VI), flow index (FI) and vascularizationflow index (VFI), were auto-calculated. The means and standard deviation values of three vascular indices per fetus were calculated and regression analysis of the vascular indices as a function of GA was performed in twin pregnancies. The vascular indices of twin and singleton pregnancies were compared using independent *t*-test.

Results: There were no significant differences in VI, FI or VFI among the fetuses of twins ($p > 0.05$). These vascular indices increased over the course of pregnancy ($p < 0.05$). We obtained the regression equations for the indices as a function of GA in days: VI = exp. (4.369–28.533/GA) ($R^2 = 0.699$, $p < 0.05$), FI = exp. (3.916–13.003/GA) ($R^2 = 0.511$, $p < 0.05$), and VFI = exp. (3.577–37.468/GA) ($R^2 = 0.675$, $p < 0.05$). There were no significant differences in three vascular indices between MCDA twin and singleton groups ($p > 0.05$).

Conclusions: 3D-PD placental data using sonobiopsy technique could reflect the placental blood flow of each twin, which could be applied to the study of placental perfusion in MCDA twin pregnancies. This study also presented the vascular indices distribution with GA in normal twin pregnancies, which might be useful for early detection of MCDA complications.

Keywords: Monochorionic, Three-dimensional power Doppler, Twin, Prenatal ultrasound, Placenta

* Correspondence: caiailu1224@126.com
[1]Department of Sonography, Shengjing Hospital of China Medical University, Shenyang, China

Background

Monochorionic diamniotic (MCDA) twin pregnancies are at higher risk of adverse outcomes than single or dichorionic diamniotic twin pregnancies, which are attributed to the influence of placental morphology in MCDA twins [1]. The complications of MCDA twin pregnancies include twin-to-twin transfusion syndrome, selective intrauterine growth restriction, twin anemia polycythemia sequence and intra-uterine demise due to uneven blood flow across placental inter-twin vascular anastomoses and/or unequal placental share [2]. Therefore, MCDA twin pregnancies need more monitoring for early detection of complications.

The placenta is an important organ to maintain pregnancy. Monitoring of placental function is an important index for clinical decisions [3]. A number of Doppler studies of placental circulation in normal and pathological pregnancies have been performed. Due to the low velocity of blood flow in the placental vascular villi, conventional color Doppler may lose some blood flow signals to reflect the placental internal perfusion. The pathological basis of abnormal blood flow in umbilical artery is the reduction of the number of placental villi. Reduction of placental blood perfusion comes earlier than the umbilical resistance index. Three-dimensional power Doppler (3D-PD) ultrasound has been used to monitor the placental perfusion, which is not affected by the angle of ultrasound detection or blood flow velocity [4]. 3D-PD, which displays vascular patterns and Doppler signals within tissues, provides estimates of three vascular indices: vascularization index (VI), flow index (FI), and vascularizationflow index (VFI) [5, 6].

3D-PD has been widely used in quantitative assessment of fetal/placental blood perfusion of singleton pregnancies [7–11], with little information in twin pregnancies due to the complexity of the placenta. In our study, we prospectively acquired the volume data of twin pregnancies using sonobiopsy technique and evaluate the vascular indices distribution with gestational age (GA), then we compared the vascular indices with those of singleton pregnancies to show the effectiveness of 3D-PD ultrasound in evaluation of placental blood flow in MCDA twin pregnancies.

Methods

MCDA twin pregnancies (GA range, 14–32 weeks) were included in this prospective study in Shengjing hospital from August 2015 to February 2018. Chorionicity was based on first-trimester ultrasound findings and confirmed by postpartum placental pathology. GA was confirmed by last menstruation and early pregnancy ultrasound examination. Exclusion criteria were as follows: unclear display of umbilical cord insertion site; placenta previa; velamentous cord insertion; the distance between the umbilical cord insertions ≤5 cm; fetal malformations or complications; fetal abdominal circumference and/or estimated fetal weight below the tenth percentile for GA; pregnant women with obvious abnormalities or hereditary diseases. The MCDA twins that meet the criteria were included in our study. The twin pregnancies were divided into 19 subgroups according to GA; each group included 5–7 cases. Accordingly, we collected the similar number of singleton fetuses in each GA. A control group was selected from low-risk singleton pregnancies attending our hospital between gestational weeks 14 and 32 for routine ultrasound scan. After delivery, only cases with uneventful pregnancy course were considered for comparison.

This study was approved by the hospital ethics committee. All individual participants included in the study signed the informed consent. All fetuses were followed up and confirmed to be normal after birth. And the placentae of twin pregnancies were confirmed MCDA.

Ultrasound examination

The Voluson E8 4D ultrasound system (GE Healthcare Austria GmbH & Co., Pfaffing, Austria) with a 4.0–8.0 MHz transabdominal transducer was used for sonographic examinations. An initial two-dimensional conventional study was conducted to obtain general fetal and placental information. At 3D acquisition, the following power Doppler settings were applied to standardize evaluations of placental blood flow: pulse repetition frequency, 0.9 kHz; frequency, low; quality, norm; balance, 170; filter, 2; wall motion filter, low-1; smooth, 4/5; artifact, on. Each fetal placental sample was examined in 3D rendering mode. The power Doppler sampling frame was placed on the connection point between the placenta and umbilical cord. Each gain value was set individually. The sub-noise gain setting was applied to allow the attenuation of power Doppler signal due to different maternal abdominal wall thicknesses and placental sites. At first, the maximum gain value was set and then lowered to a level that could eliminate artifacts and get an accurate image of placental blood vessels [12, 13]. In pregnancies with posterior placentae, the probe was inclined laterally to bring the placenta closer to the probe. The technique adopted a fixed 35° scanning angle to gather the 3D volume information close to each fetal umbilical cord insertions. If motion artifacts appeared, acquisition was repeated to obtain clear views of 3D-PD volumes.

The volumes were measured using the virtual organ computer-aided analysis (VOCAL) program (4D View; GE Healthcare Austria GmbH & Co) by one person. The technique described by Mercé et al. was used for 3D-PD evaluation of the placenta, which was a reproducible and validated method [14–16]. The obtained 3D volumes were rotated to locate the area with the highest vascular density. The sphere mode was activated to contain the placental total thickness, while excluding vessels from basal and chorionic plates (Fig. 1). Three indices (range, 0–100) were used for quantitative evaluation of placental blood perfusion of a sphere sample (Fig. 2). VI referred to the percentage of the number of color voxels in the volume of interest. FI referred to the average amplitude values of all color voxels. VFI combined the vessel presence and flow information [6]. The same 3D volume data of each twin was measured three times. The average values of VI, FI and VFI were calculated for each twin.

Data analysis

The clinical characteristics between MCDA twin and singleton groups were compared using independent *t*-test and Chi-square testing. Difference of three vascular indices between the fetuses of each twin was compared using paired samples *t*-test. Kolmogorov–Smirnov tests were used to confirm the normal distribution of three vascular indices. The means and standard deviation values of three vascular indices per fetus were calculated and regression analysis of the vascular indices as a function of GA was performed in twin pregnancies. The vascular indices of two groups were compared using independent *t*-test. We performed a test–retest series to assess the intraobserver and interobserver variation in measurements. Thirty MCDA twins were examined in duplicate by the same examiner and re-examined by a second examiner. All examiners were blinded to all previous results. All data processing was performed with SPSS 23.0 statistical software (SPSS, Inc., Chicago, IL, USA). $P < 0.05$ was considered statistical significance.

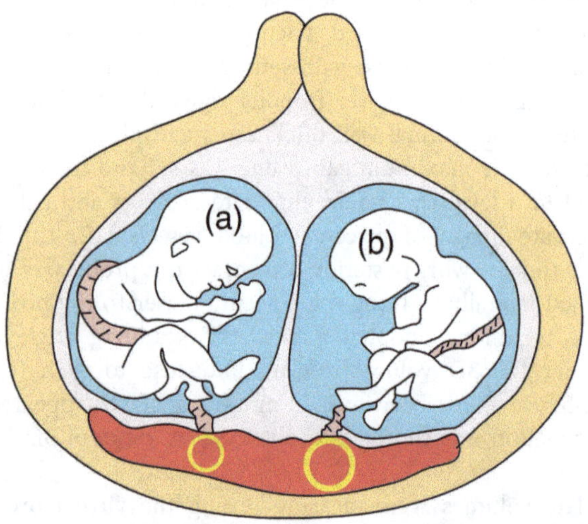

Fig. 1 Schematic representation of three-dimensional power Doppler of each fetal placental volume in twin pregnancy. The sphere (yellow sphere frame) included placental tissue between the chorionic and basal plate close to each fetal (fetus **a** and fetus **b**) umbilical cord insertion site

Results

A total of 121 MCDA twin pregnancies and 119 singleton pregnancies (GA range, 14–32 weeks) were included in the study. The volume acquisition of 17 twins and 13 singleton fetuses was unsuccessful because of fetal shadowing or frequent fetal movement. The acquisition was successful in 86% (104/121) / 89% (106/119) of twin/singleton pregnancies.

There were no significant differences in maternal age, parity and BMI between the two groups ($p > 0.05$). Table 1 presented the comparative characteristics of subjects between the MCDA twin and singleton groups. There were no significant differences in VFI, FI, and VI between the fetuses of normal MCDA twins ($p > 0.05$). The vascular indices, VI, FI and VFI were plotted as a function of GA on a curve. The scatterplots revealed a positive relationship between the three indices and GA. The regression equations for three indices as a function of GA in days were as follows: VI = exp. (4.369–28.533/GA) ($R^2 = 0.699$, $p < 0.05$), FI = exp. (3.916–13.003/GA) ($R^2 = 0.511$, $p < 0.05$), and VFI = exp. (3.577–37.468/GA) ($R^2 = 0.675$, $p < 0.05$) (Fig. 3). Table 2 listed the mean values and standard deviations of the three vascular indices of MCDA fetuses by GA from week 14 to 32. There were no significant differences in three vascular indices between MCDA twin and singleton groups ($p > 0.05$). Line charts displayed the comparisons of vascular values between two groups (Fig. 4).

Intra-observer variations for measurements of placental VI, FI and VFI were 5.7, 15.5 and 9.1%, respectively, and inter-observer variations were 7.9, 17.8 and 8.1%, respectively.

Discussion

MCDA twins required more attention for early detection of complications. The placental 3D-PD indices acquired by sonobiopsy technique could reflect the placental blood flow of each twin in MCDA twin pregnancies. Our study provided reference ranges for the placental indices VI, FI, VFI in MCDA twins between gestational weeks 14 and 32, measured using 3D-PD combined with VOCAL.

Many previous reports on measurement of placental blood flow focused on singleton pregnancies. Our study showed the vascular indices increased as pregnancy progressed, consistent with some of them [14, 17]. Some scholars reported different results, due to different analytical methods. De Paula et al. analyzed the vascular indices by 3D-PD scanning the whole placental volume and presented consistent distributions throughout gestational period [16]. This method was more suitable for

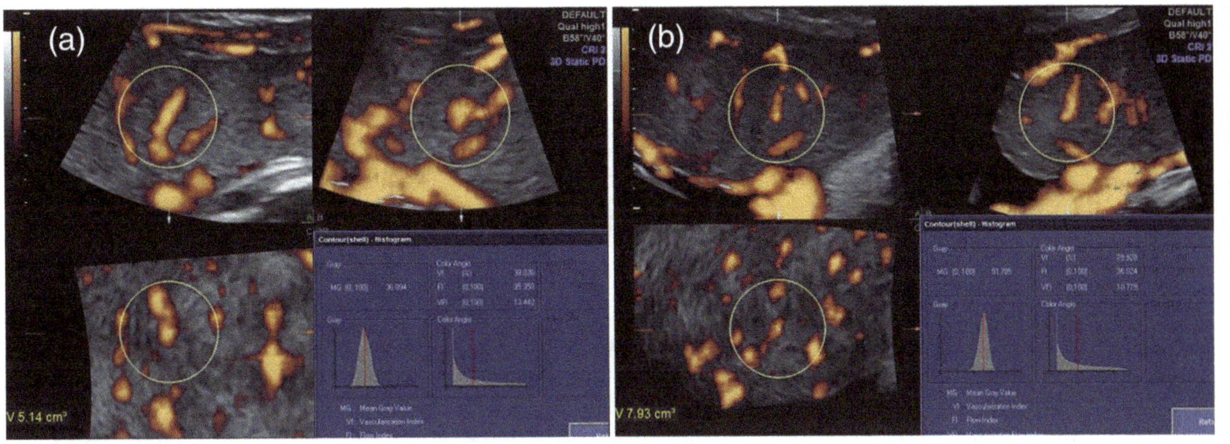

Fig. 2 Acquisition of placental volumes with three-dimensional power Doppler in twin pregnancy. The volume data was acquired close to the umbilical cord implantation site of a normal monochorionic diamniotic twin pregnancy (fetus **a** and fetus **b**) at gestational week 32^{+6}. The sphere volume (yellow sphere frame) varied according to placental thickness. Placental indices of fetus **a**: volume 5.14 cm^3; VI 38.026; FI 35.35; VFI 13.442. Placental indices of fetus **b**: volume 7.93 cm^3; VI 29.92; FI 36.024; VFI 10.779. FI, Flow index; VFI, Vascularizationflow index; VI, Vascularization index

study of small placentae, such as early pregnancies [18, 19]. MCDA twins shared one placenta; it was difficult to distinguish the placental part of each twin. It was uneasy to scan the whole placental volume in late pregnancy with fetal shadowing. However, it was feasible to catch the site of the umbilical cord insertions of each twin. In our study, we acquired the 3D-PD placental data with Mercé's sonobiopsy at the site of each fetal umbilical cord insertion [13]. This method could be used throughout the gestational period. There were no significant differences in VI, FI and VFI of fetuses among MCDA twin and singleton pregnancies. 3D-PD placental data using sonobiopsy technique could reflect the placental blood flow of each twin, which could be applied to the study of placental perfusion in MCDA twin pregnancies.

All MCDA placentae had inter-twin anastomoses. Three principal types of these anastomoses existed, including arteriovenous anastomoses (AVAs), arterioarterial anastomoses (AAAs) and venovenous anastomoses (VVVs). AAAs and VVVs connections were superficial without interposed villous vascular trees. During volume acquisition, we excluded the blood vessels from basal and chorionic plates. Thus, AAAs and VVVs connections had no effect on the results. AVAs ended in a shared cotyledon and existed in the vascular equator between the twins, often far from the umbilical cord insertion site. The sample volume varied according to placental thickness. In this study, placental thickness was less than 5 cm in all cases. MCDA twins with an umbilical cord entrance distance of less than 5 cm were excluded to ensure each fetal independent volume measurements.

Some reports emphasized that the application of 3D-PD should consider the impact of depth of measurement due to acoustic attenuation [20–22]. However, in some clinical studies, there were no significant differences in vascular indices based on placental position, despite the expected attenuation [6, 23, 24]. The signal loss due to attenuation by depth might be compensated by the false Doppler signal generated by the time gain control setting [25]. However, we could not calculate the amount of difference between loss of signal with attenuation and false Doppler signal. There were 18 twin pregnancies with posterior placentae, 7 twin pregnancies with fundal wall placentae in our research. These 25 twin pregnancies had a good visualization of each fetal umbilical cord insertion. We applied some methods to reduce the impact of depth. The probe was inclined laterally to bring the placenta closer to the probe. Individual adjustments of PD were applied for adequate assessment of placental blood flow [12, 13, 25]. From the third trimester on, it was hard to display the umbilical cord insertion sites of MCDA twins in fundal wall or posterior placentae. Therefore, in the third trimester, only the MCDA twins with anterior placentae were enrolled in the study.

Table 1 Comparative characteristic of subjects between the MCDA twin and singleton groups

	MCDA twin group ($n = 104$)	Singleton group ($n = 106$)
Maternal age (years old)	29.2 ± 6.2	27.7 ± 3.4
Parity (primapara/multipara)	61 (58.7%)/43 (41.3%)	56 (53.3%)/50 (46.7%)
BMI	29.9 ± 4.3	27.6 ± 4.0
Gestational age at time of delivery (weeks)	35 ± 3.4[a]	38 ± 2.2

BMI body mass index, *MCDA* monochorionic diamniotic, [a], $p < 0.05$, data were presented compared with the singleton group

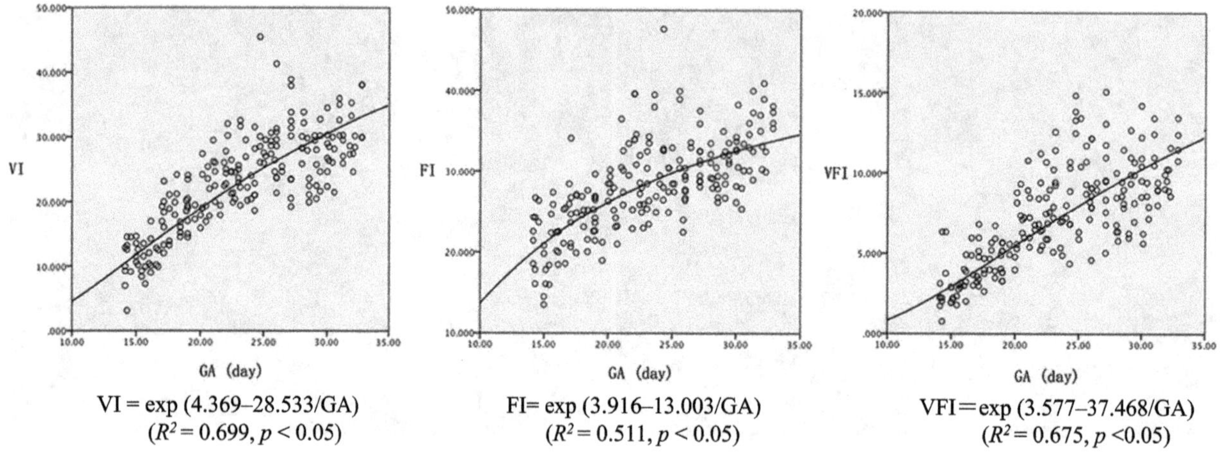

Fig. 3 Scatterplots of vascularization index, flow index and vascularizationflow index versus gestational age. Curve regression lines indicate the mean values. VI = exp. (4.369–28.533/GA) (R^2 = 0.699, p < 0.05); FI = exp. (3.916–13.003/GA) (R^2 = 0.511, p < 0.05); VFI = exp. (3.577–37.468/GA) (R^2 = 0.675, p < 0.05). GA, Gestational age; FI, Flow index; VFI, Vascularizationflow index; VI, Vascularization index

3D-PD could display intra-placental vascular tree and quantitatively assessment of placental blood flow [14],which could not be done by 2D Doppler. The vascular indices obtained by sonobiopsy technique showed good intraclass and interclass correlation in our study. It was easy to master the 3D-PD acquisition method. Data post-analysis required time and expertise. However, time would be shortened as experience increased. Therefore, the 3D-PD technique could be applied to traditional ultrasound for monitoring placental blood perfusion in twin pregnancies.

There were some limitations to this study. It was hard to display the umbilical cord insertion sites at an older GA because of the shadowing of twins and crowed

Table 2 Sonographic measurements of placental indices of monochorionic diamniotic twins by gestational age

GA (week)	Number of fetuses	VI			FI			VFI		
		M	-SD~ + SD	-2SD~ + 2SD	M	-SD~ + SD	-2SD~ + 2SD	M	-SD~ + SD	-2SD~ + 2SD
14~	10	10.6	7–14.2	3.4–17.8	22.2	18.5–25.9	14.8–29.6	3.1	1.2–5	−0.7-6.9
15~	12	11.1	8.9–13.3	6.7–15.5	19.8	15.2–24.4	10.6–29	2.5	2–3	1.5–3.5
16~	10	11.8	9.4–14.2	7–16.6	21.7	19.2–24.2	16.7–26.7	3.9	2.7–5.1	1.5–6.3
17~	12	17.2	13.7–20.7	10.2–24.2	25.4	21.5–29.3	17.6–33.2	4.2	2.9–5.5	1.6–6.8
18~	10	18.4	15.4–21.4	12.4–24.4	24.2	21.8–26.6	19.4–29	4.9	3.9–5.9	2.9–6.9
19~	10	18.9	15.7–22.1	12.5–25.3	24.2	20.9–27.5	17.6–30.8	4.6	3.6–5.6	2.6–6.6
20~	12	20.7	17–24.2	13.3–28.1	26.3	23.4–29.2	20.5–32.1	6.7	5.1–8.3	3.5–9.9
21~	10	23.4	19.8–27	16.2–30.6	29.4	25.3–33.5	21.2–37.6	7.5	5.9–9.1	4.3–10.7
22~	14	24.6	21–28.2	17.4–31.8	30.6	25.4–35.8	20.2–41	7.6	5.7–9.5	3.8–11.4
23~	12	25.1	20.8–29.4	16.5–33.7	30.3	25–35.6	19.7–40.9	8.1	5.6–10.6	3.1–13.1
24~	12	26.5	19.2–33.8	11.9–41.1	31	25.2–36.8	19.4–42.6	9.8	6.5–13.1	3.2–16.4
25~	10	27.7	25.9–29.5	24.1–31.3	30.5	24.8–36.2	19.1–41.9	9.2	6.8–11.6	4.4–14
26~	10	28	22.2–33.8	16.4–39.6	29.4	27–31.8	24.6–34.2	9	6.8–11.2	4.6–13.4
27~	10	29.1	22–36.2	14.9–43.3	31.6	28.5–34.7	25.4–37.8	9.8	6.8–12.8	3.8–15.8
28~	12	26.9	22.5–31.3	18.1–35.7	29.4	27.3–31.5	25.2–33.6	8.2	6.5–9.9	4.8–11.6
29~	10	26.5	22.3–30.7	18.1–34.9	31.2	28.8–33.6	26.4–36	9.1	6.9–11.3	4.7–13.5
30~	12	27.3	23.7–30.9	20.1–34.5	31.1	27.3–34.9	23.5–38.7	9.2	6.7–11.7	4.2–14.2
31~	10	30.2	26.8–33.6	23.4–37	34.4	31–37.8	27.6–41.2	10.2	8.5–11.9	6.8–13.6
32~	10	31.5	27–36	22.5–40.5	35.3	31.6–39	27.9–42.7	10.7	9.2–12.2	7.7–13.7

FI flow index, *GA* gestational age, *M* mean, *SD* standard deviation, *VFI* Vascularizationflow index, *VI* Vascularization index

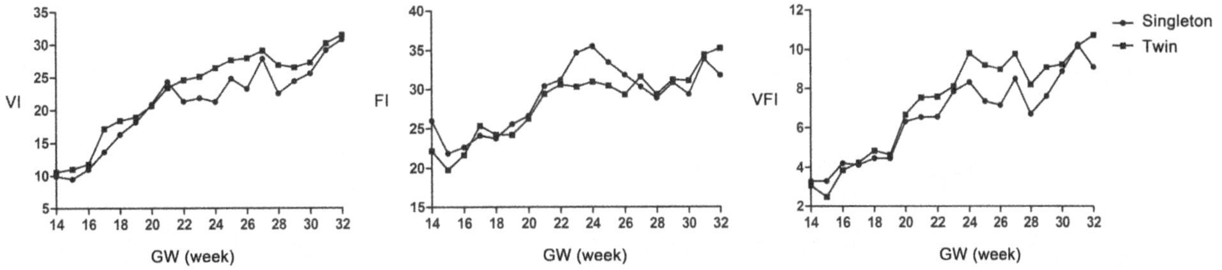

Fig. 4 Comparisons of vascularization index, flow index and vascularizationflow index between twin and singleton pregnancies. Dots represented the mean values at each GA of singleton pregnancies. Squares represented the mean values at each GA of monochorionic diamniotic twin pregnancies. There were no significant differences of VI, FI, and VFI between MCDA twin and singleton pregnancies ($p > 0.05$). GW, Gestational week; FI, Flow index; VFI, Vascularizationflow index; VI, Vascularization index

space. We didn't get a certain amount of volume data beyond 32 weeks of gestation. Nevertheless, complications of MCDA twin pregnancies mostly occured between 15 and 26 weeks of gestation [2]. There were some limitations in the study of changes of 3D-PD placental indices in the third trimester of MCDA twin pregnancies, thus further studies with larger cohorts of women in late pregnancy were needed to confirm these results. There were 25 twin pregnancies with posterior or fundal wall placentae in our research. To some extent, the inclusion of twin pregnancies with posterior or fundal wall placentae made the result about the changes in VI, FI and VFI before GA 28 might be inaccurate due to depth attenuation.

Conclusions

3D-PD placental data using sonobiopsy technique could reflect the placental blood flow of each twin, which could be applied to the study of placental perfusion in MCDA twin pregnancies. This study also presented the vascular indices distribution with GA in normal twin pregnancies, which might be useful for early detection of MCDA complications.

Abbreviations

3D-PD: Three-Dimensional Power Doppler; AAAs: Arterioarterial Anastomoses; AVAs: Arteriovenous Anastomoses; FI: Flow Index; GA: Gestational Age; MCDA: Monochorionic Diamniotic; VFI: Vascularizationflow Index; VI: Vascularization Index; VOCAL: Virtual Organ Computer-Aided Analysis; VVs: Venovenous Anastomoses

Acknowledgements

We thank for all the medical specialists who helped collecting the experimental data. We gratefully acknowledge Prof. Weidong Ren and Prof. Limei Xie for their constructive comments on the design and results of our study.

Funding

We would like to thank Outstanding Scientific Fund of Shengjing Hospital of China Medical University (No. 201209) for funding this study in the collection of data.

Authors' contributions

WS, AIC designed the study. WS, SwY, YZ, ZyY collected the data. WS, QjW, AIC, YW, WjL performed the data analyses. YZ, ZyY, AIC, QjW revised the article critically. All authors read and approved the final manuscript.

Competing interests

The authors declare that they have no competing interests.

Author details

[1]Department of Sonography, Shengjing Hospital of China Medical University, Shenyang, China. [2]Department of Obstetrics and Gynecology, Shengjing Hospital of China Medical University, Shenyang, China. [3]Department of Obstetrics and Gynecology, the University of Tennessee Health Science Center, Memphis, TN, USA.

References

1. Akkermans J, Peeters SH, Klumper FJ, Lopriore E, Middeldorp JM, Oepkes D. Twenty-five years of Fetoscopic laser coagulation in twin-twin transfusion syndrome: a systematic review. Fetal Diagn Ther. 2015;38(4):241–53.
2. Benoit RM, Baschat AA. Twin-to-twin transfusion syndrome: prenatal diagnosis and treatment. Am J Perinatol. 2014;31(7):583–94.
3. Taguchi T, Ishii K, Hayashi S, Mabuchi A, Murata M, Mitsuda N. Clinical features and prenatal risk factors for hypertensive disorders in twin pregnancies. J Obstet Gynaecol Res. 2014;40(6):1584–91.
4. Sciaky-Tamir Y, Cohen SM, Hochner-Celnikier D, Valsky DV, Messing B, Yagel S. Three-dimensional power Doppler (3DPD) ultrasound in the diagnosis and follow-up of fetal vascular anomalies. Am J Obstet Gynecol. 2006;194(1): 274–81.
5. Raine-Fenning N. The role of three-dimensional ultrasound in assisted reproduction treatment. Ultrasound Obstet Gynecol. 2004;23(4):317–22.
6. Guimaraes Filho HA, Araujo Junior E, Mattar R, Da Costa LL, de Mello Junior CF, Nardozza LM, Moron AF. Placental blood flow measured by three-dimensional power Doppler ultrasound at 26 to 35 weeks gestation in normal pregnancies. J Matern Fetal Neonatal Med. 2010;23(1):69–73.
7. Collins SL, Stevenson GN, Al-Khan A, Illsley NP, Impey L, Pappas L, Zamudio S. Three-dimensional power Doppler ultrasonography for diagnosing abnormally invasive placenta and quantifying the risk. Obstet Gynecol. 2015; 126(3):645–53.
8. Mansour GM, El-Mekkawi SF, Akl SA, Abd El Khalek SY. Three-dimensional power Doppler indices of preeclamptic placentas correlated to umbilical artery Doppler and albuminuria. J Matern Fetal Neonatal Med. 2015;28(2): 149–52.
9. Suranyi A, Kozinszky Z, Molnar A, Nyari T, Bito T, Pal A. Placental three-dimensional power Doppler indices in mid-pregnancy and late pregnancy complicated by gestational diabetes mellitus. Prenat Diagn. 2013;33(10): 952–8.

10. Noguchi J, Hata K, Tanaka H, Hata T. Placental vascular sonobiopsy using three-dimensional power Doppler ultrasound in normal and growth restricted fetuses. Placenta. 2009;30(5):391–7.
11. Sato M, Noguchi J, Mashima M, Tanaka H, Hata T. 3D power Doppler ultrasound assessment of placental perfusion during uterine contraction in labor. Placenta. 2016;45:32–6.
12. Collins SL, Stevenson GN, Noble JA, Impey L, Welsh AW. Influence of power Doppler gain setting on virtual organ computer-aided AnaLysis indices in vivo: can use of the individual sub-noise gain level optimize information? Ultrasound Obstet Gynecol. 2012;40(1):75–80.
13. Pomorski M, Zimmer M, Florjanski J, Michniewicz J, Wiatrowski A, Fuchs T, Milnerowicz-Nabzdyk E. Comparative analysis of placental vasculature and placental volume in normal and IUGR pregnancies with the use of three-dimensional power Doppler. Arch Gynecol Obstet. 2012;285(2):331–7.
14. Merce LT, Barco MJ, Bau S, Kupesic S, Kurjak A. Assessment of placental vascularization by three-dimensional power Doppler "vascular biopsy" in normal pregnancies. Croat Med J. 2005;46(5):765–71.
15. Tuuli MG, Houser M, Odibo L, Huster K, Macones GA, Odibo AO. Validation of placental vascular sonobiopsy for obtaining representative placental vascular indices by three-dimensional power Doppler ultrasonography. Placenta. 2010;31(3):192–6.
16. de Paula CF, Ruano R, Campos JA, Zugaib M. Quantitative analysis of placental vasculature by three-dimensional power Doppler ultrasonography in normal pregnancies from 12 to 40 weeks of gestation. Placenta. 2009; 30(2):142–8.
17. Yu CH, Chang CH, Ko HC, Chen WC, Chang FM. Assessment of placental fractional moving blood volume using quantitative three-dimensional power doppler ultrasound. Ultrasound Med Biol. 2003;29(1):19–23.
18. Demers S, Girard M, Roberge S, Tetu A, Giguere Y, Forest JC, Bujold E. First-trimester placental and myometrial blood perfusion measured by three-dimensional power Doppler in preeclampsia. Am J Perinatol. 2015;32(10): 920–6.
19. Rizzo G, Capponi A, Pietrolucci ME, Aiello E, Arduini D. First trimester placental volume and three dimensional power doppler ultrasonography in type I diabetic pregnancies. Prenat Diagn. 2012;32(5):480–4.
20. Noguchi J, Tanaka H, Koyanagi A, Miyake K, Hata T. Three-dimensional power Doppler indices at 18-22 weeks' gestation for prediction of fetal growth restriction or pregnancy-induced hypertension. Arch Gynecol Obstet. 2015;292(1):75–9.
21. Jones NW, Hutchinson ES, Brownbill P, Crocker IP, Eccles D, Bugg GJ, Raine-Fenning NJ. In vitro dual perfusion of human placental lobules as a flow phantom to investigate the relationship between fetoplacental flow and quantitative 3D power doppler angiography. Placenta. 2009;30(2):130–5.
22. Raine-Fenning NJ, Nordin NM, Ramnarine KV, Campbell BK, Clewes JS, Perkins A, Johnson IR. Evaluation of the effect of machine settings on quantitative three-dimensional power Doppler angiography: an in-vitro flow phantom experiment. Ultrasound Obstet Gynecol. 2008;32(4):551–9.
23. Rizzo G, Capponi A, Cavicchioni O, Vendola M, Arduini D. Placental vascularization measured by three-dimensional power Doppler ultrasound at 11 to 13 + 6 weeks' gestation in normal and aneuploid fetuses. Ultrasound Obstet Gynecol. 2007;30(3):259–62.
24. Guiot C, Gaglioti P, Oberto M, Piccoli E, Rosato R, Todros T. Is three-dimensional power Doppler ultrasound useful in the assessment of placental perfusion in normal and growth-restricted pregnancies? Ultrasound Obstet Gynecol. 2008;31(2):171–6.
25. Martins WP, Raine-Fenning NJ, Ferriani RA, Nastri CO. Quantitative three-dimensional power Doppler angiography: a flow-free phantom experiment to evaluate the relationship between color gain, depth and signal artifact. Ultrasound Obstet Gynecol. 2010;35(3):361–8.

16

Factors influencing the quality of life of pregnant women

Nolwenn Lagadec[1], Magali Steinecker[1], Amar Kapassi[1], Anne Marie Magnier[1], Julie Chastang[1], Sarah Robert[2], Nadia Gaouaou[1] and Gladys Ibanez[2*]

Abstract

Background: Pregnancy is a period of transition with important physical and emotional changes. Even in uncomplicated pregnancies, these changes can affect the quality of life (QOL) of pregnant women, affecting both maternal and infant health. The objectives of this study were to describe the quality of life during uncomplicated pregnancy and to assess its associated socio-demographic, physical and psychological factors in developed countries.

Methods: A systematic review was performed according to the PRISMA guidelines. Searches were made in PubMed, EMBASE and BDSP (Public Health Database). Two independent reviewers extracted the data. Countries with a human development index over 0.7 were selected. The quality of the articles was evaluated on the basis of the STROBE criteria.

Results: In total, thirty-seven articles were included. While the physical component of QOL decreased throughout pregnancy, the mental component was stable and even showed an improvement during pregnancy. Main factors associated with better QOL were mean maternal age, primiparity, early gestational age, the absence of social and economic problems, having family and friends, doing physical exercise, feeling happiness at being pregnant and being optimistic. Main factors associated with poorer QOL were medically assisted reproduction, complications before or during pregnancy, obesity, nausea and vomiting, epigastralgia, back pain, smoking during the months prior to conception, a history of alcohol dependence, sleep difficulties, stress, anxiety, depression during pregnancy and sexual or domestic violence.

Conclusions: Health-related quality of life refers to the subjective assessment of patients regarding the physical, mental and social dimensions of well-being. Improving the quality of life of pregnant women requires better identification of their difficulties and guidance which offers assistance whenever possible.

Keywords: Quality of life, Pregnancy, Primary care, Health-related quality of life, Measurement

Background

According to the World Health Organization, quality of life (QOL) is defined as "*individuals' perception of their position in life in the context of the culture and value systems in which they live and in relation to their goals, expectations, standards and concerns. This is a very broad concept, and one that can be influenced in a complex way by the physical health of the subject, his or her psychological state and level of independence, social relations and relationship with the essential elements of his or her environment*" [1]. It is therefore founded on several objective factors (linked to the quality of the environment and living conditions), and subjective factors (linked to the personal sphere and measurable in terms of satisfaction and well-being). Health status as an essential component of quality of life is referred to as health-related quality of life (HRQOL) [2].

Pregnancy is a period of transition with important physical and emotional changes [3]. Even in uncomplicated pregnancies, these changes can affect the quality of life of pregnant women and affect both maternal and infant health (pregnancy monitoring, pregnancy

* Correspondence: gladys.ibanez@upmc.fr
[2]Sorbonne Universités, UPMC Univ Paris 06, INSERM, Institut Pierre Louis d'épidémiologie et de Santé Publique (IPLESP UMRS 1136), F75012 Paris, France

outcomes, maternal postpartum health, and the psychomotor development of the infant) [4–8]. Health professionals in the field of prenatal maternal and child health try to satisfy their patients with respect to their experience during preconception and pregnancy periods [2]. Traditionally used pregnancy outcome measures, such as morbidity and mortality rates, remain essential. However, they are not sufficient on their own because population health should be assessed, not only on the basis of saving lives, but also in terms of improving quality of life [2, 9].

Over the past decades, numerous instruments have been developed to measure HRQOL in various patient populations, with 2 basic approaches: generic and disease-specific [10]. While generic measures (for example the SF-36 Short-Form Item 36 and WHOQOL-BREF World Health Organization's Quality of Life Scale) have broad application across different types and severity of diseases, disease-specific measures are designed to assess particular diseases or patient populations. To our knowledge, there is no review of the literature to describe the quality of life of pregnant women in primary care. The objectives of this study were to describe the quality of life during uncomplicated pregnancy and to assess its associated socio-demographic, physical and psychological factors in developed countries.

Methods

Type of study

The study consisted of a systematic review of the literature in the PUBMED, EMBASE and BDSP databases (BDSP is the French Public Health Database). The search was performed according to the Preferred Reporting Items for Systematic Reviews and Meta-Analyses (PRISMA) criteria.

Inclusion and exclusion criteria

The search strategy and inclusion/exclusion criteria were developed by the whole group of authors after which two authors (LN and IG) individually conducted the literature search. Key search terms included "Pregnancy", "Quality of life", or "Health related quality of life". Search terms were selected with reference to relevant index terms (MeSH, Emtree or Thesaurus). All observational studies (e.g., cohort, cross-sectional, case-control) which were published in English and French prior to March 2016 have been considered (no restriction in the starting date). Developed countries were chosen as a basis for the research to ensure epidemiological uniformity. In order to define a list of developed countries comparable to France, countries with a human development index (HDI) of over 0.7 were selected. This list, provided by the United Nations (UN), is available online [11]. Studies measuring quality of life with a single question were excluded [12, 13]. Studies on specific populations (women with complicated pregnancy) or on a specific scale of quality of life (sexual HRQOL or HRQOL in relation to faecal incontinence, etc.) were also excluded, as it is not possible to compare patients with different pathologies.

HRQOL measurement

The most frequently used HRQOL instruments during pregnancy are the Medical Outcomes Study Short Form 36 survey (SF-36), the Medical Outcomes Study Short Form 12 survey (SF-12), the World Health Organization's Quality of Life Scale (WHOQOL) and the World Health Organization's Quality of Life Scale – BREF (WHOQOL – Bref).

The SF-36 includes 36 items and collects information on eight health concepts including, physical functioning, role limitations due to physical and emotional health, mental health, bodily pain, general health, vitality and social functioning. These items are scored providing a component summary scale score for both mental (SF36-MCS) and physical (SF36-PCS) HRQOL (from 0 to 100) [14]. The SF-12 is a validated shortened version of the SF-36. A lower score on the summary scales represents a poorer HRQOL.

The WHOQOL includes 100 questions grouped into 6 categories (physical, psychological, independence, social, environmental and spiritual) (from 0 to 100). The WHOQOL-BREF instrument comprises 26 items and is a validated shortened version of the WHOQOL. A lower score on the summary scales represents a poorer HRQOL.

Article selection and quality assessment

A preliminary selection was made from the titles, then another on reading the summaries and a lastly on a reading of the entire article. Publications "related" to the selected articles as well as the bibliography of the selected articles were also examined. Two independent reviewers extracted the data (LN and IG). Disagreement between reviewers was resolved by consensus. The quality of the articles was evaluated using the STROBE criteria (STrengthening the Reporting of OBservational studies in Epidemiology) [15].

Analysis

The results were organised in two sections: first, a description of the quality of life of pregnant women in developed countries and second, by the socio-demographic, physical and psychological factors associated with their quality of life. When the study compared two quality of life scales, we used only the "Gold Standard" scale. In the case-control studies where the controls were a particular subgroup, we have retained the "control" group that was most representative of the general population of pregnant women, where all subjects in the study would have resulted in a serious selection bias.

Results

Article selection

The article selection is described in Fig. 1. Of the 1487 articles retrieved, 37 were selected for our analysis (Fig. 1 and Table 1). The methodological quality was rated from 11 to 22 in the selected articles. The selected articles were published between 2001 and 2016. The samples of pregnant women included in the studies varied between 55 and 12,056 women. Concerning the design of the selected studies, twenty were cross-sectional studies [16–35], four were case-controlled studies [36–38], and fourteen were longitudinal cohort studies [14, 39–51]. Thirteen studies were conducted during the first trimester of pregnancy [17, 20, 22, 23, 26, 30, 38–40, 44–47], eleven were from the second trimester [14, 16, 24, 35, 38–41, 45, 46, 48], eighteen were from the 3rd trimester [14, 18, 19, 27, 29, 31, 33, 34, 37–42, 46, 48–50] and six studies focused on the entire pregnancy [25, 28, 32, 36, 43, 51]. In measuring the quality of life, nineteen studies used SF-36 [14, 17–19, 21, 22, 25–27, 30, 33, 34, 38–41, 44, 46, 51], twelve studies used SF-12 [16, 20, 23, 24, 28, 29, 35, 42, 43, 46, 48, 50], two studies used the WHOQOL Brief [32, 47], one study used The Duke Health Profile [49], and another Nottingham Health Profile [31].

The quality of life of pregnant women

Comparison with the general population

The quality of life of pregnant women was generally lower than that of the general population. Two studies explicitly compared their results with those of non-pregnant women of the same age. On the SF-36

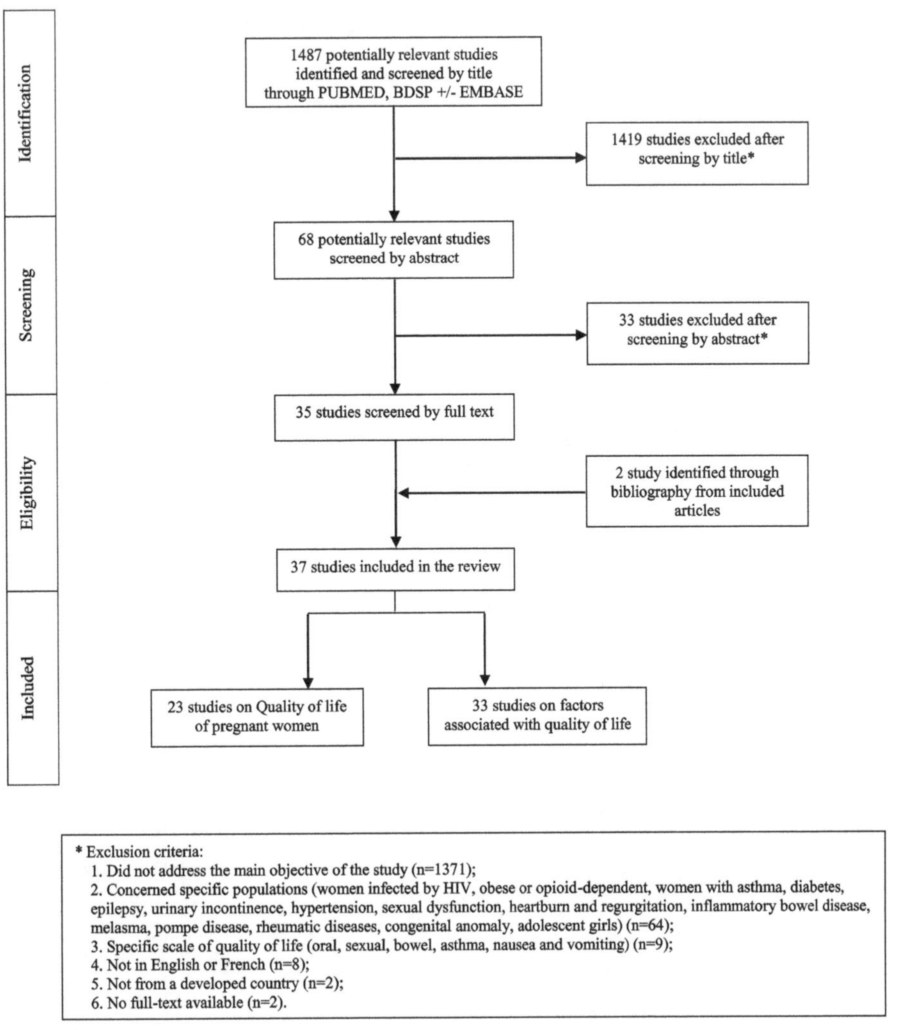

Fig. 1 Flow chart of the study selection

Table 1 Studies characteristics

Author,Year, Reference	Study design	Number of participants	Response rate	QOL scale used	STROBE rate
Abbasi M. et al.(2013) Iran [38][a]	Prospective cohort study	1550	66%	Medical Outcomes Study Short Form 36 (SF-36)	20
Aquino NM (2009) Brasil [15][b]	Cross-sectional study	179	99,40%	Standard Short Form 12 Health Survey (SF-12)	18
Chan OK et al. (2010) China [16][a,b]	Cross-sectional study	418	94,70%	Medical Outcomes Study Short Form 36 (SF-36)	17
Chang et al. (2014) Taiwan [40] [a,b]	Longitudinal cohort study	410	83,30%	Medical Outcomes Study Short Form 36 (SF-36)	19
Coban A. et al. (2011) Turkey [36][b]	Case-controlled study	100	–	WHO-QOL-BREF Questionnaire	13
Da Costa D et al. (2010) Canada [18] [a,b]	Cross-sectional study	245	66,60%	Medical Outcomes Study Short Form 36 (SF-36)	17
Dall'Alba V et al. (2015) Brasil [18][b]	Cross-sectional study	82	–	Medical Outcomes Study Short Form 36 (SF-36)	13
De Pascalis L. et al. (2012) Italy [40][a,b]	Case-controlled study	115	87,79	Medical Outcomes Study Short Form 36 (SF-36)	19
Elsenbruch S. et al. (2006) Germany [19][a,b]	Cross-sectional study	978	91,60%	Medical Outcomes Study, Short Form 12 (SF-12)	19
Emmanuel EN et al. (2012) Australia [50][a, b]	Longitudinal cohort study	630	77%	Medical Outcomes Study Short Form 12 (SF-12) Version 2	17
Emmanuel EN et Sun J. (2014) Australia [42] [a,b]	Longitudinal cohort study	605	60%	Medical Outcomes Study, Short Form 12 (SF-12)	18
Fatemeh A et al. (2010) Iran [32][a,b]	Cross-sectional study	600	–	Medical Outcomes Study Short Form 36 (SF-36)	12
Gezginç K et al., (2008) Turkey [35][b]	Cross-sectional study	55	–	WHO-QOL-BREF Questionnaire	14
Gharacheh M. et al., (2015) Iran [20][b]	Cross-sectional study	328	96%	Medical Outcomes Study Short Form 36 (SF-36)	19
Haas JS et al. (2004) USA [42][a, b]	Longitudinal cohort study	2854	63%	Medical Outcome Study Short Form-36 (SF-36)	20
Hama K et al. (2008) Japan [51][b]	Longitudinal cohort study	190	83%	Medical Outcomes Study Short Form 36 (SF-36) version 2	14
Jomeen J., Martin CR; (2005) United Kingdom [21][a,b]	Cross-sectional study	129	–	Medical Outcomes Study Short Form 36 (SF-36) Version 2	15
Lacasse A et al. (2008) Canada [23] [a,b]	Cross-sectional study	507	77%	Medical Outcomes Study, Short Form 12 (SF-12)	18
Lau Y et al. (2011) China [23][b]	Cross-sectional study	1151	71,4%	Standard Short Form 12 Health Survey (SF-12)	18
Li J et al. (2012) China [24][b]	Cross-sectional study	454	79%	Medical Outcomes Study Short Form 36 (SF-36) version 2	17
Liu L et al.(2013) USA [25][b]	Cross-sectional study	195	88%	Medical Outcomes Study Short Form 36 (SF-36)	19
Mckee MD et al (2001) USA [26][b]	Cross-sectional study	114	74%	Medical Outcomes Study Short Form 36 (SF-36)	18
Mota N. et al. (2008) Canada [27][a]	Cross-sectional study	12,056	81,20%	Medical Outcomes Study, Short Form 12 (SF-12)	19
Moyer CA et al. (2009) USA, China, Ghana [29] [a,b]	Cross-sectional study	251 Chine, 311 USA	–	Medical Outcomes Study, Short Form 12 (SF-12)	14
Nakamura Y. et al. (2012) Japan [38] [a,b]	Case-controlled study	692	66,10%	Medical Outcomes Study Short Form 36 (SF-36) Version 2	16
Ngai FW, Ngu SF. (2013) Hong Kong [43] [a]	Prospective cohort study	256	79,3%	Medical Outcomes Study, Short Form 12 (SF-12)	17

Table 1 Studies characteristics *(Continued)*

Author,Year, Reference	Study design	Number of participants	Response rate	QOL scale used	STROBE rate
Nicholson WK (2006) USA [29][b]	Cross-sectional study	221	79%	Medical Outcomes Study Short Form 36 (SF-36)	19
Olsson C, Nilsson-Wikmar L.(2004) Sweden [31] [b]	Cross-sectional study	136	85%	Nottingham Health Profile	22
Ramirez-Vélez R (2011) Colombia [34][a, b]	Cross-sectional study	64	–	Medical Outcomes Study, Short Form 12 version 2 (SF-12 V2)	17
Setse R et al. (2008) USA [44][b]	Prospective cohort study	200	81%	Medical Outcomes Study Short Form 36 (SF-36)	20
Shishehgar S. et al. (2014) Iran [31][a, b]	Cross-sectional study	210	–	WHO-QOL-BREF Questionnaire	15
Tavoli Z et al. (2016) Iran [33][a, b]	Cross-sectional study	266	86,5%	Medical Outcomes Study Short Form 36 (SF-36)	19
Tendais I et al. (2011) Portugal [45][b]	Prospective cohort study	56	56%	Medical Outcomes Study Short Form 36 (SF-36)	16
Tsai SY et al. (2016) Taiwan [46][a, b]	Prospective cohort study	172	95,3%	Medical Outcomes Study, Short Form 12 version 2 (SF-12 V2)	18
Vachkova E et al. (2013) Czech Republic [47][a]	Prospective cohort study	225	90,60%	WHO-QOL-BREF Questionnaire	11
Vinturache A. et al. (2015) Canada [48][a, b]	Prospective cohort study	3388	99%	Medical Outcomes Study, Short Form 12 (SF-12)	18
Wang P et al.(2013) Taiwan [49][a, b]	Prospective cohort study	265	78,86%	Duke Health Profile (DUKE)	20

List of abbreviations: *QOL* Quality of life, [a]First research question: quality of life of pregnant women in developed countries; [b]second research question: factors associated with their quality of life

scale, Da Costa et al. found physical activity and physical pain values equal to 56.7 and 61.7; these values were 90.9 and 75.0 for non-pregnant Canadian women of the same age [18]. Similarly, Nakamura et al. made similar comparisons in Japan [38]. The Chan et al. study in 2010 also found that pregnant women had, on average, statistically lower QOL scores ($p < 0.001$) compared to the general population, excepting general health ($p = 0.1$) [17, 18]. Similarly, Elsenbruch et al. [20] found a reduced quality of life, physically, when compared to German women of the same age ($p < 0.001$).

The progression of the quality of life during the trimesters

Of the 23 studies selected, 20 (86,9%) described the progression of QOL using SF-36 or SF-12 (Figs. 2, 3). The study of the SF-36 PCS and MCS aggregate scores revealed that there were significant variations during the trimesters (Fig. 2).

The PCS values ranged from 48 to 61 during the 1st trimester; between 39 and 55 during the 2nd trimester; between 37.5, and 47.5 during the 3rd trimester. For SF-12, values ranged from 44 to 46 in the 1st trimester, 43 and 50 in the 2nd trimester and 41 and 45 in the 3rd trimester. The results of the studies indicated a decrease in physical quality of life throughout pregnancy, particularly related to decreased physical activity and functional limitations (related to physical health and physical pain). In terms of prevalence, the Haas et al. study in 2005 showed an increase in pregnant women with poor physical quality of life during pregnancy: 9% of pregnant women in the second trimester, and 13% in the third trimester [14]. The proportion of pregnant women reporting generally poor health (score 0 to 50) increased from 15.5 to 20.1 and 26.9% and then decreased to 21% in the postpartum period [49].

The MCS values were as follows for the SF-36: in the 1st trimester values between a minimum of 51 and a maximum of 58; in the 2nd trimester between 49 and 62; in the 3rd trimester between 49.5 and 66. In parallel with SF-12, the MCS was between 47 and 48 in the first trimester, between 49 and 52 in the second trimester and 50 and 54 in the third trimester. In five studies, the quality of mental life of the pregnant women increased or remained stable over the course of the trimesters (Fig. 2).

The evolution of the 8 dimensions of SF-36 during the quarters is presented in Fig. 3. The following domains had the lowest scores: role limitations due to physical problems (RP) and vitality (VT). The following domains had the highest scores: general health perceptions (GH) and bodily pain (BP). The results concerning the role limitations due to emotional problems (RE) varied across studies.

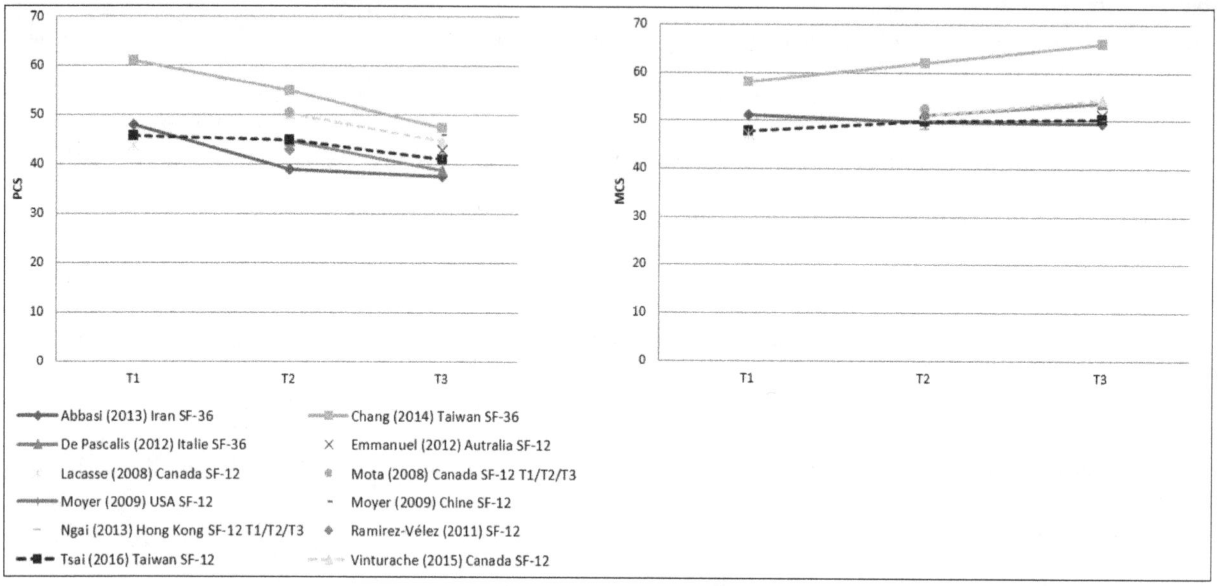

T1 : first trimester ; T2 : second trimester ; T3 : third trimester ; PCS : Physical Component Summary; MCS : Mental Component Summary

Fig. 2 Changes in PCS and MCS over trimesters

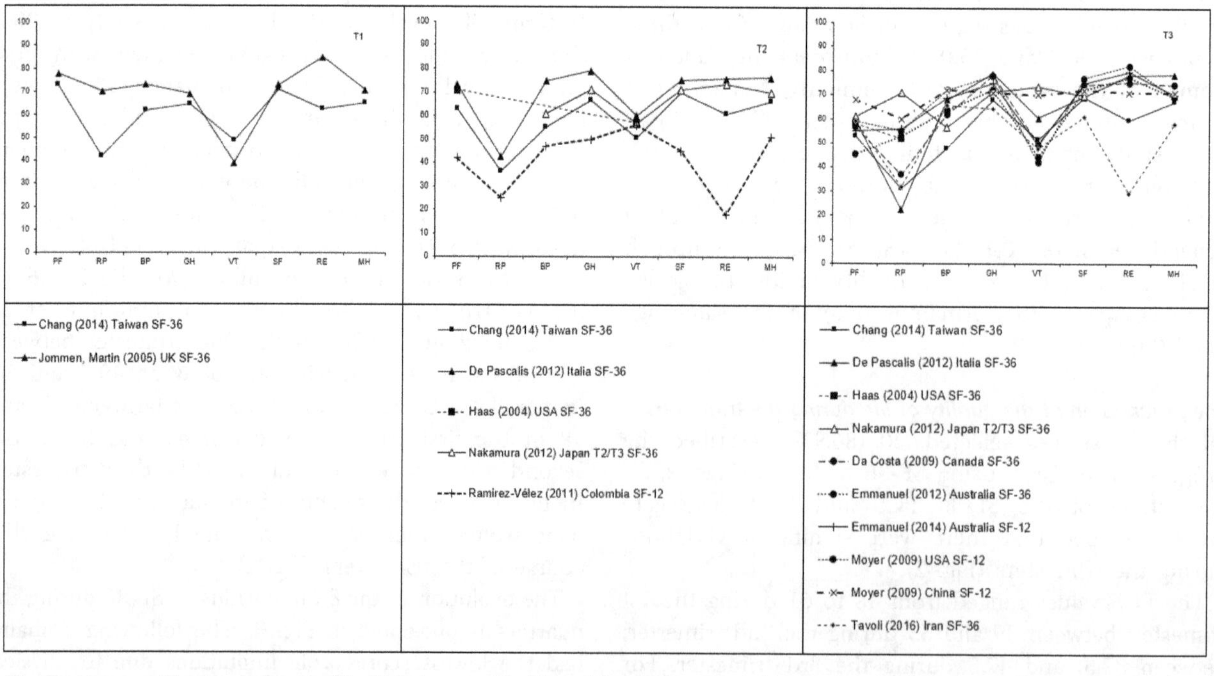

T1 : first trimester ; T2 : second trimester ; T3 : third trimester ; PF : Physical Functioning ; RP : Role Limitations due to Physical Problems ; BP : Bodily Pain ; GH : General Health Perceptions ; VT : Vitality ; SF : Social Functioning ; RE : Role Limitations due to Emotional Problems ; MH : General Mental Health

Fig. 3 Evolution of the 8 dimensions of SF-36 during the trimesters

Table 2 Factors significantly associated with poor quality of life according to the studies ($p < 0.05$)

Risk factors	Protective Factors
Socio-demographic characteristics	
Older pregnant women [18, 23, 25, 42]	
Economic difficulties [14, 30, 32, 35]	
Low level of education [18, 25, 33, 35, 49]	
Unemployment [25, 49]	Occupation (housewife) [35]
Ethnic minority [30]	Ethnic minority [23, 42]
Isolation	
Single [18, 35, 42]	Single [25]
No partner support [18]	
No social support [18, 20, 30]	
Little / no partner support [18]	
Medical characteristics	
Adverse medical history [18]	
Obesity [14, 48]	Obesity [25]
Bad physical condition prior to conception [43, 49]	
Smoking prior to conception [14]	
Addiction to alcohol prior to conception [14]	
Practicing physical exercise [14, 23, 45]	
Obstetrical characteristics	
Experience of infertility [16]	
Primiparity [48, 51]	Primiparity [18, 33, 40, 49]
More advanced in weeks pregnant [16, 28, 33]	More advanced in weeks pregnant [39-mcs]
Hospitalisation during pregnancy [25]	
Medically assisted reproduction [14, 40, 41]	Medically assisted reproduction [48]
Obstetric Complications [18, 21, 40]	
Psychological characteristics	
Prenatal depressive symptoms [18, 22, 25, 30, 44]	
Stress, prenatal anxiety [18, 22, 24, 32, 42]	
History of sexual violence [16]	
History of domestic violence [21, 34]	
Difficult life events [18]	
	Wanted pregnancy [25, 33, 40]
	Happy being pregnant [49]
	Optimistic [29] Life Satisfaction [33]
Symptoms during pregnancy	
Nausea / vomiting [14, 17, 23]	
Epigastralgia / reflux [19]	
Back pain [14, 31]	
Sleep disorder [14, 18, 46]	
Comfort [38]	

Factors influencing quality of life

The results of studies on the factors associated with the quality of life of pregnant women are presented in Tables 2 and 3. Thirty-three articles were selected for this section.

Socio-demographic factors

The following socio-demographic factors were strongly associated with a better quality of life in 15 studies: mean maternal age, primiparity, early gestational age, the absence of economic problems, a high educational level, being employed, being married, having family and friends. With less consensus, belonging to an ethnic minority and alcohol consumption have also been associated in 2 studies with a poorer quality of life.

Physical factors

Medically assisted reproduction, obstetric complications, medical history, possible hospitalisation and obesity were factors frequently indicating a poor quality of life during pregnancy (in 9 studies). Physical symptoms associated with pregnancy such as nausea and vomiting, epigastralgia, reflux, shortness of breath, dizziness, back pain and sleep problems affected women's quality of life. Exercise was a factor that improved the quality of life of pregnant women. With less consensus, we found other factors associated with a poorer QOL such as smoking during the months prior to conception, a history of alcohol dependence and poor comfort.

Psychological factors

Eight studies have shown that symptoms of depression, anxiety, and stress were factors that had a strong negative impact on the quality of life of pregnant women. Sexual and domestic violence was linked to a lower quality of life, as well as the experience of life-threatening events and the experience of infertility. Happiness at being pregnant and being optimistic were factors related to a better quality of life.

Discussion

Summary of results

Pregnant women, especially during the third trimester, had significantly lower quality of life scores than non-pregnant women of the same age. Physically, the quality of life decreased significantly during the course of the trimesters. On a psychological level, several studies reported an increase in quality of life relative to mental health during pregnancy, and in others psychological stability was seen. Many factors were associated with the quality of life in pregnant women. Some factors associated with higher well-being were socio-demographic (first-time pregnancy, a favourable socio-economic status, social support, partner support). Similarly, the desire to be pregnant and moderate physical activity were factors associated with a positive quality of life. A lesser quality of life was attributed to physical factors, (such as complications during pregnancy, medically assisted reproduction, obesity prior to conception, physical symptoms such as nausea and vomiting, sleep difficulties), and otherwise attributed to psychological factors, (such as anxiety and stress during pregnancy and depressive symptoms).

Strengths and limitations of the study

To our knowledge, this is the only systematic review of international literature aimed at synthesizing data regarding the quality of life of pregnant women. Many factors have been studied, considering the different dimensions of the quality of life, for pregnant women in general good health. This work also has its limitations: the research only included articles written in English or French. Therefore, the issue of generalizability should be discussed. In addition, two other articles could not be read in their entirety. Within the selected studies, few studies were multi-centric and only one study used information from a large national survey. In addition, we found a high degree of heterogeneity in the methodology for population selection, in choosing the quality of life scale, as well as in the results presented (dimensions of SF-36, composite scores, etc) complicating the synthesis study. Specific HRQOL questionnaires were not included because they are focused more on specific problems in pregnancy (such as nausea and vomiting) rather than on women's overall well-being and their quality of life. With regard to the quality of these studies, three studies did not explicitly take into account the confounding factors in the presentation of the results [22, 38, 47], which may lead to confusion bias. In addition, a large number of studies were cross-sectional. These studies did not establish an associative cause-and-effect relationship.

Research and policy implications

In some countries, the quality of life of pregnant woman has been little studied. In France, for example, only one study provided information on pregnant women well-being [6] (study not included in our analysis – cf. exclusion criteria). In this study, the mental health of pregnant women was measured through the following question: "On a psychological level, how did you feel during your pregnancy? Well, Quite well, Quite poor, Poor". Of the 14,326 women interviewed, 8.9% reported poor self-rated mental health during pregnancy. Moreover, sociodemographic characteristics indicative of social disadvantage were associated with a higher-risk of poor quality of life; sometimes, a social gradient was observed. [6, 52]. Since SF-36 is a generic scale, it allows

Table 3 Factors Associated with Quality of Life During Pregnancy

Author, Year, Country	Factors related to QOL *	Key Results
Aquino NM (2009) [17]	Sexual Violence *	Women who had experienced sexual violence had significantly lower PCS and MCS (PCS 42.2, SD = 5.3 and MCS 37.4, SD = 11.2) than women who had no history of sexual violence (PCS 51.0, SD = 7.5 and MCS 48.1, SD = 10.2, $p < 0.001$).
Chan OK (2010) [18]	Nausea and vomiting*	PW without symptoms of NVP: PCS: 67.92; MCS 68.36; PW with moderate symptoms: PCS: 56.93; MCS 60.86; PW with severe symptoms: PCS: 50.01; MCS: 50.23 The variations between the PCS and MCS of the 3 groups are all significant. ($P < 0.01$). All QOL dimensions are affected by NVP ($p < 0.05$)
Chang SR (2014) [39]	Pregnancy stage *, Experience of infertility *, Medically Assisted Reproduction *, Number of Pregnancies, Spontaneous Abortions, Parity *, Medical Condition *, Pregnancy wanted *	Factors associated with PCS: Pregnancy stage (beta = – 7.79, p < 0.001), experience of infertility (beta = – 6.39, $p = 0.03$). Factors associated with MCS: stage of pregnancy (beta = 3.31, p < 0.001), number of pregnancies (beta = – 7.12, $p = 0.01$), medical condition beta = – 4.08, $p = 0.04$). Factors associated with overall QOL: Pregnancy stage (beta = 1.64, p = 0.01), desired pregnancy (beta = 5.52, p = 0.04), medical condition (beta = – 5.29, p < 0.001).
Coban A. (2011) [35]	Back pain	No significant difference between PBP and NBP in the different areas of WHO-QOL-BREF: physical health $p = 0.229$; psychological health $p = 0.069$; Social relationship $p = 0.125$; Environment $p = 0.790$
Da Costa D (2009) [19]	Age* , Education *, Income*, Professional status* , Marital status * , Parity * , Weeks pregnant , Medical history* , Medical complications during pregnancy * , Anxiety related to pregnancy * Partner Support * , Social Support * , Sleep Problems * , Depressive symptoms * , Life Events *	Multivariable analysis: Sleep problems affected most QOL components (PF: b = – 0.17, $p < 0.007$; PR: b = – 0,19, $p = 0.002$; BP: b = – 0,35, $p < 0.0001$; GH: b = – 0.21, p < 0.0001; VT: b = – 0.25, p < 0.0001; SF: b = – 0.26, p < 0.0001, MH: b = – 0.20, p < 0.0001). A depressive mood was an independent determinant in 6/9 of the QOL dimensions (BP: b = – 0.13, p = 0,.039, GH: b = – 0.28, p < 0.0001, VT: b = – 0.40, $p < 0.0001$, SF = – 0.27, p < 0.0001; ER: b = – 0.50, $p < 0.0001$, MH: b = – 0.59, $p < 0.0001$), and anxiety also affected physical activity and limitations due to physical state. The life experience of the past year had a negative impact on physical activity, social functioning and mental health scores. Having complications during pregnancy affected physical activity and social functioning. Age, professional status, educational level and medical problems were linked to only one parameter of SF36.
Dall'Alba V (2015) [20]	Epigastralgia *, Gastroesophageal Reflux *	Epigastralgia: significant decrease in PR ($p = 0.009$) and of SF ($p = 0.020$); RGO: significant decrease in PR ($p = 0.004$) and of ER ($p = 0.002$)
De Pascalis L. (2012) [40]	Medically assisted fertility*	PW having a medically assisted pregnancy: PCS: 40.0 then 35.97; MCS: 52.32 then 53.02; PW having conceived spontaneously: PCS: 44.78; then 38.86. MCS: 51.08 then 53.65 Physical well-being scores significantly lower in the medically assisted pregnancy group than in the spontaneous conception group ($P = 0.033$) in the categories: physical health limitations, vitality, social functioning. Physical well-being scores of PW with medically assisted pregnancy decreased during pregnancy, more significantly than spontaneously conceived PW. ($P = 0.008$)
Elsenbruch S. (2006) [21]	Social support*	Low social support was statistically associated with a reduced QOL (For PCS: F = 11.53, $P < 0.001$, For MCS: F = 90.60, P < 0.001). On the contrary, the group where social support was high had better QOL. (P < 0.001)
Emmanuel EN (2012)	Age, Relationship status, Length of relationship, Level of education, Parity, Timing of first antenatal visit, Social upport	Social support: beta = 0.21 [– 0.04,0.47] was not significant during pregnancy
Emmanuel EN (2014) [41]	Age *, Number of pregnancies *, Marital status *, Ethnicity *, Maternal stress *	PW between 25 and 29 years of age had a better RF, PR, BP than the others (PF: F = 11.07 $P = 0.001$; PR: F = 5,17 p = 0,006; BP: F = 11.01 $p = 0.001$) Caucasian and Asian PW had higher SF and MH scores than other ethnic groups (SF: F = 2.65, $p = 0.02$; MH: F = 2.42 $p = 0.03$) Single PW had higher SF and MH scores than other ethnic groups (SF: F = 2.65, p = 0.02; MH: F = 2.42 p = 0.03) A significant relationship is found between the different components of SF12 and maternal stress except for BP (PH $r = – 3.87$; PR $r = – 7.79$; BP: r = – 7.79; GH:

Table 3 Factors Associated with Quality of Life During Pregnancy *(Continued)*

Author, Year, Country	Factors related to QOL *	Key Results
		$r = -6.63$; VT = − 7.70; SF: $r = -12.61$; ER: $r = -12.66$; MH: r-12.80 $p < 0.01$)
Fatemeh A (2010) [32]	Age*, Gestational age*, Gravidity*,Education*, Wanted pregnancy*, life satisfaction*, Income	Age: < 25 years: GH = 63.68; PF = 64.71; SF = 66.37; MH = 68.33; > 25 years: GH = 60.44 p = 0.009; PF = 20.60 $p = 0.010$; SF = 61.47 p = 0.009; MH = 64.81 $p = 0.018$ Gestationnal age: < 20 weeks: PF = 65.51; BP = 56.89; > 20 weeks: PF = 60.72 $p = 0.013$; BP = 57.22 $p = 0.022$ Gravid 1 N: GH = 63.23; PF = 62.93; RP = 56.86; SF = 65.35; MH = 67.73; VT = 56.97; > 2 N: GH = 55.42 p = 0 .000; PF = 56.16 $p = 0.011$; RP = 52.09 $p = 0.038$; SF = 56.52 p = 0.002; MH = 60.09 $p = 0.000$; VT = 52.56 $p = 0.048$ Significant association between levels of education and PF and MH, between wanted pregnancy and RE and MH, life satisfaction and SF and MH (figures not available)
Gezginç K (2008) [34]	Obsessive Compulsive Disorder	Patients with OCD: Physical health: 49.92 +/− 15.44 Mental health: 46.20 +/− 15.98 Social relationships 44.96 +/− 15.00 Environment 50.32 +/− 9.88 PW control group: Physical health: 61.96 /− 10.08 and p = 0.002; Mental health: 66.32 +/− 10.47and $p < 0.0001$; Social relations: 67.12 +/− 11.92 and p < 0.0001; Environment 69.60 +/− 10.23 and p < 0.0001
Gharacheh M. (2015) [22]	Domestic violence*	6 SF36 sub-scales are lower for abused women than for non-abused women: PR (p = 0,041) GH ($p = 0.003$) PCS (p = 0.009) VT (p = 0.011) SF ($p = 0.05$) ER ($p = 0.037$) MH ($p = 0.035$) MCS ($p = 0.07$)
Haas JS (2004) [42]	Age, Ethnicity, Marital Status, Level of Education, Body Mass Index, Obesity * , Financial problems*, Physical exercise *, Depressive Symptoms *, Pre-conception smoking *, History of alcohol addiction *, Symptoms associated with pregnancy *, Medical background, Medical complications	Factors associated with poor health: financial problems (OR = 2.11, IC (1.49–2.98)), low physical function before pregnancy (OR = 1.99, IC (1.37–2.88)), depressive symptoms (OR = 2.30; IC (1.61–3.29)), obesity = (OR = 1.70; IC (1.16–2.48), lack of physical exercise, (OR = 1.12; IC (0.77–1.63) Smoking during the 3 months prior to conception (OR = 1.04; IC (0.65–1.68)), History of alcohol dependence (OR = 1.55, IC (1.00–2.39)) Indigestion was associated with poor physical function (OR = 1.49; IC (1.04–2.13)). Dizziness (OR = 2.06; IC(1.57–2.71), back pain (OR = 1.71; IC(1.27–2.31)), breathlessness (OR = 1.32; IC(1.02–1.71)) were associated with a low vitality score. Dizziness, indigestion, shortness of breath and sleep disorders were associated with depressive symptoms.
Hama K (2008) [51]	Number of pregnancy*	PF, RP, GH: no significant differences between nulliparous and multiparous women BP and VT: scores higher in multiparous in the 3rd and 4th monthes of pregnancy, and lower in the 9th month of pregnancy; SF: higher in multiparous from the 3th month to the 7th month and lower in the 9th month; RE and MH: scores higher in multiparous up to 6th month pregnancy (p < 0,05) (no figures avalaible)
Jommen J (2005) [23]	Depression*, Anxiety*.	The PW group with depression had significantly lower QOL scores for all SF36 parameters ($p < 0.05$) except for physical function ($p = 0.73$) and vitality ($p = 0.09$). The PW group with clinically significant anxiety levels had significantly lower QOL scores in terms of physical pain ($p = 0.02$) and general health ($p < 0.001$)
Lacasse A (2008) [24]	Nausea and Vomiting *, Ethnicity *, Age *, Medical Insurance, employment, Educational level, Income, Physical exercise *, Alcohol and tobacco *	PW without NVP: PCS = 49,5; MCS = 49; PW with NVP: PCS = 43; MCS = 46 $P < 0.001$ AND $P = 0.003$ PCS age: b = − 0.32 $p = 0.006$; Country of birth MCS: b = 3.02 $P = 0.035$; Hispanic ethnicity MCS: b = 4.88 p = 0.035 Physical exercise: PCS: b = 3.47 $p = 0.001$ MCS: b = 2.17 $p = 0.031$; Coffee: PCS: b = 2.84 p = 0.006; Alcohol:: PCS: b = 3.38 $p = 0.045$
Lau Y (2011) [25]	Perceived Stress *	Significant association between perceived stress and PCS (beta = − 0.501, p < 0.001) and MCS (b = − 0.115, p < 0.001)
Li J (2012) [26]	Depression*, Age*, Body Mass Index*, Educational Level* Physical exercise, History of smoking, History of alcohol abuse, Income*, Wanted pregnancy, Weeks pregnant*, Parity, History of abortion, Pregnancy complications	The PW group presenting depression had significantly lower QOL scores for all SF36 parameters ($p < 0.002$) PW not depressed: PCS = 49.13 (6.95); MCS = 48.67 (7.33)) (p < 0.001); PW depressed: PCS = 46.43 (7.42); MCS = 39.62 (7.94) (p < 0.001) Age: PCS $r = -0.170$ (p < 0.001); MCS: $r = 0.108$ ($p < 0.05$); BMI: MCS: $r = 0.114$ (p < 0.05); Education level: MCS $r = 0.203$ (p < 0.001) Monthly income: MCS $r = 0.183$ (p < 0.001); Week of pregnancy: PCS: $r = 0.145$ (p < 0.001); MCS $r = 0.118$ (p < 0.05) Multivariable: PCS: EPDS: beta = − 0.232 ($p < 0.0001$); Age: beta = − 0.179 (p < 0.0001); WP: beta = − 0.129 ($p = 0.004$); Employment: beta = − 0.111 ($p = 0.012$); Marital status: beta = − 0.107 ($p = 0.017$); MCS: EPDS: beta = − 0.662 (p < 0.0001);

Table 3 Factors Associated with Quality of Life During Pregnancy *(Continued)*

Author, Year, Country	Factors related to QOL *	Key Results
		BMI: beta = 0.129 (p < 0.0001); Wanted pregnancy: beta = 0.086 (*p* = 0.018)
Liu L (2013) [27]	Ethnicity	Black patients: PF = 58; PR = 52; BP = 69; GH = 71; VT = 47; SF = 72; ER = 63; MH = 79; White patients: PF = 77; PR = 78; BP = 83; GH = 83; VT = 58, SF = 87; ER = 89; MH = 83. Black women had significantly lower QOL scores in physical activity (*p* < 0.001), physical limitation (p < 0.001), physical pain (p = 0.02) (*P* = 0.01), social functioning (*p* = 0.002), limitations related to mental state (p < 0.001). After adjusting for depressive symptoms, social support and BMI, these differences become no longer statistically significant.
Mckee MD (2001) [28]	Depression* Social support*	Depression is strongly and negatively correlated with all subscales of SF 36 MH (r = – 0,69), VT (r = – 0,63), SF (*r* = – 0.62), and ER (*r* = – 0.54) Social support was related to MH (*r* = 0.24), ER (*r* = 0.19), and SF (r = 0.14).
Moyer CA (2009) [30]	Optimism*	Optimism is positively associated with MCS (*p* = 0.001), VT (*p* = 0.041), and MH (p < 0.001)
Nakamura Y (2012) [36]	Comfort*, Hospitalisation*	The sense of comfort and the 6 areas of HRQOL were significantly lower for inpatients than for ambulatory PW and non-pregnant women (*p* < 0.05 and p = 0.001). A significant correlation was found between subjective comfort and QOL in vitality (p < 0.001) and mental health (p < 0.001)
Nicholson WK (2006) [31]	Ethnicity*, Income*, Social Support* Depressive Symptoms*, Multi-parity* Chronic illness	Ethnicity: African Americans / Whites: PF: – 15 (– 22;-8) RP: – 28 (– 41, – 15), GH: – 11 (– 19; – 13)(, VT: – 13(– 28;-3): SF: – 7 (– 8; – 6), Income: GH -10 (– 17; – 3), SF -4 (– 5, – 3), MH -9 (– 15; – 4); Social support: PR: 30 (6,55) GH: 9 (5,15), MH: 14 (12; 16) Multi-parity (> 2 previous deliveries): PR: 18 (7;30), SF: 17 (16, 18); Depressive symptoms: PR: – 50 (p = 0.006); BP: – 12 (*p* = 0.01); GH: – 10 (p = 0.01); VT = – 20 (*p* > 0.001); SF = – 38 (*p* < 0.01); ER: – 40 (p < 0.01); MH = – 24 (p < 0.01); Still significant in multivariable analysis
Olsson C (2004) [32]	Back pain	The QOL was lower in the PW group with back pain group (16 ± 16) (*p* = 0.000), also found in the sleep subcategories (P = 0.003), energy (*p* = 0.024), pain (p = 0.000) and physical mobility (p = 0.000). The PW group with back pain had a higher rate of occupational withdrawal (57%, *p* = 0.005), aptitude for household work (62%, p = 0.002), Social life (35%, *p* = 0.007) and leisure time (68%, *P* = 0.001)
Ramirez-Vélez (2011) [34]	Age*, Educational Status*, Socioeconomic levels*, Work status*, Marital Status*, Gestational weeks	Age: PF: r = – 0.17 (p < 0.05); Educational Status: GH: *r* = 0.34 (p < 0.001) Socioeconomic levels: PR *r* = 0.17 (p < 0.05); GH *r* = 0.29 (p < 0.001); SF: r = 0.19 (p < 0.05); ER: *r* = 0.27 (p < 0.01); MH: *r* = 0.22 (p < 0.01) Occupation (housewife): PR: r = 0.20 (p < 0.01); GH: r = 0.19 (p < 0.05); Marital Status (Being married or cohabiting): PF: *r* = 0.15 (p < 0.05) PR: *r* = 0.16 (p < 0.05) GH: *r* = – 0.22 (p < 0.01) VT: r = 0.19 (p < 0.05) SF: *r* = – 0.23 (p < 0.01) ER: *r* = – 0.19 (p < 0.01) MH: *r* = – 0.25 (p < 0.01)
Setse R (2008) [43]	Depressive symptoms*	In the 1st trimester: PW not depressed: PF = 82; PR = 59; BP = 77; GH = 65; VT = 47; SF = 81; ER = 87; MH = 79 Depressed PW: PF = 78; PR = 39; BP = 59; GH = 51; VT = 35; SF = 54; RE = 41; MH = 57 Depressed PW had a significantly worse QOL on the following SF36 conditions: physical pain, vitality, social functioning, functioning related to mental health, mental health. These PW had QOL scores of 10–23 points and 19–31 points lower in the 2nd and 3rd trimester
Shishehgar S (2014) [33]	Perceived stress during pregnancy *	Significant relationship between QOL and stress rate (*p* = 0.026, *r* = 0.007)
Tavoli Z (2016)	Domestic violence*	Non-abused women: PF = 68.7; RP 43.2; BP = 70.7; GH = 69.5; VT = 55.6; SF = 70.5; RE = 46.0; MH = 63.5; Abused women: PF = 53.9 (p < 0.0001); RP = 25.8(p < 0.0001); BP = 64.2 (NS); GH = 61.4 (p < 0.01); VT = 43.5(p < 0.0001); SF = 55.8 (p < 0.0001); RE = 20.1 (p < 0.0001); MH = 55.3(*p* < 0.003); General Health: physical violence OR = 2.13 (*p* = 0.03), Mental Health: psychological violence OR = 1.24 (p = 0.04)
Tendais I (2011) [44]	Physical activity*	PW who had low physical activity before and 1st trimester had better mental health at 19–24 WP than active PW who became less active 10–15 PW (*p* = 0.015).
Tsai SY (2016) [45]	Sleep patterns	Pittsburgh Sleep Quality Index: T1: MCS b = – 1.40 PCS b-1.07; T2: MCS b = – 0.74 PCS b = – 0.88; T3: MCS b = – 1.42 PCS b = – 0.68; *P* < 0.01

Table 3 Factors Associated with Quality of Life During Pregnancy *(Continued)*

Author, Year, Country	Factors related to QOL *	Key Results
Vinturache A (2015) [47]	Medically assisted reproduction*, Maternal age Gravidity, Pre-pregnancy BMI*, Physical function before pregnancy*, Mental function before pregnancy	Prior to 25 WP, AC women (who had MAR) had better mental QOL ($p > 0.05$) but a lower physical health score ($p = 0.031$) than SC women (spontaneous conception). At 34–36 WP, one difference persisted for the physical symptoms between the 2 Groups ($p < 0.05$). No post-partum health-related QOL differences.
Wang P (2013) [48]	Employment *, Happy being pregnant *, Education *, Primipara *, Age	Employment: $b = -4.05$, $p < 0.001$ for mental health; $B = -3.06$ $p = 0.002$ for social health; $B = -3.39$, $p = 0.001$ for general health; Happy being pregnant: $b = 8.70$, $p = 0.01$ in the mental health component and $b = 6.94$, $p = 0.03$ for general health; level of education $b = -2.10$, $p = 0.04$ for the mental health component Primipara: $b = 0.04$, $p = 0.04$ for general health

*Significantly associated with the quality of life of pregnant women ($p < 0.05$). Abbreviations: *PW* Pregnant women, *QOL* Quality of life, *WP* Weeks of pregnant, *PCS* Physical Component Summary, *MCS* Mental Component Summary, *T1* First trimester, *T2* Second trimester, *T3* Third trimester, *PP* Postpartum, *PF* Physical Functioning, *PR* Physical role, *BP* Bodily Pain, *GH* General Health, *VT* Vitality, *SF* Social Functioning, *ER* Emotional role, *MH* Mental Health

comparisons with chronic pathologies such as diabetes. The results obtained concerning physical activity and pain in pregnant women can be compared to those obtained for chronic diseases such as cardiovascular diseases, diabetes and cancer [18]. A study by Sprangers et al. in 2000 found an average value of 58 in the "Physical Functions" and 64 in the "Bodily Pain" categories concerning diabetic patients [53]. In comparison, we found values between 53 and 77 for "Physical Functions" and between 48 and 74 for "Bodily Pain" in pregnant women. Moreover, quality of life refers to subjective elements that may vary from one culture to another. In the Coban et al. study undertaken in three countries over three continents: China, Ghana, USA [25], the subjective concepts of "well-being" or "vitality" were perceived and measured in very different ways on the three continents. This study did not focus on the quality of life of fathers. According to the *Abassi* et al. study, the quality of life of fathers was significantly higher during pregnancy and postpartum than that of their partner [39]. Specifically, their physical quality of life was significantly higher. Their mental quality of life was close, and there was no significant difference between them and their partner in two studies where this was studied [41, 43]. Finally, we believe that it is necessary to systematically screen women having a poor quality of life during pregnancy. Studies have to determine whether a single question is sufficient in clinical practice or whether it is preferable to have a more specific questionnaire before the follow-up consultation.

Conclusions

Health-related quality of life refers to the subjective assessment of patients regarding the physical, mental and social dimensions of well-being. Women's subjective perception of their health-related quality of life is an essential measure of the quality and effectiveness of maternal and child health interventions. However, few women (less than 20%) speak spontaneously about their psychological ill-health to a health professional. Health authorities' recommendations are needed to better detect a poor quality of life of pregnant women and to evaluate the impact of care in terms of quality of life of pregnant women. Then, given the diversity of factors associated with the quality of life, the medical and paramedical professions need to work in cohesion with social agencies, networks, and associations.

Acknowledgements
None.

Funding
None.

Authors' contribution
Conception and design: NL, GI. Collection and assembly of data: NL, NG, MS, SR, GI. Data analysis and interpretation: NL, NG, MS, SR, GI, AK, JC. Coordination of the research project, conception and interpretation of data: AMM. Substantial contributions to the first draft of the article: NL, NG, MS, SR, GI, AMM, AK, JC. Work on the revised version of the manuscript: MS and NG. Final approval of manuscript: All authors.

Competing interests
None of the authors have any competing interests.

Author details
[1]Department of Education and Research in General Medicine, Faculty of Medicine Pierre et Marie Curie, 27, rue Chaligny - 75571, cedex 12 Paris, France. [2]Sorbonne Universités, UPMC Univ Paris 06, INSERM, Institut Pierre Louis d'épidémiologie et de Santé Publique (IPLESP UMRS 1136), F75012 Paris, France.

References

1. Programme on Mental Health, Worl Health Organization. WHOQOL Measuring Quality of Life. 1997 [cited 2017 May 23]. Available from: http://www.who.int/mental_health/media/68.pdf
2. Mogos MF, August EM, Salinas-Miranda AA, Sultan DH, Salihu HMA. Systematic review of quality of life measures in pregnant and postpartum mothers. Appl Res Qual Life. 2013;8:219–50.
3. Bourgoin E, Callahan S, Séjourné N, Denis A. Image du corps et grossesse : vécu subjectif de 12 femmes selon une approche mixte et exploratoire. Psychol Fr. 2012;57:205–13.

4. Da Costa D, Dritsa M, Larouche J, Brender W. Psychosocial predictors of labor/delivery complications and infant birth weight: a prospective multivariate study. J Psychosom Obstet Gynaecol. 2000;21:137–48.
5. Diego MA, Field T, Hernandez-Reif M, Cullen C, Schanberg S, Kuhn C. Prepartum, postpartum, and chronic depression effects on newborns. Psychiatry. 2004;67:63–80.
6. Ibanez G, Blondel B, Prunet C, Kaminski M, Saurel-Cubizolles M-J. Prevalence and characteristics of women reporting poor mental health during pregnancy: findings from the 2010 French National Perinatal Survey. Rev Epidemiol Sante Publique. 2015;63:85–95.
7. Graignic-Philippe R, Tordjman S. Effets du stress pendant la grossesse sur le développement du bébé et de l'enfant. Arch Pédiatrie. 2009;16:1355–63.
8. Chang S-R, Kenney NJ, Chao Y-MY. Transformation in self-identity amongst Taiwanese women in late pregnancy: a qualitative study. Int J Nurs Stud. 2010;47:60–6.
9. World Bank. World Dev Report 1993: Investing in Health. New York: Oxford University Press. © World Bank; 1993. Available from: https://openknowledge.worldbank.org/handle/10986/5976
10. Wells GA, Russell AS, Haraoui B, Bissonnette R, Ware CF. Validity of quality of life measurement tools—from generic to disease-specific. J Rheumatol Suppl. 2011;88:2–6.
11. Rapport sur le développement humain. Pérenniser le progrès humain: réduire les vulnérabilités et renforcer la résilience. New York: Programme des Nations Unies pour le Développement; 2014. p. 2014.
12. Debout C. Le concept de qualité de vie en santé, une définition complexe. Soins. 2011;56:32-4.
13. Guyatt GH, Feeny DH, Patrick DL. Measuring health-related quality of life. Ann Intern Med. 1993;118:622–9.
14. Haas JS, Jackson RA, Fuentes-Afflick E, Stewart AL, Dean ML, Brawarsky P, et al. Changes in the health status of women during and after pregnancy. J Gen Intern Med. 2005;20:45–51.
15. The Strengthening the Reporting of Observational Studies in Epidemiology (STROBE) Statement: guidelines for reporting observational studies | The EQUATOR Network. [cited 2017 Oct 8]. Available from: http://www.equator-network.org/reporting-guidelines/strobe/
16. de Aquino NMR, Sun SY, de Oliveiraw EM, Martins MG, da Silva JF, Mattar R. Sexual violence and its association with health self-perception among pregnant women. Rev Saude Publ. 2009;43:954–60.
17. Chan OK, Sahota DS, Leung TY, Chan LW, Fung TY, Lau TK. Nausea and vomiting in health-related quality of life among Chinese pregnant women. Aust N Z J Obstet Gynaecol. 2010;50:512–8.
18. Da Costa D, Dritsa M, Verreault N, Balaa C, Kudzman J, Khalifé S. Sleep problems and depressed mood negatively impact health-related quality of life during pregnancy. Arch Womens Ment Health. 2010;13:249–57.
19. Dall'alba V, Callegari-Jacques SM, Krahe C, Bruch JP, Alves BC, de Barros SGS. Health-related quality of life of pregnant women with heartburn and regurgitation. Arq Gastroenterol. 2015;52:100–4.
20. Elsenbruch S. Social support during pregnancy: effects on maternal depressive symptoms, smoking and pregnancy outcome. Hum Reprod. 2007;22(3):869–77.
21. Gharacheh M, Azadi S, Mohammadi N, Montazeri S, Khalajinia Z. Domestic violence during pregnancy and Women's health-related quality of life. Glob. J. Health Sci. 2015;8(2):27–34.
22. Jomeen J, Martin CR. The factor structure of the SF-36 in early pregnancy. J Psychosom Res. 2005;59:131–8.
23. Lacasse A, Rey E, Ferreira E, Morin C, Bérard A. Nausea and vomiting of pregnancy: what about quality of life? BJOG Int J Obstet Gynaecol. 2008; 115:1484–93.
24. Lau Y, Yin L. Maternal, obstetric variables, perceived stress and health-related quality of life among pregnant women in Macao, China. Midwifery. 2011;27:668–73.
25. Li J, Mao J, Du Y, Morris JL, Gong G, Xiong X. Health-related quality of life among pregnant women with and without depression in Hubei, China. Matern Child Health J. 2012;16:1355–63.
26. Liu L, Setse R, Grogan R, Powe NR, Nicholson WK. The effect of depression symptoms and social support on black-white differences in health-related quality of life in early pregnancy: the health status in pregnancy (HIP) study. BMC Pregnancy Childbirth. 2013;13:125.
27. Mckee MD, Cunningham M, Jankowski KR, Zayas L. Health-related functional status in pregnancy: relationship to depression and social support in a multi-ethnic population. Obstet Gynecol. 2001;97(6):988–93.
28. Mota N, Cox BJ, Enns MW, Calhoun L, Sareen J. The relationship between mental disorders, quality of life, and pregnancy: findings from a nationally representative sample. J Affect Disord. 2008;109:300–4.
29. Moyer CA, Yang H, Kwawukume Y, Gupta A, Zhu Y, Koranteng I, et al. Optimism/pessimism and health-related quality of life during pregnancy across three continents: a matched cohort study in China, Ghana, and the United States. BMC Pregnancy Childbirth. 2009;9:39.
30. Nicholson WK, Setse R, Hill-Briggs F, Cooper LA, Strobino D, Powe NR. Depressive symptoms and health-related quality of life in early pregnancy. Obstet Gynecol. 2006;107:798–806.
31. Olsson C, Nilsson-Wikmar L. Health-related quality of life and physical ability among pregnant women with and without back pain in late pregnancy. Acta Obstet Gynecol Scand. 2004;83:351–7.
32. Shishehgar S, Dolatian M, Majd HA, Bakhtiary M. Perceived pregnancy stress and quality of life amongst Iranian women. Glob J Health Sci. 2014;6:270–7.
33. Fatemeh A, Azam B, Nahid M. Quality of life in pregnant women results of a study from Kashan, Iran. Pak J Med Sci. 2010;26(3):692–7.
34. Tavoli Z, Tavoli A, Amirpour R, Hosseini R, Montazeri A. Quality of life in women who were exposed to domestic violence during pregnancy. BMC Pregnancy Childbirth. 2016;16:19.
35. Ramírez-Vélez R. Pregnancy and health-related quality of life: a cross sectional study. Colomb Med. 2011;42(4):476–81.
36. Gezginc K, Uguz F, Karatayli S, Zeytinci E. The impact of obsessive-compulsive disorder in pregnancy on quality of life. Int J Psychiatry Clin Pract. 2008;12:134–7.
37. Coban A, Arslan GG, Colakfakioglu A, Sirlan A. Impact on quality of life and physical ability of pregnancy-related back pain in the third trimester of pregnancy. J Pak Med Assoc. 2011;61(11):1122–4.
38. Nakamura Y, Takeishi Y, Atogami F, Yoshizawa T. Assessment of quality of life in pregnant Japanese women: comparison of hospitalized, outpatient, and non-pregnant women. Nurs Health Sci. 2012;14:182–8.
39. Abbasi M, Van den Akker O, Bewley C. Persian couples' experiences of depressive symptoms and health-related quality of life in the pre- and perinatal period. J Psychosom Obstet Gynaecol. 2014;35:16–21.
40. Chang S-R, Chen K-H, Lin M-I, Lin H-H, Huang L-H. Lin W-A. a repeated measures study of changes in health-related quality of life during pregnancy and the relationship with obstetric factors. J Adv Nurs. 2014;70:2245–56.
41. De Pascalis L, Agostini F, Monti F, Paterlini M, Fagandini P, La Sala GB. A comparison of quality of life following spontaneous conception and assisted reproduction. Int J Gynaecol Obstet Off Organ Int Fed Gynaecol Obstet 2012;118:216–219.
42. Emmanuel EN, Sun J. Health related quality of life across the perinatal period among Australian women. J Clin Nurs. 2014;23:1611–9.
43. Ngai F-W, Ngu S-F. Quality of life during the transition to parenthood in Hong Kong: a longitudinal study. J Psychosom Obstet Gynaecol. 2013;34: 157–62.
44. Setse R, Grogan R, Pham L, Cooper LA, Strobino D, Powe NR, et al. Longitudinal study of depressive symptoms and health-related quality of life during pregnancy and after delivery: the health status in pregnancy (HIP) study. Matern Child Health J. 2009;13:577–87.
45. Tendais I, Figueiredo B, Mota J, Conde A. Physical activity, health-related quality of life and depression during pregnancy. Cad Saude Publica. 2011;27:219–28.
46. Tsai S-Y, Lee P-L, Lin J-W, Lee C-N. Cross-sectional and longitudinal associations between sleep and health-related quality of life in pregnant women: a prospective observational study. Int J Nurs Stud. 2016;56:45–53.
47. Vachkova E, Jezek S, Mares J, Moravcova M. The evaluation of the psychometric properties of a specific quality of life questionnaire for physiological pregnancy. Health Qual Life Outcomes. 2013;11:214.

48. Vinturache A, Stephenson N, McDonald S, Wu M, Bayrampour H, Tough S. Health-related quality of life in pregnancy and postpartum among women with assisted conception in Canada. Fertil Steril 2015;104:188–195.e1.
49. Wang P, Liou S-R, Cheng C-Y. Prediction of maternal quality of life on preterm birth and low birthweight: a longitudinal study. BMC Pregnancy Childbirth. 2013;13:124.
50. Emmanuel E, St John W, Sun J. Relationship between social support and quality of life in childbearing women during the perinatal period. J Obstet Gynecol Neonatal Nurs. 2012;41:E62–70.
51. Hama K, Takamura N, Honda S, Abe Y, Yagura C, Miyamura T, et al. Evaluation of quality of life in Japanese Normal pregnant women. Acta Med Nagasakiensa. 2007;52(4):95–9.
52. Ibanez G. Santé mentale des femmes enceintes et développement de l'enfant. Thèse de doctorat en santé publique. Paris. Thèse de doctorat en santé publique; 2014.
53. Sprangers MA, de Regt EB, Andries F, van Agt HM, Bijl RV, de Boer JB, et al. Which chronic conditions are associated with better or poorer quality of life? J Clin Epidemiol. 2000;53:895–907.

17

Labour Q1 pain – poorly analysed and reported

Hans Järnbert-Pettersson[1*] and Linda Vixner[2]

Abstract

Background: Modelling and analysing repeated measures data, such as women's experiences of pain during labour, is a complex topic. Traditional end-point analyses such as t-tests, ANOVA, or repeated measures [rANOVA] have known disadvantages. Modern and more sophisticated statistical methods such as mixed effect models provide flexibility and are more likely to draw correct conclusions from data. The aim of this study is to study how labour pain is analysed in repeated measures design studies, and to increase awareness of when and why modern statistical methods are suitable with the aim of encouraging their use in preference of traditional methods.

Methods: Six databases were searched with the English language as a restriction. Study eligibility criteria included: Original studies published between 1999 and 2016, studying pregnant women in labour with the aim to compare at least two methods for labour pain management, with at least two measurements of labour pain separated by time, and where labour pain was analysed.

After deduplication, all records ($n = 2800$) were screened by one of the authors who excluded ineligible publication types, leaving 737 records remaining for full-text screening. A sample of 309 studies was then randomly selected and screened by both authors.

Results: Among the 133 (of 309) studies that fulfilled the study eligibility criteria, 7% used mixed effect models, 20% rANOVA, and 73% used end-point analysis to draw conclusions regarding treatment effects for labour pain between groups. The most commonly used end-point analyses to compare groups regarding labour pain were t-tests (57, 43%) and ANOVA (41, 31%). We present a checklist for clinicians to clarify when mixed effect models should be considered as the preferred choice for analysis, in particular when labour pain is measured.

Conclusions: Studies that aim to compare methods for labour pain management often use inappropriate statistical methods, and inaccurately report how the statistical analyses were carried out. The statistical methods used in analyses are often based on assumptions that are not fulfilled or described. We recommend that authors, reviewers, and editors pay greater attention to the analysis when designing and publishing studies evaluating methods for pain relief during labour.

Keywords: Labour pain, Repeated-measures data, Longitudinal study, Mixed models, Mixed effect models, Repeated measure ANOVA, Statistical analysis, CONSORT, STROBE

Background

Women's experiences of pain during labour are highly variable [1] and are related to women's overall assessments of childbirth [2]. A painful labour may have long-term consequences for women's health and wellbeing [3]. Most women in labour require pain relief, which can be administered in either pharmacological or non-pharmacological form [4].

Comparing labour pain between different treatment groups needs consideration, both regarding when and how often pain assessments are made, and how statistical analyses have been conducted to reflect the reality of women's pain varying during labour. Women's pain varies both between individual women and within the same woman over time as well as between different treatment groups. The mean intensity of labour pain is closely

* Correspondence: Hans.pettersson@ki.se
[1]Karolinska Institutet - Department of Clinical Science and Education, Södersjukhuset, Stockholm, Sweden

related to the progression of labour and increases with greater cervical dilatation [5–10]. In addition, labour pain correlates with the intensity, duration, and frequency of uterine contractions [1, 8]. Furthermore, although pain increases with time, individual progression can differ from woman to woman as a result of both biological factors and the interventions that are administered.

When pain assessments are made more than once for each woman, conclusions made on the management of labour pain will be based on repeated measures data. The most common research questions (and corresponding statistical test) for these study designs are; *1) Is there any difference in mean pain between the treatment group and the control group(s) over all time-points?* (overall treatment effect between groups), 2) *If so, are the differences in labour pain between groups equal or do they differ at different time-points?* (interaction between treatment and time), and 3) *is there a difference in pain within each group?* (within group effect). In these cases, appropriate statistical methods for repeated measures data should be used (rANOVA or mixed models). This is in contrast to analyses in studies where only one time-point is of interest. In such cases, end-point analyses such as t-tests or ANOVA could be used.

The most commonly used methods to measure labour pain are verbal reports with standardised instruments such as the Visual Analogue Scale (VAS), the McGill Pain Questionnaire (MPQ), the Short-Form MPQ, verbal rating scales, or simple ordinal scales [1]. Although there are many studies that consider how labour pain should be assessed [1] in trials evaluating methods for pain relief during labour, to our knowledge there are no studies that have studied how these assessments are analysed and reported.

The purpose of this paper is to study how labour pain is analysed in studies with a repeated measures design, and to increase awareness of when and why modern statistical methods are suitable, so as to encourage their use over traditional methods. This paper will briefly review the most frequently occurring methods of repeated measures analysis for continuous outcomes when means are compared. A summary of aspects to consider when studies with an emphasis on labour pain are planned and analysed and the potential consequences of the choice of statistical method are presented in Table 1, (modified from [11, 12]).

Traditional methods

End-point analysis compares mean pain between treatments and control groups at one specific time-point, or a difference between two specific time-points (e.g. baseline versus last measurement). Independent t-tests assume that two groups are compared while ANOVA or ANCOVA are used if three or more groups are compared, and these are often followed by independent t-tests to study pairwise comparisons. This approach tests the mean difference between groups at a specific time-point rather than testing whether there is a general difference between the groups over all relevant time-points. Although easy to understand and implement, it is well known that the probability of a type I error (false positive) increases when using this approach if comparisons are done at each time-point, which implies that the conclusion might falsely be that a treatment has an effect on labour pain). Furthermore, it is not possible to formally test if there are any interactions between time and treatment since only one time-point is considered at a time.

In contrast to end-point analysis, repeated measures ANOVA (rANOVA) includes data from all time-points in the analysis. It makes it possible for the total increase in mean pain to be equal between baseline and the final measurement in both groups, even though there is a difference in mean pain score among the groups at earlier time-points. In such cases, an end-point analysis will find differences at the final time point but not at earlier time-points. Thus, end-point analysis cannot, in contrast to rANOVA, give any answer to if there is an overall difference in mean pain between the groups with respect to all time points, which is often the research question. In addition, rANOVA can formally find if the differences are similar at all time-points by using the statistical test for interactions between treatment and time.

There are, however, disadvantages in using rANOVA in the context of analysing labour pain. The assumptions for this model to make appropriate conclusions regarding treatment effects are rarely met in practice. Firstly, rANOVA requires the same number of repeated measurements to be made for all women. Hence, even one missing pain measurement at one time point for one woman, would lead to all data collected from this woman to be lost, i.e. each woman with missing data will be excluded from the analyses. There are two ways to circumvent this missing data problem when using rANOVA; either data need to be imputed, which in turn might lead to an estimation bias, or analyses could be conducted only on data from the group of women with complete data sets, which might introduce a sample bias since these women may not be representative for the whole population. In addition, statistical power will be reduced.

Secondly, an assumption that is implicit for rANOVA is the sphericity assumption, which implies that variance is assumed to be equal at all times (constant variance) and that the covariance (correlation) between any two time-points is equal. These assumptions are usually not met when labour pain is analysed since consecutive pain measurements on the same woman tend to be more correlated than measurements taken further away in time.

Table 1 Comparison of traditional and mixed-effect approaches and questions to answer when choosing a statistical method for the analysis of labour pain in repeated measures data

Questions to ask when you choose statistical method	Statistical property	Statistical method		
		End-point Analysis	rANOVA	Mixed effect models
1. What do you want to compare?	Research question	Compares mean labour pain between groups at one time-point	Compares mean labour pain between groups at several time-points Study interactions between time[a]treatments	a. Compares mean labour pain between groups at several time-points b. Study interactions between time and treatment c. Study individual women's pain changes over time
2. Do you have measurements of labour pain at all time-points for all women?	Missing data	Excludes woman with missing measurements	Excludes woman with missing measurements	Use all available measurements under the assumption of missing at random (MAR)
	Possible effect of omitting women with missing values?	Sample bias	Sample bias	Not applicable
	Possible effect of imputation of missing data?	Estimation bias	Estimation bias	Not applicable
3. Can you assume that correlation of pain is equal between all time-points?	Assumption on the between woman pain correlation	Independent	Independent	Independent
Are the labour pain assessments made with unequal distances, e.g. at baseline, and after 2 and 6 h?	Assumption on the individual woman pain correlation or covariance matrix	Independent	Compound symmetry	Allow a variety of covariance structures, e.g. Independence, Compound symmetry, AR [1], Unstructured
4. Can you assume that the variance of labour pain is equal at all time-points?	Assumption on the variance of pain at different time-points	Constrained to be equal at all time-points	Constrained to be equal at all time-points	Allowed to vary
5. Are measurements of labour pain normally distributed?	Assumption of normal distribution	Normality assumption	Normality assumption	Normality assumption
6. What requirements do you have on your statistical model to model the pain over time?	Description of time effect	Simple	Flexible	Flexible
7. Would you like to consider labour pain traits for individual women over time?	Estimation of individual trends	No	No	Yes
8. Do you need to adjust labour pain for factors that vary during labour, e.g. cervical dilatation and use of other pain relief?	Time dependent covariates	No	Yes	Yes
9. Do you have knowledge of applied statistics?	Ease of implementation	Very easy	Easy	Complex
10. Do you have access to a good computer?	Computational complexity	Low	Low	High

For example, the correlation between a woman's pain assessments at the two first measurements (which are often measured with a short time interval between them) are often higher than the correlation between the first and last pain measurement. When rANOVA is used despite not fulfilling the assumptions, there is a risk for type I errors when the interaction between treatment and time is tested, which in turn might lead to incorrect conclusions about the question of whether there is a difference in labour pain at different time-points .

Modern methods

Using mixed effect models is a more flexible method of analysing labour pain than traditional methods as they allow correlated data, variances that differ between time-points and have greater flexibility in handling missing data [13, 14]. They have a number of advantages, the first being that mixed effect models can account for the correlation between measurements, which implies that mixed effect models can handle uneven time intervals between measurements, such as when pain is measured more frequently during the first hour after an intervention than in the later stages of labour (e.g. at 15, 30, 45, 60, 90, 150 min). These correlations can be modelled, which implies that, for example, the assumption of data sphericity in rANOVA does not need to be met. In addition, the variance is also allowed to vary between time-points that enable the model to allow for greater variance in labour pain at time-points closer to birth.

The second advantage is that mixed effect models can use all available measurements for all women and therefore handle missing data more appropriately – as long as they meet the missing-completely-at-random definition [15]. Data are missing completely at random (MCAR) if the occurrence of missing data is independent of both observed and unobserved outcomes. If a woman drops out of a study due to treatment-related adverse effects, any lacking measurements of pain for this patient is classified as missing-at-random (MAR). Mixed effect models can take care of missing data as long as they meet the assumptions of MCAR. In contrast, in these cases traditional methods require the exclusion of all data from a woman with partially missing data in the analysis.

The third advantage is that mixed models can manage between-individual heterogeneity and that pain for each individual woman will deviate randomly from the overall average pain (random intercept), and that the treatment effect also will differ among the women (random treatment effect). This is in contrast to traditional models, which assume that average pain is equal for all women at baseline (i.e. no random intercept) and that the treatment effects are equal for all women (i.e. no random effect of treatment) in all groups.

Methods

Study selection

We followed the preferred reporting standard for systematic reviews (PRISMA) [16] to review studies with a repeated measures design and with labour pain analysed as a continuous outcome. Our searches were limited by date (published between Jan 1, 1999, and March 7, 2016) and included the following databases: Medline (OVID), Cinahl (Ebsco), Cochrane (Wileys), Embase (Embase.com), PubMed (complement), and WoS (Thomson Reuters). The search was conducted by librarians at Karolinska Institutet's University Library. Search terms used for each database can be found in Additional file 1: Appendix S1. Inclusion criteria were: original studies, studying pregnant women in labour intending a vaginal birth (any parity or risk status), with the aim to compare at least two methods for labour pain management, with at least two measurements of labour pain at different time points, and where labour pain was analysed or presented as a mean.

The total number of studies after deduplication was 2800, which were all screened by one of the authors to exclude ineligible publication types (including, letters, editorials, and reviews), animal or in vitro research, and studies published in a language other than English (Fig. 1). After the screening process, 737 studies remained eligible for full-text screening.

A sample size calculation were performed to assure that we could estimate the proportion of studies that used mixed models with a high precision (95% confidence interval with a precision of plus-minus 4 percentage points). We assumed that the proportion of studies that used mixed effect models, would be 5%. The sample size calculation gave 150 studies; in addition, we assumed that approximately 50% would fulfil our inclusion and exclusion criteria. A sample of 309 studies were therefore randomly selected from the 737 studies assessed eligible for full-text screening.

Data collection process

Of the 309 selected studies that were read in full-text, 175 did not fulfil the inclusion criteria, leaving 133 that were included (Fig. 1) from 54 different journals (Additional file 2: Table S1). We developed a data extraction sheet, Additional file 3: Appendix S2, with items modified from the CONSORT [17] and STROBE [18] checklists. In addition, information on study design, instruments for pain assessment including anchor labels, time-points, and intervals for pain assessments, number of comparison groups, effect measure for labour pain, number of observations in the analysis, tests for normality, and management of missing data were recorded in the data extraction sheet. We also examined if there were any discrepancies between the statistical method section and the reporting in the result section.

Both authors pilot-tested the sheet on 30 randomly selected included studies. Thereafter, both authors independently read all the studies and assessed the most advanced statistical method used in the following order: mixed-effect model, rANOVA, ANOVA, and end-point analysis. Disagreements between the authors' assessments

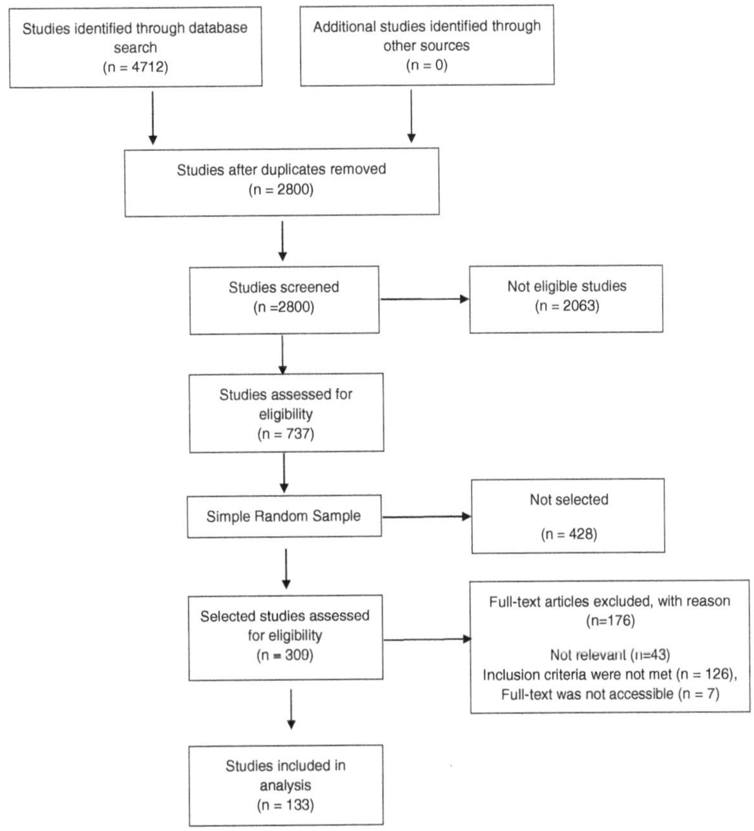

Fig. 1 Flow chart for inclusion of studies

were resolved by reading the studies again followed by a discussion between the two review authors.

Statistical methods

We present data from our sample as frequencies and percentages that represent an estimate of the occurrence in the population from which the sample of studies intends to generalize the results to. To illustrate the precision in the estimates (highest uncertainty around 50% and lowest close to 0%), we generated binomial exact confidence intervals (Clopper Pearson) for the following percentages: 1, 5, 10, 20, 50, and 90% presented in Tables 2 and 3. Analysis was conducted using SPSS version 23, and the pre-specified sample size calculation was conducted using Sample Power 3.0.

Results

The most commonly used study design was a randomised controlled trial (87%) with two or three experiment groups (Table 2). Analyses of labour pain were conducted including $\geq$51 women in 66% of the studies. Measurements of labour pain were made repeatedly for each woman between 3 and 10 times in 90% of the studies, and the time intervals between each measurement was equal in 31% of the studies. Labour pain was rarely explicitly defined as a primary or secondary outcome.

A Visual Analog Scale (VAS) [19] was the most-often used tool to measure labour pain (used in 110 studies [83%]), although the description of the scale differed among the studies, or the scale was not clearly described. The maximum anchor labels of VAS were in 60% (66/110) of the studies. Among these 66 studies, we found 23 different definitions. The most commonly used anchor labels for maximum pain were "worst pain imaginable" ($n = 17$), "worst possible pain" ($n = 10$), "worst pain" ($n = 10$), "worst imaginable pain" ($n = 9$), "unbearable pain" ($n = 4$), and "severe pain" ($n = 3$). For the minimum anchor label of VAS, we found four definitions among the 67 studies where it was defined, with the most common definitions being "no pain" ($n = 60$) and "no pain at all" ($n = 4$).

Statistical methods used to compare labour pain between treatment groups are presented in Table 3. Among the 133 included studies, Mixed effect models were the most advanced statistical method found in 9 studies (7%), rANOVA in 26 studies (20%), and end-points analysis in 97 studies (73%). The most frequently used statistical methods to analyse repeated measures data were t-tests and ANOVA.

Table 2 Repeated measures designs in 133 labour pain studies

		Number	Percent (%)
Study Design	Experiment - randomised	116	87.2
	Experiment - not randomised	13	9.8
	Observational - Cohort	3	2.3
	Not clear	1	0.8
Number of groups compared	2	96	72.2
	3	24	18.0
	> 4	13	9.8
Total number of women included in analysis	20–30	10	7.5
	31–50	32	24.1
	51–100	55	41.4
	101–500	32	24.1
Pain - number of time points measured	2	14	10.5
	3–5	48	36.1
	6–10	56	42.1
	> 10	15	11.3
Equally spaced time intervals	No	92	69.2
	Yes	40	30.1
	Not clear	1	0.8
Pain - outcome measure	Primary outcome	11	8.3
	Secondary outcome	4	3.0
	Not explicit	118	88.7
Pain - measurement Instrument[a]	VAS (Visual analogue scale)	110	82.7
	NRS (numeric rating scale)	6	4.5
	MPQ, short version	1	0.8
	Verbal rating scale	14	10.5
	Other	2	1.5

[a]Anchor labels for the instruments were specified in 65% (67/133)
Illustrative binomial exact 95% confidence intervals for percentages when sample size is 133: 1% (0 to 4%); 5% (2 to 10%); 10%(5 to 16%); 25%(18 to 33%); 50%(40 to 58%); 90(84 to 95%)

Table 3 Statistical methods and presentation of results in 133 labour pain studies with repeated measures design

		Number	Percent (%)
Most advanced statistical method to analyse labour pain	End-point analysis[a]	97	72.9
	rANOVA	26	19.5
	Mixed effect models	9	6.8
	Not clear	1	0.8
Clear how between-groups comparisons are conducted?	No	34	25.6
	Yes	99	74.4
Are comparison conducted within groups (between time points)?	No	87	65.4
	Yes	46	34.6
Clear how within group comparisons are conducted?	No	19	41.3
	Yes	27	58.7
Are numbers of valid observations used in analysis for each group and time-point stated?	No - only number of individuals at one time-point, e.g. baseline is stated	112	84.2
	Yes - number of individuals/valid measurements at each time-point is stated	21	15.8
Is normality assumption tested/mentioned?	No	120	90.2
	Yes	13	9.8
Clear agreement between statistical methods and results presented?	No	77	57.9
	Yes	56	42.1

[a]Several end-point analyses could be used in each of these 97 studies: t-tests were used in 59 (44%) studies, ANOVA in 41 studies (31%), Mann-Whitney in 20 studies (15%), Wilcoxon in 6 studies (5%), and ANCOVA in 1 study (1%)
Illustrative binomial exact 95% confidence intervals for percentages when sample size is 133: 1% (0 to 4%); 5% (2 to 10%); 10%(5 to 16%); 25%(18 to 33%); 50%(40 to 58%); 90(84 to 95%)

Among the 123 studies that used end-point or rANOVA to analyse labour pain, the specific number of observations used in the analysis at each time-point were stated in only 16% of the studies. In 85 of the 123 studies (69%), pain was assessed at time-points with unequal distances between them. It was not clear whether there were missing data, and/or if the measurements of labour pain were made at time-points with unequal distances in 108 of the 123 studies (88%), which used end-point analysis or rANOVA.

There was no clear presentation of how between-group comparisons were made in 34 of the 133 studies (26%). In the 46 of the 133 studies (35%) where within-group comparisons were made (i.e. comparison within a group between time-points), it was not clear how these comparisons had been made in 19 (41%) of them.

There was clear agreement between the statistical methods presented in the method section of the paper and the result section in only 42% of the studies. For example, the method section might state that ANOVA was used to compare labour pain between the groups; however p-values in the results section did not specify at which time points comparisons were made, or whether the p-value corresponded to an overall test between three groups made by an ANOVA or by a post-hoc t-test between two specific groups. How, or if, assumptions regarding normality were examined was reported in only 10% of the studies.

Discussion

This systematic review found that studies aiming to compare at least two methods of labour pain management often use inappropriate statistical methodology, and inaccurately report how the statistical analyses were conducted. In particular:

(1) Statistical models used in the analyses were more often than not based on incorrect assumptions to give an appropriate answer to the research question. End-point analysis or ANOVA were used to test for differences between groups over time, though these methods only formally test for differences at a specific time-point.
(2) How the analyses were conducted was often not clearly described. This means that the reader has to make assumptions about how the analyses have been carried out. In particular, missing data at different time-points were rarely reported.
(3) The verbal anchor descriptors of the end-points of VAS, time intervals between each pain assessment, and the number of pain assessments varied largely in the studies.

Problems associated with the poor application and reporting of statistical methods are not new. Altman (1982) [20] noted decades ago that researchers both use the wrong techniques (wilfully or in ignorance) and use the right techniques incorrectly. Our study supports this finding, as the quality of the studies included here makes it difficult for readers to assess the value of the conclusions regarding labour pain management.

The use of more advanced statistical methods has increased in recent decades, and continues to do so [21–23]. In general, there is a natural time lag between new statistical methods being developed and being used and applied in research. Mixed models were developed during the 1980s and implemented in statistical software programs such as SAS, STATA, SPSS and R in the following decades. In contrast to other research areas where there has been a debate on methodological aspects regarding how to analyse data that is measured repeatedly with mixed models [11], we have found no such debate in the area of labour pain research.

Thus, the prerequisites for using mixed models in the context of measuring labour pain in this study show that analyses are rarely carried out using an approach that reflects how data are collected. If and how the conclusions regarding the management of labour pain would change if appropriate analyses were conducted remains unknown.

Statements such as CONSORT [17] and STROBE [18] give recommendations on how statistical methods and results should be reported with the principle to follow; *"Describe statistical methods with enough detail to enable a knowledgeable reader with access to the original data to verify the reported results (www.icmje.org)"* [17]. In this study we did not only assess whether the statistical methods used were clearly described in the methods section (CONSORT, item 12a), but we also assessed if there was a clear agreement between the methods section and the results section, and whether the choice of statistical methods was appropriate for answering the research question in the context of repeated measured data. Our results should be interpreted with this in mind, and for clarity we would like to emphasise the following points. A clear description of the statistical methods used in the methods section does not necessarily mean that those methods were actually used, or that these methods were used appropriately. Also, a clear description of the method and clear agreement in the results section does not necessarily mean that the used method was appropriate to answer the research question.

We noted a few typical reporting errors, for example that the statistical method section described several methods that had been used, however, as a reader, when reading the results section you needed to make assumptions as to which test or model had been used. The method section could describe both t-tests and Mann-Whitney U-tests, but in the results section there was no information as to which of the methods had been used for specific results. Other examples such as the use of ANOVA without a description of which model was used (e.g. with/without interactions, adjusted/not adjusted for confounders), commonly occurred. We also found studies where the method section seemed to be completely independent from the results section, as if the method section appertained to another study, and was not in accordance with the study's research question at all. In addition, we found studies that we suspected contained simple misspellings or typos, for example, a methods section could describe that a dependent t-test was used to compare differences between groups, which raises the question whether this was the case, or if actually it was an ***in***dependent t-test that had been used.

The problem of using inappropriate statistical methods even though the statistical methods were clearly described was also quite common. For example, the methods section could describe that a t-test was used, which was also in clear agreement with the results section (which is often the case if a single method is used), but this occurred in cases where the method was not appropriate. One might argue that a "simple test" need not be presented in detail, which motivates the use of sentences such as "t-tests, rANOVA and Mann Whitney U tests were used as appropriate". The problem is that what "appropriate use" is according to professional statisticians and applied researchers seems to differ somewhat.

Although most of the included studies were randomised and should follow the CONSORT statement for reporting, the recommendation to describe statistical methods in detail was not followed. One explanation for this lack of detail could be that not all journals have yet endorsed CONSORT, or had not endorsed CONSORT at the time of the publication of the included study. It has been shown that journal endorsement of CONSORT may benefit the completeness of the reporting of randomised trials [24].

A strength of this study is that generalizations can be made to all studies that compare the management of labour pain between groups over time with a continuous outcome, i.e. studies with a repeated measures design. In contrast to studies that investigate methodological aspects of analysis and design, we did not include studies from specific journals [21–23, 25] or conduct our search strategy with keywords only regarding study design. Only 13% (17/133) of our included studies had the keywords "longitudinal" or "repeated measures". Instead, we conducted our search with a subject of medical research interest, i.e. pain among women in labour, and then manually classified the studies with regard to study design, which implies that this systematic review reflects how studies in general analyse and report labour pain, not how this is done in specific journals or in studies with a specified study design based on search words such as "longitudinal" which we believe are more aware of the analysis of repeated measures [12].

Women's perceptions of labour pain intensity vary greatly during labour, and the pattern of pain differs between women for a number of reasons, e.g. it differs between nulliparous and multiparous women and between women in early and later stages of labour [1]. Most methods for labour pain relief are safe for both mother and baby, however, their efficacy is unclear due to limited methodological quality. The way pain has been assessed differs considerably among the studies and it is not always clear which tool was used to assess pain or how the extremes of the scales were marked (anchor labels). In addition, information about pain relief at different stages of labour are also lacking [4]. The findings in our study confirm that end-points on the pain assessment scales differ considerably, which has been confirmed elsewhere [26]. High-quality systematic reviews and other synthesized research evidence compiled by HTA (Health Technology Assessment) organisations around the world, is the base for clinicians to make informed health decisions. As noted by others, to assess and analyse labour pain without considering the aspects of variability during labour, limitations in more traditional statistical methods, and without considering the fact that there are no specific recommendations with respect to anchor labels makes compiling evidence in e.g. systematic reviews challenging [4].

To improve design, analysis and reporting we recommend that authors, reviewers, and editors:

1. In addition to e.g. CONSORT and STROBE checklists, use extraction sheet Additional file 3: Appendix S2, the questions 7–22 to check if your article answer these questions.
2. Use Table 1 to choose statistical method and to check if the analysis is appropriate reported with respect to your research question and design. Consult a professional statistician if you are insecure about the answers and which statistical method that is appropriate and why.
3. Don't forget point 1 and 2. You should be aware of the questions (and answers) already in the design of your study. To press buttons in a statistical software program is not a valid foundation for the results if you are not aware about the assumptions underlying the results. The statistical analysis is the foundation for your results and, in turn, your conclusions about treatments of labour pain – don't forget that.

Conclusions

Studies aiming to compare at least two methods for labour pain management often use inappropriate statistical methods, and inaccurately report how statistical analyses were carried out. The verbal anchor descriptors of pain assessments, the time intervals between each pain assessment, and the number of pain assessments made varies largely among the studies. The statistical methods used in the analyses are often based on assumptions that are either not fulfilled or not described, or both. We recommend that authors, reviewers, and editors pay greater attention to method choice and use when designing, reviewing, and publishing studies evaluating methods for pain relief during labour.

Additional files

Additional file 1: Appendix S1. Search strategy for the six databases.

Additional file 2: Table S1. Included Journals.

Additional file 3: Appendix S2. Data extraction sheet used to collect data.

Abbreviations

ANCOVA: Analysis of covariance; ANOVA: Analysis of variance; AR: Auto Regressive; CONSORT: Consolidated standards of reporting trials; MAR: Missing at random; MCAR: Missing completely at random; MPQ: McGill Pain Questionnaire; NRS: Numeric rating scale; PRISMA: Preferred reporting standard for systematic review; rANOVA: Repeated measure ANOVA; STROBE: Strengthening the Reporting of observational studies in Epidemiology; VAS: Visual analogue scale

Acknowledgements

We thank Gun Brit Knutssön and Susanne Gustafsson, librarians at Karolinska Institutet's University Library, for their valuable help with the data base searches.

Funding

None.

Disclosure of interests

None.

Authors' contributions
Both authors designed the study, reviewed the articles, analysed the data, and wrote the article. Both authors read and approved the final manuscript.

Authors' information
HJP is an Associate professor in medical statistics with a PhD in statistics and is interested in methodological research. LV has a PhD in medical science and has performed labour pain research. We noted a gap between applied researchers that not are aware of the problems with the statistical methods they use. Statisticians are aware of the problem but are used to present these knowledge in mathematical terms that clinicians not are used to. This article is a bridge between the sciences of medical research and statistics to improve applied research.

Competing interests
The authors declare that they have no competing interests.

Author details
[1]Karolinska Institutet - Department of Clinical Science and Education, Södersjukhuset, Stockholm, Sweden. [2]Dalarna University- School of Education, Health and Social Studies, Falun, Sweden.

References
1. Lowe NK. The nature of labor pain. Am J Obstet Gynecol. 2002;186(5):S16–24. https://doi.org/10.1067/mob.2002.121427.
2. Waldenstrom U, Schytt E. A longitudinal study of women's memory of labour pain-from 2 months to 5 years after the birth. Bjog. 2009;116(4):577–83. https://doi.org/10.1111/j.1471-0528.2008.02020.x.
3. Gottvall K, Waldenstrom U. Does a traumatic birth experience have an impact on future reproduction? Bjog. 2002;109(3):254–60. https://doi.org/10.1016/s1470-0328(02)01200-4.
4. Jones L, Othman M, Dowswell T, et al. Pain management for women in labour: an overview of systematic reviews. Cochrane Database Syst Rev. 2012;3. https://doi.org/10.1002/14651858.CD009234.pub2.
5. Melzack R. The myth of painless childbirth (the bonica,john j. Lecture). Pain. 1984;19(4):321–37. https://doi.org/10.1016/0304-3959(84)90079-4.
6. Rowlands S, Permezel M. Physiology of pain in labour. Baillieres Clin Obstet Gynaecol. 1998;12(3):347–62. https://doi.org/10.1016/s0950-3552(98)80071-0
7. Lowe NK. Differences in 1st and 2nd stage labor pain between nulliparous and multiparous women. J Psychosom Obstet Gynecol. 1992;13(4):243–53. https://doi.org/10.3109/01674829209009197.
8. Melzack R, Kinch R, Dobkin P, et al. Severity of labor pain - influence of physical as well as psychologic variables. Can Med Assoc J. 1984;130(5):579–84.
9. Brown ST, Campbell D, Kurtz A. Characteristics of labor pain at 2 stages of cervical-dilation. Pain. 1989;38(3):289–95. https://doi.org/10.1016/0304-3959(89)90215-7.
10. Vixner L, Schytt E, Stener-Victorin E, et al. Acupuncture with manual and electrical stimulation for labour pain: a longitudinal randomised controlled trial. BMC Complement Altern Med. 2014;14(1):187.
11. Gueorguieva R, Krystal JH. Move over ANOVA: progress in analyzing repeated-measures data and its reflection in papers published in the Archives of General Psychiatry. Arch Gen Psychiatry 2004;61(3):310–317. https://doi.org/10.1001/archpsyc.61.3.310 [published Online First: 2004/03/03].
12. Liu C, Cripe TP, Kim MO. Statistical issues in longitudinal data analysis for treatment efficacy studies in the biomedical sciences. Mol Ther 2010;18(9): 1724–1730. https://doi.org/10.1038/mt.2010.127 [published Online First: 2010/07/01].
13. Diggle PJ. Analysis of longitudinal data. 2. ed. New York: Oxford University Press; 2002.
14. Brown H, Prescott R. Applied mixed models in medicine. Third;3; ed. New York: John Wiley & Sons Inc; 2015.
15. Little RJA, Rubin DB. Statistical analysis with missing data. 2 ed. Newy York: Wiley-Interscience; 2014.
16. Liberati A, Altman DG, Tetzlaff J, et al. The PRISMA statement for reporting systematic reviews and meta-analyses of studies that evaluate healthcare interventions: explanation and elaboration. BMJ. 2009;339. https://doi.org/10.1136/bmj.b2700.
17. Moher D, Hopewell S, Schulz K, et al. CONSORT 2010 Explanation and Elaboration: updated guidelines for reporting parallel group randomised trials. BMJ. 2010;340(mar23 1):c869–c79.
18. von Elm E, Altman DG, Egger M, et al. The strengthening the reporting of observational studies in epidemiology (STROBE) statement: guidelines for reporting observational studies. Lancet. 2007;370(9596):1453–7. https://doi.org/10.1016/s0140-6736(07)61602-x.
19. Price DD, McGrath PA, Rafii A, et al. The validation of visual analog scales as ratio scale measures for chronic and experimental pain. Pain. 1983;17(1):45–56. https://doi.org/10.1016/0304-3959(83)90126-4.
20. Altman DG. Statistics in medical journals. Stat Med 1982;1(1):59–71. [published Online First: 1982/01/01].
21. Sato Y, Gosho M, Nagashima K, et al. Statistical Methods in the Journal - An Update. N Engl J Med 2017;376(11):1086–1087. https://doi.org/10.1056/NEJMc1616211 [published Online First: 2017/03/16].
22. Arnold LD, Braganza M, Salih R, et al. Statistical trends in the Journal of the American Medical Association and implications for training across the continuum of medical education. PloS one 2013;8(10):e77301. https://doi.org/10.1371/journal.pone.0077301 [published Online First: 2013/11/10].
23. Yi D, Ma D, Li G, et al. Statistical Use in Clinical Studies: Is There Evidence of a Methodological Shift? PloS one 2015;10(10):e0140159. https://doi.org/10.1371/journal.pone.0140159 [published Online First: 2015/10/09].
24. Turner L, Shamseer L, Altman DG, et al. Does use of the CONSORT Statement impact the completeness of reporting of randomised controlled trials published in medical journals? A Cochrane review. Syst Rev 2012;1:60. https://doi.org/10.1186/2046-4053-1-60 [published Online First: 2012/12/01].
25. Welch GE, 2nd, Gabbe SG. Review of statistics usage in the American Journal of Obstetrics and Gynecology. Am J Obstet Gynecol 1996;175(5): 1138–1141. [published Online First: 1996/11/01].
26. Hjermstad MJ, Fayers PM, Haugen DF, et al. Studies comparing numerical rating scales, verbal rating scales, and Visual analogue scales for assessment of pain intensity in adults: a systematic literature review. J Pain Symptom Manag. 2011;41(6):1073–93. https://doi.org/10.1016/j.jpainsymman.2010.08.016.

Changes in serum prolactin level during intracytoplasmic sperm injection, and effect on clinical pregnancy rate

Ahmed Kamel[1*], Ayman A. Halim[1], Mohamed Shehata[2], Salwa AlFarra[1], Yahia El-faissal[1], Wafaa Ramadan[1] and Ahmed M. Hussein[1]

Abstract

Background: Transient hyperprolactinemia was proven to adversely affect the outcome of IVF. We aimed to identify changes in serum prolactin levels in patients undergoing ICSI, and to evaluate the effect of these changes on the clinical pregnancy rate.

Methods: A prospective observational study included 90 patients scheduled for ICSI cycles. In each case 4 serum samples were collected during the cycle (midluteal, before ovum pick up procedure (OPU), 2 h after OPU, and before embryo transfer). Serum prolactin level was determined by immunoassay each time.

Results: The sample collected 2 h after OPU had a mean difference of 25.8 ± 2.8 ng/ml compared to the basal serum prolactin ($p < 0.01$). In comparison to other samples, this highlighted a significant hyperprolactinemia occurring after OPU, and resolving before embryo transfer. No statistically significant difference between the different serum prolactin samples amongst the pregnant and non pregnant patients. There was a significant positive pearson correlation between the prolactin levels before OPU, and the presence of higher quality embryos ($r = 0.274$, $p = 0.019$).

Conclusion: In normoprolactinemic women transient hyperprolactinemia is identified in patients undergoing ICSI, and it doesn't affect the clinical pregnancy rates. A positive correlation was identified between higher quality embryos, and serum prolactin level before OPU.

Keywords: Embryo quality, Intracytoplasmic sperm injection, Hyperprolactinemia, Prolactin

Background

Prolactin (PRL) is a 198 amino acid polypeptide hormone secreted in a pulsatile manner from the anterior pituitary, and is synthesized by lactotroph cells. It weighs 23 kDa, and its secretion is affected by many factors which include stress, sleep, pregnancy, ingesting food, and chest wall stimulation (trauma, or pain). Prolactin has a primary role in the regulation of reproductive functions. While the elevation of its level beyond normal (hyperprolactinemia) can be either physiological, pathological, or idiopathic; its clinical manifestations can vary from severe to none [1].

Prolactin receptors have been found on endometrial cells. The secretion of endometrial prolactin helps in maintaining endometrial receptivity, and has been shown to provide an optimal environment for the implanting blastocyst transferred during in-vitro fertilization (IVF) cycles. A high enough prolactin level can inhibit the proliferation of luteinizing granulosa cells, and can also interfere with corpus luteum function resulting in luteal phase defect, as well as abnormal implantation, and embryo development [2]. Different studies have proven the existence of a state of hyperprolactinemia during IVF/Intracytoplasmic sperm injection (ICSI) cycles [3, 4].

* Correspondence: dr.ahmed.m.kamel@gmail.com
[1]Obstetrics and Gynecology Department, Cairo University, P.O. Box: 11562, KasrAlainy St., Garden City, Cairo, Egypt

Transient hyperprolactinemia has been proven to adversely affect the outcome of IVF, and studies have concluded that patients with normal serum prolactin levels had higher fertilization and cleavage rates [5–7]. While other researchers found the effect of increased serum prolactin during IVF to be insignificant [8–10], subsequent studies [11–14] found a positive effect of transient hyperprolactinemia on the outcome of ovarian simulation in IVF.

The aim of this study was to identify changes in serum prolactin levels in patients undergoing ICSI, and to evaluate the effect of these changes on the clinical pregnancy rate.

Methods

Experimental design & sample size

An internal review board "The Scientific & Ethics committee" of the OBGYN department, Cairo University approved this study protocol on the fifth of October 2014. One hundred two normo-prolactinemic patients were recruited in the study while attending the assisted reproduction clinic in Kasr Alainy, Cairo university hospital. All enrolled subjects were already scheduled for ICSI. Each participant was subjected to investigations which included follicle stimulating hormone (FSH), Luteinizing hormone (LH), thyroid stimulating hormone (TSH), prolactin, and semen analysis for the husband.

The sample size was calculated using an online calculator [15] where the measured outcome was the difference of serum prolactin levels between samples. The confidence level was set at 95%, and the margin of error at 10.4%, in a 50% response distribution, giving us 90 patients in a population more than 20,000.

Inclusion Criteria for the study included an age range between 20 and 38 years, women with either 1ry or 2ry infertility scheduled for ICSI. Exclusion from the study was due to hyperprolactinemia (high basal serum prolactin), uterine anomalies, repeated ICSI failure (3 or more failed trials), embryo transfer beyond day 3, frozen – thawed cycles, or had any contraindications for pregnancy (serious uncontrolled medical diseases such as diabetes, heart disease, hypertension, or ovarian tumors (cancer of any location). Patients were also excluded if they were on any medication that is known to alter prolactin levels e.g. antipsychotics and risperidone, or had a history of thyroid dysfunction (e.g. low TSH), or had any medical disorders that affect serum prolactin e.g. acromegaly and chronic renal failure.

After applying inclusion and exclusion criteria, the patients were scheduled to start ICSI cycle at Kasr Alainy assisted reproduction unit. Patient counseling and informed consent was taken regarding all blood samples that will be drawn, and permission for publishing this data was granted.

The first baseline serum prolactin level was recorded in the mid-luteal phase of the cycle preceding ICSI. The second blood sample was taken in operating room just before induction of anesthesia for OPU. A Third blood sample was taken two hours after aspiration of the last follicle in recovery room post-operatively. A Fourth and final blood sample was taken before embryo transfer. To avoid fluctuations in serum prolactin levels, all OPU and embryo transfers (ET) was scheduled at 9:00 am after fasting for 8 h. The blood samples were immediately sent to central laboratory of Kasr Alainy Cairo university hospital after retrieval. Serum prolactin was analyzed each time though immunoassay by ADVIA Centaur Immunoassay System (CP Immunoassay System ®, SIEMENS AG, Munich, Germany).

Intracytoplasmic sperm injection

The standard long gonadotrophin-releasing hormone (GnRH) agonist protocol was used for all patients where 0.1 mg of Triptorelin daily S.C injection *(Decapeptyl ®FERRING PHARMACEUTICALS, Switzerland)* was applied from the mid-luteal phase onward till the day of human chorionic gonadotropin (hCG) injection. When the serum estradiol (E2) level was < 50 pg/ml, gonadotropins in the form of human menopausal gonadotropin (HMG) (Merional ®, IBSA, InstitutBiochimique SA, Lugano, Switzerland) were given IM from the 3rd day of menstruation. The starting dose of HMG was set from 150 to 300 IU according to the patient's age, basal FSH level, antral follicular count (AFC), and body mass index (BMI).

The stimulation was monitored by transvaginal ultrasonography, and serial E2 measurements starting from the seventh day of the cycle, and the HMG dose was adjusted individually according to follicular response. After the development of three or more follicles ≥18 mm, 10,000 unit of hCG (Choriomon, IBSA, Institut Biochimique SA) was given IM, and trans-vaginal ultrasound guided ovum pick up procedure (OPU) was scheduled 36 h later. ICSI was performed as described by *Mansour* et al. [16].

Progesterone 100 mg IM daily injections (Prontogest ® *IBSA, InstitutBiochimique SA, Lugano, Switzerland*) were given as luteal support starting from the day of ET, and continued for 16 days. Pregnancy was recorded when β-HCG > 10 IU on day 14 after ET, and a second higher value 48 h later. This was followed by ultrasonography for confirmation of fetal pole and cardiac activity at 7 weeks of gestation.

Descriptive data such as age, cause and type of infertility, the number of oocytes retrieved at OPU, and embryo grading were recorded as well as the result of every serum prolactin sample.

Statistical analysis

Continuous data were expressed as mean ± SD (95% confidence interval [CI]), and were compared using Student t test or Mann-Whitney U test as appropriate. General linear model for repeated measures was used to evaluate the mean pair wise comparison between different prolactin levels where Bonferroni adjustment was used in the estimated marginal means. Correlation between various variables was done using Pearson moment correlation equation. Statistical analysis was performed using the Statistical Package for the Social Sciences program, v20.0 (SPSS Inc., Chicago, IL, USA). A two-tailed P value < 0.05 was considered statistically significant.

Results

The total number of participants in our study was 102 patients. During the course of our study twelve cases were excluded as the embryo transfer procedure was cancelled. Three of cancelled cases were identified as high risk for ovarian hyperstimulation, and had their embryos frozen for transfer in another cycle. In four cases, no oocytes were retrieved, and in another four cases only germinal vesicles (GV) were retrieved, and not injected. There was a single case of failed fertilization. Recruitment then continued till 90 patients were enrolled.

Descriptive data

33 patients out of 90 got pregnant (36%), only 27 of which were clinical pregnancies, giving us 30% clinical pregnancy rate. The implantation rate was 19.3%, and the live birth rate was 23.3%. Primary infertility represented 61.1% of cases, tubal factor comprised 40% of the cases, unexplained infertility was 26.6%, male factor was 20%, and unovulatory polycystic ovarian syndrome (PCOS) was 13.4%. Endometriosis was identified in 17% of cases with tubal factor.

Descriptive statistics are illustrated in Table 1, where the ovarian reserve of the participants appears normal as denoted by the AFC, serum FSH and LH. The mean BMI was 29.1 ± 1.5 kg/m^2, and there was no statistical significance in the BMI between the patients that got pregnant and those that didn't ($p = 0.846$).

Transient hyperprolactinemia

The mean level of prolactin before OPU was within the normal range, while the level after OPU was elevated beyond normal reaching a maximum of 93.2 ng/ml. However the mean levels of PRL before embryo transfer did fall back to normal levels and a maximum value of 73.6 ng/ml was recorded.

The difference between the mean basal prolactin levels and the other serum samples collected is shown in Table 2. The sample collected 2 h after OPU had a statistically significant mean difference of 25.8 ± 2.8 ng/ml in comparison to the basal level of serum prolactin ($p < 0.01$). This helps highlight a significant hyperprolactinemia occurring after OPU, and resolving before embryo transfer. There was no statistical difference between the other samples, and the basal prolactin level as shown in Table 2.

Table 1 Descriptive statistics showing different hormone levels & factors affecting ICSI outcome

	Minimum	Maximum	Mean ± SD
Age (years)	20	38	29.6 ± 5.4 (28.7–30.6)
AFC (follicles)	2	32	13 ± 6.3 (11.7–14.4)
FSH (IU/mL)	1.89	16.4	6 ± 2.9 (6–7.2)
LH (IU/mL)	1.1	13.9	5.2 ± 2.8 (4.7–5.8)
TSH (mIU/L)	0.7	4.1	2.01 ± 0.84 (1.83–2.18)
BMI (kg/m^2)	25.1	33	29.1 ± 1.5 (28.8–29.4)
Basal PRL level (ng/ml)	1.1	28	13.7 ± 6.6 (12.3–15.1)
PRL before OPU (ng/ml)	0.4	46.2	16.8 ± 11. 6 (14.4–19.2)
PRL after OPU (ng/ml)	0.5	93.2	39.5 ± 25.4 (34.2–44.8)
PRL before ET (ng/ml)	0.1	73.6	11. 5 ± 10 (9.4–13.6)
Number of oocytes retrieved in OPU	2	44	17.3 ± 10.7 (15–19.5)
Number of metaphase II oocytes	1	13	5.7 ± 2.9 (5.1–6.4)
Fertilization rate (%)	40	100	81.5 ± 16 (78.2–85)
Number of embryos transferred	1	5	3.2 ± 1.1 (3–3.4)
Number of high quality embryos	0	5	2.9 ± 1.3 (2.6–3.1)
Number of low quality embryos	0	2	1.1 ± 0.3 (1–1.2)

Values are given in given in numbers, & mean ± SD (95% CI)
SD standard deviation

Table 2 The mean difference between different levels of serum prolactin compared to the basal level

	Mean Prolactin level ng/ml	Mean difference from basal PRL level ng/ml	95% confidence interval		*p*-value
			Lower bound	Upper bound	
PRL before OPU	16.8 ± 11.6	3.1 ± 1.4	0.556	6.816	0.146
PRL after OPU	39.5 ± 25.4	25.8 ± 2.8	18.205	33.391	< 0.01*
PRL before ET	11.5 ± 10	2.2 ± 1.1	0.852	5.29	0.326

Values are given as mean ± standard error (95% CI)
*Statistically significant result $p < 0.05$
($F = 406.9$, $p < 0.001$)

Table 3 compares the mean prolactin levels between patients who had a clinical pregnancy to those who didn't. There was also no statistically significant difference between the different prolactin samples amongst the two groups even though there was a statistically significant rise in serum prolactin in the sample taken 2 h after OPU.

Relationship between PRL samples and other parameters

Table 4 shows a statistically significant positive pearson correlation between the prolactin level before OPU, and the number of higher quality embryos ($p = 0.019$). Higher quality embryos were defined as embryos with equal blastomeres, and fragmentation less than 30%. Figure 1 shows a scatter plot which illustrates the correlation between high quality embryos and serum PRL before OPU. There were no other correlations between the remaining prolactin samples, and higher, or lower quality embryos (unequal blastomeres, fragmentation ˃30%, multinucleation or other cytoplasmic defects).

There was also a statistically significant negative relationship between the number of oocytes retrieved, and serum prolactin level before embryo transfer as shown by pearson correlation. The same sample also showed a statistically significant positive correlation with fertilization rate. There were no other significant correlations between any other serum prolactin sample and fertilization rate, or the number of oocytes retrieved. The clinical application of this correlation is not of value, as chronologically the number of oocytes retrieved is already known, and the fertilization rate can be calculated before this sample can be drawn at a later time (before ET).

Discussion

Serum prolactin levels vary in the body according to different stimuli, including sleep, pregnancy, stress, chest

Table 3 Comparison between the clinical parameters, and mean levels of serum prolactin in the pregnant and non pregnant groups

	Pregnant	Non pregnant	*P*-value
Age (years)	29.2 ± 6 (26.9–31.6)	29.8 ± 5.2 (28.7–31.1)	0.644
AFC (follicles)	15.1 ± 7.2 (12.3–17.9)	12.1 ± 5.7 (10.7–13.5)	0.101
FSH (IU/mL)	7 ± 3.4 (5.7–8.3)	6.4 ± 2.6 (5.8–7.1)	0.403
LH (IU/mL)	5.5 ± 2.6 (4.5–6.6)	5.1 ± 2.9 (4.4–5.8)	0.487
TSH (mIU/L)	2.10 ± 0.84 (1.78–2.43)	1.96 ± 0.84 (1.75–2.18)	0.467
BMI (kg/m^2)	29.1 ± 1.4(28.5–29.6)	29.1 ± 1.5 (28.7–29.5)	0.853
Basal PRL level (ng/ml)	12.8 ± 6.5 (10.3–15.3)	14.1 ± 6.8 (12.4–15.8)	0.414
PRL before OPU (ng/ml)	15.7 ± 11.2 (11.4–20.1)	17.3 ± 11.8 (14.3–20.3)	0.551
PRL after OPU (ng/ml)	35.2 ± 25.4 (25.4–45.1)	41.4 ± 25.4 (35–47.8)	0.286
PRL before ET (ng/ml)	9.7 ± 7.6 (6.7–12.6)	12.3 ± 10.9 (9.5–15)	0.254
Number of oocytes retrieved in OPU	22.8 ± 9.6 (19.1–26.6)	14.8 ± 10.3 (12.2–17.4)	0.001*
Number of metaphase II oocytes	7.3 ± 2.6 (6.3–8.3)	5.1 ± 2.8 (4.4–5.8)	0.001*
Fertilization rate (%)	82 ± 13.1 (76.87–87.03)	81.4 ± 17.2 (77–85.7)	0.954
Number of embryos transferred	3.7 ± 0.7 (3.4–4)	3 ± 1.1 (2.7–3.2)	0.001*
Number of high quality embryos	3.5 ± 6.9 (3.1–3.8)	2.6 ± 1.3 (2.3–2.9)	0.002*
Number of low quality embryos	1.2 ± 0.4 (0.8–1.6)	1.1 ± 0.2 (0.9–1.2)	0.391

Values are given as mean ± SD (95% CI)
*Statistically significant result $p < 0.05$

Table 4 Correlation between serum prolactin levels, embryo quality & fertilization rate

	Higher quality embryos		Lower quality embryos		Number of retrieved oocytes		Fertilization rate	
	PC	*p*-value	PC	*p*-value	PC	*p*-value	PC	*p*-value
Basal PRL level	−0.182	0.085	0.108	0.607	−0.119	0.264	0.065	0.541
PRL before OPU	0.274	***0.019****	0.245	0.237	−0.004	0.972	0.044	0.680
PRL after OPU	0.108	0.310	0.306	0.136	−0.135	0.205	−0.081	0.446
PRL before ET	−0.117	0.272	0.093	0.093	−0.218	***0.039****	0.228	***0.030****

*Statistically significant result $p < 0.05$
PC Pearson Correlation

wall stimulation, food ingestion, and trauma. Stress has been shown to be a common cause for raising serum prolactin levels [1]. This may explain the significant rise in serum PRL after OPU. Many studies has documented the poor effect stress has on the success of IVF/ICSI [17–20]. Our study has clearly documented a state of transient hyperprolactinemia which was also documented by other authors [3, 4].

This rise in serum prolactin peaked after the ovum pickup procedure with some readings reaching a maximum recorded value of 93.2 ng/ml, but returning to normal levels before ET.

Boyers et al. [4] had similar results where the mean basal level of serum prolactin was comparable to ours. They had a mean increase in serum prolactin during OPU reaching values higher than we recorded. The level decreased after OPU but remained above the baseline. Their results also showed a return of serum prolactin to normal before embryo transfer.

Our results showed that elevated serum prolactin identified after OPU had no significant impact on pregnancy, as did the results from previous work by Doldi et al. [21] This was contradictory to the work presented by Zhong et al. [3] which stated that the rise in serum prolactin level ≥ 90 ng/ml dramatically affected pregnancy rate, by modulating the hypothalamo-pituitary ovarian axis, corpus luteum function and endometrial receptivity. Other studies [8–10] had findings similar to our own, confirming the presence of hyperprolactinemia without recording any deleterious effects on pregnancy.

In the study by Doldi et al. [21] they divided the patients into two groups and attempted to treat hyperprolactimenia in one group with cabergoline (Dostinex®; pharmacia and Upjohn; 500 μg per week), or bromocriptine (Parlodel®;

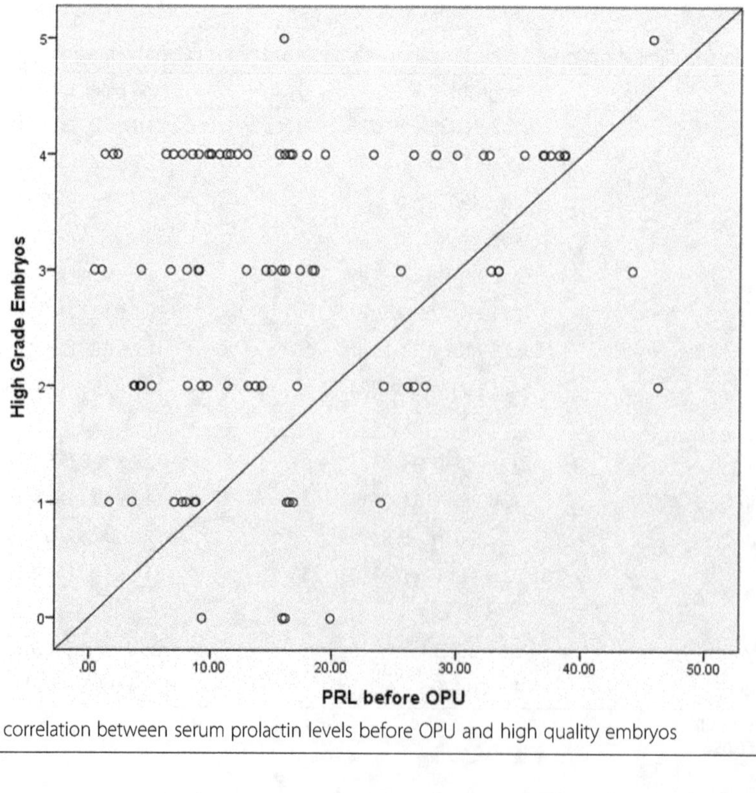

Fig. 1 Scatter plot showing correlation between serum prolactin levels before OPU and high quality embryos

Novartis; 2.5 mg per week), and placebo in the control group. The treatment started prior to ovarian stimulation, and continued till there was a decrease in plasma prolactin levels, and eventually they found no significant difference in the pregnancy rate.

We also found a positive correlation between higher quality embryo and the serum prolactin sample taken before OPU. This can theoretically help predict better embryo implantation and successful pregnancy, however the same sample failed to show statistical significance when it came to clinical pregnancy. Mendoza et al. [11] concluded that better quality oocytes and embryos resulted from follicles with higher steroid and prolactin levels.

Keeping in mind that the development of high quality embryos requires good quality oocytes, the presence of prolactin receptors or it mRNA has been detected in the matured oocyte, and its surrounding cumulus cells. Evidence also suggests that it participates in the development, and maturation of oocytes [22]. Hypoprolactinemia was reported to decrease cleavage and pregnancy rates [23]. Jinno et al. [24] studied the effect of giving bromocriptine in the cycle preceding IVF, and found that they had higher cleavage, fertilization, and pregnancy rates. They also reported a higher proportion of high quality embryos. This was attributed to better oocyte maturation which was achieved due to the rebound increase of prolactin after the discontinuation of bromocriptine, which restored post receptor responsiveness in granulosa cells. Moride et al. [25] also concluded that the bromcriptine rebound method yielded morphologically better embryos.

Zhong et al. [3] presented results stating that a higher prolactin level at the day of hCG trigger yielded more oocytes by showing a positive spearman correlation while failing to show prolactin in a multiple linear regression analysis equation, concluding that serum prolactin at the day of pick up cannot predict the number of oocytes retrieved. They also showed no marked difference in the fertilization rate. Our study showed no correlation between the serum prolactin samples drawn, and either fertilization rate or the number of oocytes retrieved in the 1st three samples.

However our study demonstrated in the sample taken before embryo transfer, a statistically significant positive pearson correlation with fertilization rate, and a negative relationship with the number of oocytes retrieved. Optimizing these results for clinical value is doubtful as the final serum prolactin sample is taken before embryo transfer, and so if any benefit is to come from their value, the sample has to predate the oocyte retrieval process or the fertilization procedure.

Some of the limitations to our study included not identifying a cut off value for PRL sample before OPU in predicting higher quality embryos. This finding was a secondary outcome, and couldn't be predicted before the statistical analysis of the results. The inclusion criteria was not specific enough to exclude all causes of low cleavage rates, and poor embryo quality e.g. older age, low ovarian reserve, PCOS, and endometriosis, which may lead to bias, and low accuracy if receiver operating characteristic (ROC) analysis was done to determine a cut off value.

Conclusions

In normoprolactinemic women a state of transient hyperprolactinemia is clearly identified in patients undergoing ICSI. Although its cause is not identified, it can be attributed to stress and anxiety. This increase appears to be harmless, and doesn't affect the outcome of ICSI. A significant positive correlation was identified between higher quality embryos and prolactin before ovum pickup. More research is warranted to help increase the predictability of better quality embryos, and hence quantification of their implantation potential. This might help with embryo selection aiming at smaller number of embryos to be transferred per cycle, with a consequent decrease in the risk of multiple pregnancies without decreasing pregnancy rates.

Abbreviations

AFC: Antral follicle count; AUC: Area under the curve; BMI: Body mass index; E2: Estradiol; ET: Embryo transfer; FSH: Follicle stimulating hormone; GnRH: Gonadotrophin-releasing hormone; hCG: human chorionic gonadotropin; HMG: Human menopausal gonadotropin; ICSI: Intracytoplasmic sperm injection; IVF: In vitro-fertilization; OPU: Ovum pick up procedure; PC: Pearson correlation; PCOS: Polycystic ovary syndrome; PRL: Prolactin; ROC: Receiver operating characteristic; β-HCG: beta chorionic gonadotrophin

Funding

This work was funded by Cairo University, and they had no role or influence in conducting the actual work.

Authors' contributions

The idea was conceived and study design was made by AK & AAH. The clinical aspect (folliculometry, ovum pick & embryo transfer) of the study was done by AK & SA. MS was responsible for supervising sample collection and lab work. SA did all data collection. YEF, AMH and WR revised the collected data and did the statistics. Drafting was written by AK and AMH, revision was done by WR & MS. Final approval & revision by AAH & YEF. All authors read and approved the final manuscript.

Authors' information

All authors of this work have years of experience in the field of ART.

Competing interests

The authors of this study declare no conflict of interest and no competing interests with respect to the research, authorship, and publication of this article.

Author details

[1]Obstetrics and Gynecology Department, Cairo University, P.O. Box: 11562, KasrAlainy St., Garden City, Cairo, Egypt. [2]Clinical and Chemical Pathology Department, Cairo University, Cairo, Egypt.

References

1. Majumdar A, Mangal NS. Hyperprolactinemia. J Hum Reprod Sci. 2013;6(3): 168–75.
2. Chawla R, Antonios T, Berhanu E, Ayana G. Detection of Macroprolactinemia and molecular characterization of prolactin isoforms in blood samples of hyperprolactinemic women. In: Journal of medical biochemistry, vol. 31; 2012. p. 19.
3. Y-p Z, Shen X-t, Ying Y, Wu H-T, Li J, Qi Q, Zhou C-Q, Zhuang G-L. Impact of transitory hyperprolactinemia on clinical outcome of in vitro fertilization and embryo transfer. In: Journal of medical biochemistry, vol. 31; 2012. p. 27.
4. Boyers SP, Lavy G, Russell JB, Polan ML, DeCherney AH. Serum prolactin response to embryo transfer during human in vitro fertilization and embryo transfer. J In Vitro Fert Embryo Transf. 1987;4(5):269–72.
5. Huang KE, Bonfiglio TA, Muechler EK. Transient hyperprolactinemia in infertile women with luteal phase deficiency. Obstet Gynecol. 1991; 78(4):651–5.
6. Reinthaller A, Deutinger J, Csaicsich P, Riss P, Muller-Tyl E, Fischl F, Janisch H. Effect of serum prolactin on cycle stimulation and fertilization of human oocytes. Geburtshilfe Frauenheilkd. 1987;47(4):246–8.
7. del Pozo E. Management of borderline hyperprolactinemia. Horm Res. 1985; 22(3):204–8.
8. Chang SP, Ng HT, Lan TL, Chao HT, Wei TC, Yang TS, Ou-Yang XR. Transient hyperprolactinemia in gonadotropin-stimulated cycles for in vitro fertilization and its effect on conception. Zhonghua Yi Xue Za Zhi. 1993; 51(6):401–6. Free China ed
9. Pattinson HA, Taylor PJ, Fleetham JA, Servis SA. Transient hyperprolactinemia has no effect on endocrine response and outcome in in vitro fertilization (IVF). J In Vitro Fert Embryo Trans. 1990;7(2):89–93.
10. Hummel WP, Clark MR, Talbert LM. Transient hyperprolactinemia during cycle stimulation and its influence on oocyte retrieval and fertilization rates. Fertil Steril. 1990;53(4):677–81.
11. Mendoza C, Cremades N, Ruiz-Requena E, Martinez F, Ortega E, Bernabeu S, Tesarik J. Relationship between fertilization results after intracytoplasmic sperm injection, and intrafollicular steroid, pituitary hormone and cytokine concentrations. Hum Reprod. 1999;14(3):628–35.
12. Jinno M, Katsumata Y, Hoshiai T, Nakamura Y, Matsumoto K, Yoshimura Y. A therapeutic role of prolactin supplementation in ovarian stimulation for in vitro fertilization: the bromocriptine-rebound method. J Clin Endocrinol Metab. 1997;82(11):3603–11.
13. Jinno M, Yoshimura Y, Ubukata Y, Nakamura Y. A novel method of ovarian stimulation for in vitro fertilization: bromocriptine-rebound method. Fertil Steril. 1996;66(2):271–4.
14. Kamel MA, Zabel G, Bernart W, Neulen J, Breckwoldt M. Comparison between prolactin, gonadotrophins and steroid hormones in serum and follicular fluid after stimulation with gonadotrophin-releasing hormone agonists and human menopausal gonadotrophin for an in-vitro fertilization programme. Hum Reprod. 1994;9(10):1803–6.
15. Raosoft Sample size calculator. http://www.raosoft.com/samplesize.html. Accessed 3 May 2018.
16. Mansour R, Fahmy I, Tawab NA, Kamal A, El-Demery Y, Aboulghar M, Serour G. Electrical activation of oocytes after intracytoplasmic sperm injection: a controlled randomized study. Fertil Steril. 2009;91(1):133–9.
17. Rockliff HE, Lightman SL, Rhidian E, Buchanan H, Gordon U, Vedhara K. A systematic review of psychosocial factors associated with emotional adjustment in in vitro fertilization patients. Hum Reprod Update. 2014; 20(4):594–613.
18. Li XH, Ma YG, Geng LH, Qin L, Hu H, Li SW. Baseline psychological stress and ovarian norepinephrine levels negatively affect the outcome of in vitro fertilisation. Gynecol Endocrinol. 2011;27(3):139–43.
19. Turner K, Reynolds-May MF, Zitek EM, Tisdale RL, Carlisle AB, Westphal LM. Stress and anxiety scores in first and repeat IVF cycles: a pilot study. PLoS One. 2013;8(5):e63743.
20. Nouri K, Litschauer B, Huber JC, Buerkle B, Tiringer D, Tempfer CB. Saliva cortisol levels and subjective stress are not associated with number of oocytes after controlled ovarian hyperstimulation in patients undergoing in vitro fertilization. Fertil Steril. 2011;96(1):69–72.
21. Doldi N, Papaleo E, De Santis L, Ferrari A. Treatment versus no treatment of transient hyperprolactinemia in patients undergoing intracytoplasmic sperm injection programs. Gynecol Endocrinol. 2000;14(6):437 41.
22. Lebedeva IY, Singina GN, Lopukhov AV, Shedova EN, Zinovieva NA. Prolactin and growth hormone affect metaphase-II chromosomes in aging oocytes via cumulus cells using similar signaling pathways. Front Genet. 2015;6:274.
23. Gonen Y, Casper RF. Does transient hyperprolactinemia during ovarian hyperstimulation interfere with conception or pregnancy outcome? Fertil Steril. 1989;51(6):1007–10.
24. Jinno M, Ubukata Y, Satou M, Katsumata Y, Yoshimura Y, Nakamura Y. A novel method of ovarian stimulation for in vitro fertilization (bromocriptine-rebound method) increases developmental potential of oocytes and pregnancy rate. Nihon Sanka Fujinka Gakkai zasshi. 1995;47(12):1337–44.
25. Moride N, Kuwahara A, Yamashita M, Tanaka Y, Matsuzaki T, Yasui T, Irahara M. Does the bromocriptine-rebound method improve embryo quality? J Med Invest. 2011;58(1–2):63–6.

19

Intermittent fetal heart rate monitoring using a fetoscope or hand held Doppler in rural Tanzania

Paschal Francis Mdoe[1,2,8*], Hege L. Ersdal[2,3], Estomih R. Mduma[1,2], Jeffrey M. Perlman[4], Robert Moshiro[2,7], Peter T. Wangwe[6] and Hussein Kidanto[5,6]

Abstract

Background: Neonatal mortality is a global challenge, with an estimated 1.3 million intrapartum stillbirths in 2015. The majority of these were found in low resource settings with limited options to intrapartum fetal heart monitoring devices. This trial compared frequency of abnormal fetal heart rate (FHR) detection and adverse perinatal outcomes (i.e. fresh stillbirths, 24-h neonatal deaths, admission to neonatal care unit) among women intermittently assessed by Doppler or fetoscope in a rural low-resource setting.

Methods: This was an open-label randomized controlled trial conducted at Haydom Lutheran Hospital from March 2013 through August 2015. Inclusion criteria were; women in labor, singleton, cephalic presentation, normal FHR on admission (120–160 beats/minute), and cervical dilatation ≤7 cm. Verbal consent was obtained.

Results: A total of 2684 women were recruited, 1309 in the Doppler and 1375 in the fetoscope arms, respectively. Abnormal FHR was detected in 55 (4.2%) vs 42 (3.1%). (RR = 1.38; 95%CI: 0.93, 2.04) in the Doppler and fetoscope arms, respectively. Bag mask ventilation was performed in 80 (6.1%) vs 82 (6.0%). (RR = 1.03; 95%CI: 0.76, 1.38) of neonates, and adverse perinatal outcome was comparable 32(2.4%) vs 35(2.5%). (RR = 0.9; 95%CI: 0.59, 1.54), in the Doppler and fetoscope arms, respectively.

Conclusion: This trial failed to demonstrate a statistically significant difference in the detection of abnormal FHR between intermittently used Doppler and fetoscope and adverse perinatal outcomes. However, FHR measurements were not performed as often as recommended by international guidelines. Conducting a randomized controlled study in rural settings with limited resources is associated with major challenges.

Keywords: Intermittent fetal heart rate monitoring, Pinard fetoscope, Doppler

Background

Globally, an estimated 1.2 million fresh stillbirths (FSB) and 2.1 early neonatal deaths (END) occurred in 2013, 98% in low and middle-income countries [1–4]. Currently, the proportion of neonatal deaths constitute 44% of under-five child mortality [5]. Intrapartum hypoxia (often defined as birth asphyxia) has been reported to be associated with as much as 70% of FSB and 60% of END [6–9]. Identification and timely management of intrapartum hypoxia is therefore a priority area for reducing perinatal mortality in low resource countries.

Intrapartum fetal heart rate (FHR) monitoring aims at recognizing the hypoxic fetus as a result of fetal interruption of placental blood flow during labor. FHR tracings can reveal specific information regarding fetal oxygenation. Thus, an abnormal FHR tracing (i.e. late deceleration, severe variability, bradycardia and tachycardia) during the first stage of labor has been associated

* Correspondence: pfmdoe@gmail.com
[1]Haydom Lutheran Hospital, Mbulu, Tanzania
[2]Department of Health Science, University of Stavanger, Stavanger, Norway
Full list of author information is available at the end of the article

with fetal hypoxia and fetal acidosis [10–12], and intermittently detected abnormal FHR has been associated with adverse perinatal outcome in a rural setting [13]. Several studies from resource replete settings have reported lower rate of operative deliveries (i.e. cesarean section, vacuum or forceps extraction) when comparing intermittent to continuous FHR monitoring, respectively [14, 15]. Importantly, in these studies, intermittent FHR assessments were performed according to recommended guidelines i.e. optimal frequency and length of measurements.

In low resource settings, FHR monitoring is mainly performed intermittently, using a Pinard fetoscope. However, in 1994 in an urban hospital in Harare, a hand-held Doppler ultrasound was found to be more effective in detecting abnormal FHR and improved perinatal outcome in low risk deliveries as compared to the Pinard fetoscope [16]. The hand-held Doppler allows the care provider to assess FHR quickly, to communicate with the mother who can hear the heart sounds of her baby hence increase maternal confidence concerning the wellbeing of her unborn baby, and it is preferred by women over the use of fetoscope [17, 18]. Main barriers toward the more widely use of Doppler in low-resource countries have been costs and lack of reliable electricity supply. Therefore, a wind-up hand-held Doppler device has been developed using a hand-crank to generate power, that last for about 2 h for every 30-s of cracking [19]. This wind-up Doppler was tested in a low resource setting and found to be accurate and acceptable to mothers as well as midwives [19]. A recent randomized controlled study, comparing the Free-Play Doppler to the Pinard fetoscope in a peri-urban setting in Uganda, reported an increased detection rate of abnormal FHR in the Doppler arm (7.6%) as compared to the Pinard arm (4.7%), but no improvement of perinatal outcome [20].

To our knowledge, intermittent FHR monitoring using Doppler or fetoscope has never been compared in a rural sub-Saharan setting that differs substantially from (peri-) urban settings. The aim of this study was to compare the Free-Play Doppler with the Pinard fetoscope for intermittent FHR monitoring, detection of abnormal FHR and impact on perinatal outcomes in a low-resource rural hospital.

Methods

We conducted a randomized control trial comparing the Pinard fetoscope and Free-Play Doppler (Free Play, Power-free Education Technology, Pet.og.za) for intermittent FHR monitoring from March 2013 through August 2015. Data collection was carried out at Haydom Lutheran Hospital (HLH), a rural referral hospital in Northern Tanzania. The hospital provides comprehensive emergency obstetric care and basic newborn care to a population of approximately 500,000 people, while the greater reference area covers about 2 million people [21]. Midwives largely conduct uncomplicated deliveries, and doctors on call for 24 h perform operative deliveries. Traditionally, FHR is routinely monitored by the attending midwife using a Pinard fetoscope. For this study, the wind-up hand-held Free-Play Doppler was introduced. All midwives and doctors were initially trained and then retrained after every six months on how to use the Doppler and simultaneously reminded about abnormal FHR patterns and its obstetrical management. Midwives were allowed to use Doppler, if available, also for deliveries not included in the study.

Study population and randomization

The inclusion criteria are listed in Table 1. Recruitment, information about the study, and verbal consent was obtained by the admitting midwife in the admission room. Women who consented were randomly allocated using sealed opaque envelops. The allocation label was stapled to the patient file, and the selected device (Doppler or fetoscope) used for that woman.

Data collection

Research assistants were continuously present in the labor ward, observing every delivery. They worked in three shifts over 24 h. Three research assistants covered each shift; two research assistants were always in the delivery rooms or in the operating theatre; one in the adjacent neonatal area. Altogether 14 research assistants were trained to observe health care workers' performance related to deliveries and newborns. Findings were recorded on a data collection form. This included labor progress information and FHR categorized as normal (120 to 160 beats/minute), abnormal (< 120 or > 160 beats/minutes), absent, or not measured; specific device used for FHR assessment; neonatal characteristics and interventions in the delivery room, and perinatal outcome (normal, admitted neonatal area, death within 24 h and FSB). The frequency of FHR monitoring was not recorded, though midwives were expected to follow WHO guidelines of monitoring FHR every 30 min during the first and after five to 15 min during the second stage of labor. Therefore, categorization of FHR was

Table 1 Inclusion criteria

• In labor (i.e. cervical dilatation ≥3 cm with uterine contractions)
• Singleton
• Cephalic presentation
• Gestation age ≥ 36 weeks
• Cervical dilatation ≤7 cm
• Normal FHR at admission
• Able to give verbal consent

based on multiple measurements throughout labor. Abnormal FHR was reached after at least one confirmed measurement at any point during labor.

Maternal age was based on self-report of the mother or close relative. Maternal gravidity was the number of pregnancies the woman had ever had including the current one. Gestational age (GA) was based on self-report of the last menstrual period and distance from symphysis pubis to fundus (on admission). Normal term GA at HLH is routinely defined as ≥ 36 weeks (Thus, preterm was defined as GA < 36 weeks and post term as > 42 weeks.

Normal perinatal outcome was defined as a live birth and included all of the following; Apgar score more than seven at one and five minutes, not admitted to the neonatal unit. Intrapartum death/FSB was defined as an Apgar score of zero at both one and five minutes with intact skin and suspected death during labor/delivery i.e. with a FHR heard on admission. Antepartum death/macerated stillbirth (MSB) was defined as an Apgar score of zero at both one and five minutes with macerated skin and suspected death before start of labor. "FHR abnormalities" included abnormal or not detected. There were some cases where the FHR was not measured. "Adverse outcome" included FSB, neonatal deaths within the first 24 h and infants still admitted in the neonatal unit after 24 h.

Quality assurance of the data

The research assistants were trained, supervised, and continuously re-trained by the first author. All data collection forms were controlled for quality issues, before entering to the computer, including missing information and potential errors, on a daily basis. Data were double entered using SPSS Version 22 by two different data clerks.

Sample size and statistical consideration

Primary outcome measure was detection of an abnormal FHR. A previous study at HLH revealed an abnormal FHR detection rate of 2.7% in the total cohort when using the Pinard fetoscope [13]. Based on this study, an 80% increase in detection rate was estimated for the Free Play Doppler arm i.e. 4.8%, equivalent to the proportion of abnormal FHR detection when using Pinard in the peri-urban setting in Uganda [20]. An estimated 1277 cases were required in each arm to achieve a power of 80% using a two-sided test with significance level 0.05. A total of 2684 cases were included, 5% more than the calculated sample, to compensate for potentially missing variables. Data was analyzed using the Statistical Package for the Social Sciences (SPSS) v.22. Chi-square calculations and Fisher's exact test were used to compare categorical variables, and independent samples t-test were used for continuous data.

Ethical considerations

Ethical clearances were granted by the Muhimbili University of Health and Allied Sciences ethics and publication committee, and the Regional Committee for Medical and Health Research Ethics, Western Norway (2013/110/REK vest). Verbal consent was approved to be used in this trial. Permission to collect data was granted by the management at HLH. The trial was registered in ClinicalTrials.gov Identifier NCT01869582.

Results

General characteristics of the whole cohort

During the study period 11,045 women delivered in HLH (Fig. 1). Mean maternal age was 25.1 ± 6.5 years. Almost 99% had attended antenatal care at least once, and 1.0% reported some type of pregnancy problems. The proportion of preterm delivery was 3.3%. Mean birth weight (BW) was 3202 ± 529 g, and 880 (8%) neonates had BW less than 2500 g. On admission, 114 (1. 0%) had an abnormal FHR, 217 (2.0%) had an undetectable FHR, and 1027 (9.3%) were not assessed. During labor, irrespective of device used, abnormal FHR was detected in 387 (3.5%) women. Overall, the mean time interval from admission to detection of an abnormal FHR was 6.5 ± 6.7 h, from the first detected abnormal FHR to birth 120 ± 210 min, and from the final recorded FHR assessment to birth was 92 ± 210 min. The majority of women delivered vaginally, i.e. 8455 (76.6%), whereas 2438 (22.1%) were delivered via caesarean section (CS). Apgar scores less than seven at one and five minutes were encountered in 392 (3.5%) and 66 (0.6%) neonates, respectively. There were150 (1.4%) MSB, 155 (1.4%) FSB, 90 (0.8%) deaths within 24 h after birth and 357 (3.2%) neonates admitted to the neonatal unit for more than 24 h.

A total of 4914 women did not meet the inclusion criteria, 20.9% (1027/4914) of these due to lack of FHR assessment on admission. A sub-population of 6131 women met the inclusion criteria for the study. Of these 3447 (56.2%) women were not included because either they refused ($n = 2952$) or consent was not taken ($n = 495$) (Fig. 1). This resulted in 2684 (43.8%) women who were randomized. A comparison of general characteristics of the women and neonates in the consented and non-consented groups is presented in Table 2. There was a significantly higher incidence of the FHR not being measured during labor in the non-consented group (1.7%) as compared to the consented (0.5%) group, and the CS and FSB rates were higher in the non-consented as compared to the consented group (Table 3).

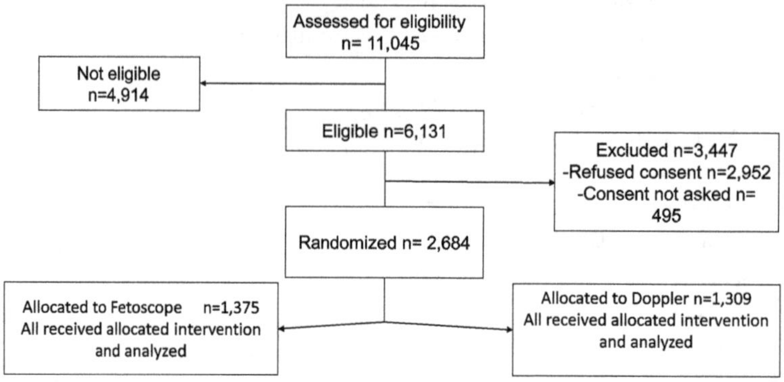

Fig. 1 Consort flow diagram

A total of 1375 and 1309 women were randomized to the fetoscope and the Doppler arm, respectively (Table 4). Maternal mean age was comparable in the two arms. There were more primigravid women in the fetoscope arm as compared to the Doppler arm, 48.5% vs. 45.2%, respectively ($p = 0.04$).

Comparison of outcome measures in the two arms are presented in Table 5. The detection of abnormal FHR was higher in the Doppler arm as compared to the fetoscope arm ($p = 0.109$). The time interval from the final recorded FHR (normal or abnormal) to birth was similar in the two arms, but much longer than recommended. The time interval from the first abnormal FHR measure to birth was comparable between the groups. Apgar scores at one and five minutes, neonates receiving bag mask ventilation, and adverse perinatal outcomes were comparable.

Among the 8361 deliveries not included in the randomization study, the type of device used for FHR assessments was noted in 6360 women. The fetoscope was preferred in 4104 (64.5%) cases and Doppler in 1036 (12.4%) cases. No device was used in 1220 (19.2%) cases.

Discussion

This trial failed to demonstrate significant differences in detection of FHR abnormalities and 24-h perinatal outcomes between Pinard fetoscope versus the Free-Play Doppler when used for intermittent FHR assessments during labor. However, several other important findings related to intermittent FHR monitoring and major challenges associated with conducting a randomized trial in such a rural setting are highlighted.

Doppler was almost 1.4 times more likely to detect abnormal FHR as compared to the fetoscope, however, this was not statistically significant, representing a potential type 2 error. Furthermore, abnormal FHR detection rates, in both arms, were lower in this study as compared to previous studies of similar design [16, 20]. Mahomed et al. reported 32% abnormal FHRs and decreased perinatal mortality when using a standard Doppler device as compared to Pinard (which had 15% abnormal FHRs) [16]. This study was conducted at the National hospital in Harare, Zimbabwe, at a time with fairly good health services (1994), and appointed research midwives were engaged in the study, increasing

Table 2 Characteristics of women and neonates included in the consented and not consented

Characteristics		Consented $n = 2684$	Not consented $n = 3447$	*P*-value
Maternal Age (Years)	Mean ± SD	25.8 ± 5.7	26.4 ± 6.6	
Maternal Gravida	1	1286 (47.9)	1603 (46.5)	0.274
	2 to 5	975 (36.3)	1276 (37.0)	0.577
	> 5	423 (15.8)	568 (16.5)	0.449
Gestational Age (Weeks)	Mean ± SD	38.3 ± 1.5	37.8 ± 1.4	
	> 40	95 (3.5)	101 (2.9)	0.179
Gender	Male	1471 (56.0)	1824 (53.6)	0.141
	Female	1213 (44.0)	1623 (46.4)	
Birth Weight (Grams)	Mean ± SD	3356 ± 463	33,804 ± 455	
	< 2500	108 (4.0)	180 (5.2)	0.028
	≥ 2500	2576 (96.0)	3267 (94.8)	

Values given are n (%) unless otherwise stated

Table 3 Comparison of fetal heart rate (FHR), newborn characteristics and perinatal outcome between the eligible women who consented to participate and those with no consent (refused or not asked for consent)

Characteristics	Eligible population		*p*-value
	Consented $n = 2684$	Not consented $n = 3447$	
FHR abnormalities	112 (4.2)	177 (5.1)	0.078
Abnormal FHR	98 (3.6)	119 (3.5)	0.676
Not measured	14 (0.5)	58 (1.7)	0.001
Time interval from admission to first abnormal FHR assessment (minutes)	466 ± 349	394 ± 357	0.173
Time interval abnormal FHR to birth (minutes)	93 ± 127	104 ± 179	0.624
Time interval last recorded FHR to birth (minutes)	79 ± 187	89 ± 194	0.059
Cesarean section	559 (20.8)	848 (24.6)	0.001
Apgar score < 7 at			
1 Minute	89 (3.3)	113 (3.3)	0.937
5 Minutes	21 (0.8)	33 (1.0)	0.466
Bag mask ventilation	162 (6.0)	239 (6.9)	0.158
Adverse neonatal outcome	67 (2.5)	111 (3.2)	0.094
Fresh stillbirths	7 (0.3)	23 (0.7)	0.023
Early neonatal deaths	14 (0.5)	17 (0.5)	0.890
Admitted neonatal area	46 (1.7)	71 (2.1)	0.471

Values given are n (%)

the ability to follow the recommended frequency for FHR measurements [16]. In 2012–13, Byaruhanga R et al. compared the same devices as used in our study in a peri-urban setting [20]. FHR abnormalities were detected in 7.6% vs 4.7% of the deliveries in the Free Play Doppler and Pinard arm, respectively, but with no differences in perinatal outcome. They speculate that there might have been an undocumented delay between recognition of fetal distress and obstetrical actions. Our study was conducted in a rural setting, and

Table 4 Characteristics of women and neonates included in the fetoscope and the Doppler arm

Characteristics		Fetoscope arm $n = 1375$	Doppler arm $n = 1309$
Maternal Age (Years)	Mean ± SD	25.4 ± 6.7	24.8 ± 6.2
Maternal Gravida	1	667 (48.5)	592 (45.2)
	2 to 5	492 (35.8)	487 (37.2)
	> 5	216 (15.7)	230 (17.6)
Gestational Age (Weeks)	Mean ± SD	38.1 ± 1.6	38.2 ± 1.7
	> 40	51 (3.7)	51 (3.9)
Gender	Male	770 (56.0)	701 (53.6)
	Female	605 (44.0)	608 (46.4)
Birth Weight (Grams)	Mean ± SD	3286 ± 473	32,804 ± 433
	< 2500	59 (4.3)	49 (3.7)
	≥ 2500	1316 (95.7)	1260 (96.3)

Values given are n (%) unless otherwise stated

intermittent FHR assessments were done by the midwives.

In addition, several other important factors may have influenced our results. Notably this was the initial time that a randomized trial was conducted in this rural hospital, with unique factors that limited the recruitment and consent seeking process. Thus in this setting women typically arrive late in labor, and many low-risk women were not eligible due to late arrival with cervical dilatation ≥7 on admission. In addition, FHR assessment was not performed in 9% of admissions, which led to the exclusion of these women. Therefore, only 55% of the total cohort fulfilled the inclusion criteria. In addition, only 44% of these eligible women agreed to participate in the study, creating a potential selection bias. There might be several reasons behind the low consent rates. First, women in labor may not be capable of receiving information and making informed decisions. Second, the midwife/patient ratio in this hospital is low, leading to a considerable time constraint for midwives on duty, which may have influenced their ability to spend adequate time recruiting women (8% of the eligible women were never approached for consent). [22, 23] Third, some midwives may have had strong preferences for which device they trusted the most, and therefore wanted to use, potentially affecting their willingness to recruit participants, and to follow the study protocol. Fourth, laboring women might have felt dependent on the midwife at the time of obtaining

Table 5 Outcomes of the Infants in the Fetoscope versus the Doppler Groups

Outcomes	Fetoscope n = 1375	Doppler n = 1309	Effect measure[a]	*p*-value
FHR abnormalities	49 (3.5)	66 (5.0)	1.42 (0.98, 2.03)	0.064
Abnormal FHR	42 (3.1)	56 (4.2)	1.38 (0.93, 2.04)	0.109
Not measured FHR	7 (0.5)	10 (0.7)	1.5 (0.57, 3.93)	0.40
Time interval admission to first abnormal FHR assessment (minutes)	520 ± 386	429 ± 321	90.2 (−63.9, 244.3)	0.248
Time interval abnormal FHR to birth (minutes)	90.8 ± 122	95.1 ± 132	−4.34 (−58.2, 49.5)	0.873
Time interval last recorded FHR to birth (minutes)	79.1 ± 185	79.5 ± 188	−0.43 (−14.6, 13.8)	0.952
Cesarean Section	286 (20.8)	273 (20.9)	1.00 (0.87, 1.16)	0.972
Bag mask ventilation	82 (6.0)	80 (6.1)	1.03 (0.76, 1.38)	0.872
Apgar Score < 7				
1 Minute	46 (3.3)	43 (3.3)	0.98 (0.65, 1.48)	0.921
5 Minutes	11 (0.8)	10 (0.8)	0.95 (0.40, 2.24)	0.914
Adverse perinatal outcome	35 (2.5)	32 (2.4)	0.96 (0.59, 1.54)	0.867
Fresh stillbirths	4 (0.3)	3 (0.2)	0.78 (0.17, 3.51)	0.527
Early neonatal deaths	5 (0.4)	9 (0.7)	1.89 (0.63, 5.63)	0.244
Admitted neonatal area	26 (1.9)	20 (1.5)	0.81 (0.45, 1.44)	0.475

Values given are n (%) unless otherwise stated
[a]Effect measure = Risk Ratio for categorical variables and Mean Difference for continuous variables

consent, and this may have influenced their free choice.

Comparing the eligible non-randomized with the randomized group, several important differences stand out. First, more non randomized women did not have FHR assessed during labor, second, time from detection of an abnormal FHR to birth was longer, and third there was a higher incidence of CS (24.6%) and FSB (0.7%) in the non-randomized group. These differences may represent a positive Hawthorne effect of being included in the study. The qualities of FHR assessments followed by timely obstetrical interventions seem to be enhanced in the trial population, with either device used, as compared to daily routine care. Interestingly, CS rate in the non-eligible sub-population, when including high-risk deliveries, was almost identical to the CS rate in the trial population, i.e. 20.9% vs 20.8%, respectively. Of the women in the not-eligible group, 2% were admitted with an absent FHR, FHR assessments were not performed in as many as 21% of admissions, time intervals from admission to birth were shorter (many of these women arrived late in labor), but time intervals from detection of an abnormal FHR to birth were considerably longer. Adverse outcomes were highest in this not-eligible group, maybe reflecting less timely expedited deliveries.

There are several limitations to this randomized trial, reflecting a typical rural sub-Saharan African setting. We report a potential selection bias and a potential positive Hawthorn effect of being enrolled in the trial. Furthermore, a 1:1 midwife/patient ratio was impossible to achieve; therefore, FHR measurements were likely not performed according to recommended guidelines, based on the fact that more than 9% of the women never had a FHR assessed, and that the mean time interval from the last FHR assessment to birth was approximately 1.5 h, much longer than recommended, a finding consistent with previous reports [22, 23]. Complying with the recommended guidelines for optimal intermittent FHR monitoring is reported to require a 1:1 midwife/patient ratio [24–26], and our findings are not representative of hospitals where FHR measurements are done according to guidelines for intermittent FHR assessments. Finally, at HLH, fetoscopes (often homemade) have been common equipment for FHR assessments for decades. Although many hand-held wind-up Dopplers were provided, available also for women not enrolled in the trial, Doppler was rarely used outside the trial. In addition, the fetoscope was used to verify FHR in the Doppler arm more often than the opposite, i.e. Doppler used to verify FHR in the fetoscope arm. This may be explained by an uncertainty related to the new device that also may have influenced the results.

The strength of the study is firstly that it represents a rural hospital with all the typical challenges related to clinical care and patient population, as in other rural low-resource settings. Secondly, at the same time, a unique research infrastructure has been established in parallel to the clinical operations, employing separate staff, not involved with clinical management. Trained research assistants have continuously observed and collected data from every birth since 2009, standard operating procedures regulate all research operations, rigorous data quality control systems involve several levels and different people (manually and electronically), and double independent entry of all data is performed locally, before external control. This comprehensive research set-up has enabled collection of high quality data obtained from all deliveries, including patients not involved in the randomized trial. Finally, a randomized trial design provides high level quality evidence.

Conclusion

This randomized trial fails to demonstrate significant differences in detection of abnormal FHRs and perinatal outcomes, comparing a fetoscope with a hand-held Doppler for intermittent FHR assessment, in a rural sub-Saharan hospital, with a low midwife/patient ratio. FHR measurements were not performed as often as recommended in the international guidelines, and we speculate that the true frequency of FHR abnormalities is higher in both arms. Conducting a randomized trial in a rural low resource setting is associated with major challenges and requires a minimum setup as described above.

Abbreviations

BW: Birth weight; CS: Cesarean section; CTG: Cardiotocograph; ENND: Early neonatal death; FHR: Fetal heart rate; FSB: Fresh stillbirth; GA: Gestation age; HLH: Haydom Lutheran Hospital; MSB: Macerated stillbirth; NIMR: National institute of medical research; REK-vest: Regional committee for medical and health research ethics western Norway; SPSS: Statistical package for the social sciences; WHO: World health organization

Acknowledgements

This study was made possible because of the research assistants at Haydom Lutheran Hospital management, Haydom Global Health Research centre and the health providers at Haydom Lutheran Hospital, Maternity Ward. We would like to give a special thanks to Anita Yeconia, Sara Lyanga, Jørgen Erland Linde, Samwel Jatosh and Ladislaus Blacy. Statistical assistance was provided by Lena Bache-Mathiesen and Ingvild Dalen, statisticians at Stavanger University Hospital.

Funding

The study was supported by the Laerdal Foundation and partly by the Research Council of Norway through the Global Health and Vaccination Programme (GLOBVAC), project number 228203. The study design, data collection, and analysis, interpretation of the data or manuscript writing do not necessarily reflect the funder's opinions.

Authors' contributions

PFM contributed to conception, study design, data collection and analysis, and prepared a first draft of the paper. HE and HK contributed to conception, study design, analysis, and interpretation of results and writing of the paper. EM contributed to study design, data collection, and interpretation of results. JP contributed to conception, study design, and interpretation of results. RM contributed to data collection and interpretation of results. PW contributed to conception, study design, and data collection. All authors critically revised the paper and approved the final manuscript for submission.

Ethics approval and consent to participate

This clinical trial was approved by both the Haydom hospital, Regional Committee for Medical and Health Research Ethics, Western Norway and the Muhimbili University of Health and Allied Sciences ethics and publication committee with clinical trial number NCT01869582. The ethics committee approved the use of verbal consent because the consent were taken from women who were in labor admitted for delivery. The verbal consent was approved aiming at reducing burden to women in labor and for those who were unable to read or write to have equal chance of participating into the study.

Competing interests

All authors declare that they have no competing interest. Although HK is a member of the editorial board of BMC Pregnancy & Childbirth journal, declares no competing interest on the review or publication of this manuscript in this journal.

Author details

[1]Haydom Lutheran Hospital, Mbulu, Tanzania. [2]Department of Health Science, University of Stavanger, Stavanger, Norway. [3]Department of Anesthesiology and Intensive Care, Stavanger University Hospital, Stavanger, Norway. [4]Department of Pediatrics, Weill Cornell, New York, USA. [5]Department of Research, Stavanger University Hospital, Stavanger, Norway. [6]Muhimbili University of Health and Allied Sciences, Dar es Salaam, Tanzania. [7]Muhimbili National Hospital, Dar es Salaam, Tanzania. [8]Obstetrics and Gynaecology, Haydom Lutheran Hospital, PO box 9000, Haydom, Mbulu, Tanzania.

References

1. Oza S, Cousens SN, Lawn JE. Estimation of daily risk of neonatal death, including the day of birth, in 186 countries in 2013: a vital-registration and modelling-based study. Lancet Glob Heal. 2014;2(11):e635–44.
2. Blencowe H, Cousens S, Oestergaard MZ, Chou D, Moller AB, Narwal R, et al. National, regional, and worldwide estimates of preterm birth rates in the year 2010 with time trends since 1990 for selected countries: a systematic analysis and implications. Lancet. 2012;379(9832):2162–72.
3. Lawn JE, Blencowe H, Waiswa P, Amouzou A, Mathers C, Hogan D, et al. Stillbirths: rates, risk factors, and acceleration towards 2030. Lancet. 2016; 6736(15):1–17.
4. Lawn JE, Kerber K, Enweronu-Laryea C, Bateman OM. Newborn survival in low resource settings - are we delivering? BJOG. 2009;116:49–59.
5. Unicef. Levels and trends in child mortality. New York: UNICEF; 2013. p. 1–30.
6. Saleem S, McClure EM, Goudar SS, Patel A, Esamai F, Garces A, et al. A prospective study of maternal, fetal and neonatal deaths in low- and middle-income countries. Bull World Health Organ. 2014;92(8):605–12.
7. Ersdal HL, Mduma E, Svensen E, Perlman J. Birth asphyxia: a major cause of early neonatal mortality in a Tanzanian rural hospital. Pediatrics. 2012;129(5): e1238–43.
8. Allanson ER, Muller M, Pattinson RC. Causes of perinatal mortality and associated maternal complications in a South African province: challenges in predicting poor outcomes. BMC Pregnancy Childbirth. 2015;15(1):37.
9. Schmiegelow C, Minja D, Oesterholt M, Pehrson C, Suhrs HE, Boström S, et al. Factors associated with and causes of perinatal mortality in northeastern Tanzania. Acta Obstet Gynecol Scand. 2012;91(9):1061–8.
10. Hadar A, Sheiner E, Hallak M, Katz M, Mazor M, Shoham-Vardi I. Abnormal fetal heart rate tracing patterns during the first stage of labor: effect on perinatal outcome. Am J Obstet Gynecol. 2001;185:863–8.
11. Verspyck E, Sentilhes L. Abnormal fetal heart rate patterns associated with different labour managements and intrauterine resuscitation techniques. J Gynecol Obstet Biol Reprod (Paris). 2008;37(Suppl 1):S56–64.
12. Xu H, Mas-Calvet M, Wei SQ, Luo ZC, Fraser WD. Abnormal fetal heart rate tracing patterns in patients with thick meconium staining of the amniotic fluid: association with perinatal outcomes. Am J Obstet Gynecol. 2009; 200(3):283.
13. Langli Ersdal H, Mduma E, Svensen E, Sundby J, Perlman J. Intermittent detection of fetal heart rate abnormalities identify infants at greatest risk for fresh stillbirths, birth asphyxia, neonatal resuscitation, and early neonatal

deaths in a limited-resource setting: a prospective descriptive observational stud. Neonatology. 2012;102(3):235–42.
14. Alfirevic Z, Devane D, Gyte GML. Continuous cardiotocography (CTG) as a form of electronic fetal monitoring (EFM) for fetal assessment during labour. Cochrane Database Syst Rev. 2006;3(3):81.
15. Herbst A, Ingemarsson I. Intermittent versus continuous electronic monitoring in labour: a randomised study. Br J Obstet Gynaecol. 1994; www.ncbi.nlm.nih.gov/pubmed/7947499
16. Mahomed K, Nyoni R, Mlambo T, Jacobus E, Kasule J. Intrapartum foetal heart rate monitoring–continuous electronic versus intermittent Doppler–a randomised controlled trial. Cent Afr J Med. 1992;38(12):458–62.
17. Mangesi L, Hofmeyr GJH, Woods DL. Assessing the preference of women for different methods of monitoring the fetal heart in labour. S Afr J Obstet Gynaecol. 2009;15(2):58–9.
18. Justus Hofmeyr G, Haws RA, Bergstrom S, Lee ACC, Okong P, Darmstadt GL, et al. Obstetric care in low-resource settings: what, who, and how to overcome challenges to scale up? Int J Gynecol Obstet. 2009;107: https://doi.org/10.1016/j.ijgo.2009.07
19. Woods D. Appropriate technology and education for improved intrapartum care in under- resourced countries; 2009. p. 78–9.
20. Byaruhanga R, Bassani DG, Jagau A, Muwanguzi P, Montgomery AL, Lawn JE. Use of wind-up fetal Doppler versus Pinard for fetal heart rate intermittent monitoring in labour: a randomised clinical trial. BMJ Open. 2015;5(1):e006867.
21. Evjen-Olsen B, Olsen OE, Kvåle G. Achieving progress in maternal and neonatal health through integrated and comprehensive healthcare services - experiences from a programme in northern Tanzania. Int J Equity Health. 2009;8:27.
22. Maaløe N, Housseine N, Bygbjerg IC, Meguid T, Khamis RS. Stillbirths and quality of care during labour at the low resource referral hospital of Zanzibar : a case-control study. BMC Pregnancy Childbirth. 2016; https://www.ncbi.nlm.nih.gov/pmc/articles/PMC5103376
23. Maaløe N, Housseine N, Meguid T, Nielsen BB, Jensen AKG, Khamis RS, et al. Effect of locally tailored labour management guidelines on intrahospital stillbirths and birth asphyxia at the referral hospital of Zanzibar: a quasi-experimental pre-post study (the PartoMa study). BJOG An Int J Obstet Gynaecol. 2018;125(2):235–45.
24. Lewis D, Downe S. FIGO consensus guidelines on intrapartum fetal monitoring: intermittent auscultation. Int J Gynecol Obstet. Elsevier B.V. 2015;131(1):9–12.
25. Committee NH, Ayres-de-campos D, Spong CY, Chandraharan E. Figo consensus guidelines on intrapartum fetal monitoring; 2015. p. 1–7.
26. Morrison JC, Chez BF, Davis ID, Martin RW, Roberts WE, Martin JN Jr, Floyd RC. Intrapartum fetal heart rate assessment: monitoring by auscultation or electronic means. Am J Obstet Gynecol. 1993;168(1 Pt 1):63–6.

20

Accelerating newborn survival in Ghana through a low-dose, high-frequency health worker training approach

Patricia P. Gomez[1*], Allyson R. Nelson[2], Amos Asiedu[3], Etta Addo[3], Dora Agbodza[3], Chantelle Allen[1], Martha Appiagyei[3], Cynthia Bannerman[4], Patience Darko[3], Julia Duodu[3], Fred Effah[3] and Hannah Tappis[1]

Abstract

Background: Newborn deaths comprise nearly half of under-5 deaths in Ghana, despite the fact that skilled birth attendants (SBAs) are present at 68% of births, which implies that evidence-based care during labor, birth and the immediate postnatal period may be deficient. We assessed the effect of a low-dose, high-frequency (LDHF) training approach on long-term evidence-based skill retention among SBAs and impact on adverse birth outcomes.

Methods: From 2014 to 2017, we conducted a cluster-randomized trial in 40 hospitals in Ghana. Eligible hospitals were stratified by region and randomly assigned to one of four implementation waves. We assessed the relative risks (RRs) of institutional intrapartum stillbirths and 24-h newborn mortality in months 1–6 and 7–12 of implementation as compared to the historical control period, and in post-intervention facilities compared to pre-intervention facilities during the same period. All SBAs providing labor and delivery care were invited to enroll; their knowledge and skills were assessed pre- and post-training, and 1 year later.

Results: Adjusting for region and health facility type, the RR of 24-h newborn mortality in the 40 enrolled hospitals was 0·41 (95% CI 0·32–0·51; $p < 0.001$) in months 1–6 and 0·30 (95% CI 0·21–0·43; $p < 0{\cdot}001$) in months 7–12 compared to baseline. The adjusted RR of intrapartum stillbirth was 0·64 (95% CI 0·53–0·77; $p < 0{\cdot}001$) in months 1–6 and 0·48 (95% CI 0·36–0·63; $p < 0{\cdot}001$) in months 7–12 compared to baseline. Four hundred three SBAs consented and enrolled. After 1 year, 200 SBAs assessed had 28% (95% CI 25–32; $p < 0{\cdot}001$) and 31% (95% CI 27–36; $p < 0{\cdot}001$) higher scores than baseline on low-dose 1 and 2 content skills, respectively.

Conclusions: This training approach results in a sustained decrease in facility-based newborn mortality and intrapartum stillbirths, and retained knowledge and skills among SBAs after a year. We recommend use of this approach for future maternal and newborn health in-service training and programs.

Keywords: Pregnancy, Labor, Birth, Stillbirth, Newborn, Resuscitation, Training, Skills, Skilled birth attendant, Mentor

* Correspondence: patricia.gomez@jhpiego.org
[1]Jhpiego/Baltimore, 1615 Thames Street, Baltimore, MD 21232, USA
Full list of author information is available at the end of the article

Background

The newborn mortality rate decreased by 47% worldwide between 1990 and 2015, from 36 to 19 deaths per 1000 live births, but the rate has declined more slowly in most low-resource settings, and is still far from the Sustainable Development Goal of less than 12 newborn deaths per 1000 live births by 2030.[1] Nearly half of newborn deaths take place during the first day of life [1]. Intrapartum-related events are now the third leading cause of all deaths among children under age 5 (U5 mortality) [2]. Rates of intrapartum stillbirths are a measure of the quality of care during labor, and newborn mortality in the 24 h following birth can reflect the quality of care during labor as well as immediate postnatal care [3].

Ghana's U5 mortality rate is 60/1000 live births and the newborn mortality rate is 29/1000 live births. Thus, newborn mortality represents 48% of U5 mortality despite the fact that 68% of births occur with a skilled birth attendant (SBA)[2] present [4]. The country's stillbirth rate is estimated at 22/1000 total births, although this estimate is not disaggregated by fetal deaths prior to labor or intrapartum stillbirths, and accurate information about the incidence of intrapartum stillbirth is lacking [5]. Two major causes of newborn deaths in Ghana, asphyxia (23%) and sepsis (32%), [6] could be prevented by increasing the use of evidence-based interventions during labor, birth, and the immediate postnatal period. The Ghana National Newborn Health Strategy and Action Plan 2014–2018 describes the country's goal to reduce institutional newborn mortality by at least 35% by 2018 through training of least 90% of SBAs in essential newborn care and basic resuscitation [6].

In-service training for SBAs is one of the most common interventions to address lack of knowledge and skills. However, these training interventions are seldom evaluated for effectiveness in improving learning or performance [7]. A literature review of effective in-service training described techniques that may improve learning outcomes and result in changes in performance [8]. The review found that didactic instruction often results in improved knowledge but no improvement in clinical practice. In contrast, the use of interactive techniques, including clinical simulation, case-based learning, hands-on practice with anatomic models, and immediate feedback on performance, results in greater improvement in knowledge and/or clinical practice than do passive techniques such as lecture or reading. Targeted, repeated training opportunities are preferable to one-time training and lead to the use of new skills in the clinical setting. Workplace learning may be superior for skill acquisition, and using multiple types of media can deliver training more efficiently. Thus, learning at the job site coupled with ongoing, repeated exposure to content is associated with greater improvement in clinical performance and health outcomes.

In collaboration with the Ghana Health Service (GHS), Jhpiego introduced interventions to reduce newborn mortality in 40 public and mission health facilities in which an ongoing quality improvement project[3] was targeting reduction of U5 mortality. Using evidence from the literature review on in-service training, we designed and tested a low-dose, high-frequency (LDHF) training approach to update hospital-based SBAs in key evidence-based intrapartum and immediate newborn care practices, using current global guidelines [9] (Table 1).

All study sites received the full LDHF intervention that included two 4-day onsite sessions (low dose) with weekly practice sessions, SMS quizzes and reminders, and mentoring via mobile phone and onsite visits between trainings (high frequency). The low-dose sessions included competency acquisition through simulation, case-based learning, and small content packages spread over short time intervals (Table 2) [7, 10]. To foster a team-centered approach, [8] we trained all SBAs providing intrapartum and immediate postpartum care in each health facility, but limited each low-dose session to no more than ten SBAs. Thus, in large facilities more than one cycle of training was conducted to accommodate all eligible SBAs. This approach was considered low dose compared to the basic emergency obstetric and newborn care (BEmONC) training that was occurring in the country at the time of this study. The BEmONC training took place away from SBAs' usual workplace, included only a few SBAs from a given facility, and lasted up to 10 days.

We hypothesized that the LDHF approach to improving clinical skills would lead to a reduction in institutional intrapartum stillbirths and newborn mortality within 24 h of birth during the year of the intervention. We also hypothesized that the approach would result in improved and retained skills and knowledge among SBAs in maternity wards in study sites after a year.

Table 1 Components of low-dose, high-frequency approach. Lists the eight components that comprised the low-dose, high-frequency approach

• Two 4-day low-dose sessions (for facility skilled birth attendants)
• 1-day peer practice coordinator training after first low-dose session
• High-frequency practice sessions using MamaNatalie® and NeoNatalie™ anatomic models
• mMentoring with SMS reminder messages and quizzes
• Mentoring calls between master mentors and peer practice coordinators, and between project staff and master mentors
• Health information officer training
• Data collection and use training
• Supply of simulators, newborn resuscitation equipment, and delivery sets provided at first low-dose training session

Table 2 Low-Dose Session Content. Lists the clinical content presented in each low-dose session

Low-Dose Session 1:

- Respectful maternity care
- Infection prevention and control
- Clinical decision-making
- Evidence-based support of normal labor and birth, including use of the partograph and active management of the third stage of labor
- Immediate newborn care
- Newborn resuscitation
- Data collection and use; reporting of data

Low-Dose Session 2:

- Antenatal corticosteroids for anticipated preterm birth
- Management of severe pre-eclampsia and eclampsia
- Management of postpartum hemorrhage, including repair of lacerations
- Prevention and treatment of maternal and newborn sepsis
- Kangaroo mother care
- Data collection and use; reporting of data

Methods

Study design

The study was a cluster-randomized trial implemented in 40 public and mission hospitals in Ghana between March 2014 and February 2017. Initial study sites included three regional hospitals, 38 district hospitals, and one polyclinic across Upper West, Central, and Western Regions of Ghana. Each facility was enrolled for 18 months. Data on institutional intrapartum stillbirths and 24-h newborn mortality were collected retrospectively for 6 months pre-intervention (i.e., baseline) and prospectively for 12 months post-intervention at each study site (Fig. 1).

All SBAs providing labor, birth, and immediate postnatal care at the selected facilities at the time of the first low-dose session were invited to participate. Four hundred and three SBAs individually consented and were enrolled in the study. All enrolled SBAs were registered or certified midwives.

Randomization and masking

Eligible facilities had at least three SBAs and an average of 30 or more births per month. These hospitals were stratified by region (three categories) and caseload (four categories), and then randomly assigned to one of four implementation waves. The pipeline randomization allowed for rigorous evaluation while the program was rolled out to all facilities. Waves 1 through 4 included eleven, seventeen, eight, and six facilities, respectively. Waves were unbalanced because of the stratification. Two hospitals were excluded at the time of implementation because they no longer met the inclusion criteria. Neither facilities nor participants were masked due to the nature of the intervention.

Procedures

Experienced SBAs were prepared as regional master mentors (MMs) through a course in targeted BEmONC and training skills. MMs conducted the onsite, low-dose sessions and follow-up mentorship activities in collaboration with project staff. Of the 40 study facilities, 19 had a MM working within the facility, while the remaining facilities received mentoring support from MMs via mobile phone and periodic visits. During the first low-dose session at each site, two to three SBAs were trained as peer practice coordinators (PPCs) to lead the high-frequency practice sessions and were oriented to their roles in a day-long session. One month later, the second 4-day low-dose session was conducted. In the month between low-dose sessions and for 11 months afterward, SBAs carried out weekly PPC-led practice sessions with simulators and participated in mMentoring, which included mobile phone–based mentoring and onsite coaching with MMs and automated SMS reminders and quiz questions about key concepts presented during the low-dose sessions (Fig. 2).

MamaNatalie® and NeoNatalie™ simulators were given to each site to enable regular practice of targeted skills. Each site also received newborn resuscitation equipment (NeoNatalie resuscitator, penguin suction [Laerdal], and basic delivery sets). SBAs and health information officers collected service delivery data. Orientation to facility-level data collection was included in the first low-dose session for all SBAs. An additional training was provided to each facility's health information officer and maternity unit in-charge to ensure a common understanding of indicators and data collection, quality, and use. Monthly service statistics were extracted from routine health information systems and a supplementary delivery register introduced by the project. All outcome data were verified using register reviews at each study site.

Objective structured clinical examination (OSCE) tools and knowledge tests, based on global and national guidelines, were developed to assess SBAs in management of normal birth, immediate newborn care, and maternal and newborn complications. These assessments were used before and immediately after low-dose sessions, and again 1 year later, to evaluate knowledge and skill acquisition and retention. Master mentors and project staff conducted and collected all OSCE and knowledge test data. Assessments were scanned into Captricity (Oakland, CA, USA) for data capture and cleaning.

Outcomes

Twenty-four hour newborn mortality was defined as the death within 24 h, or before discharge, of a newborn

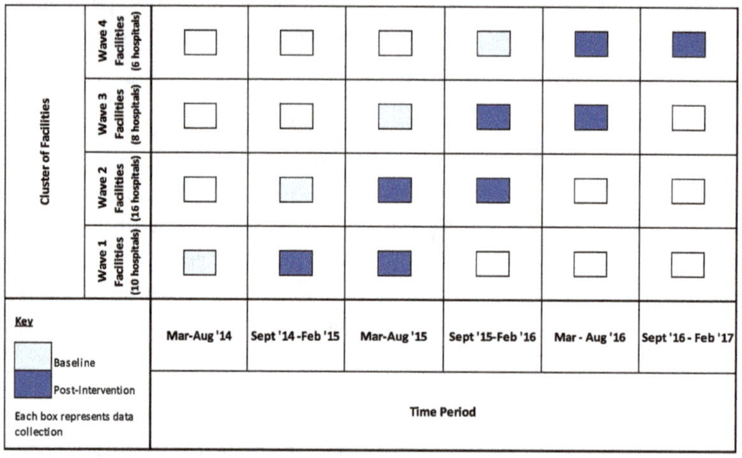

Fig. 1 Phased implementation and data collection. Describes timing of baseline and post-intervention data collection over the four waves of facility enrollment between March 2014 and February 2017

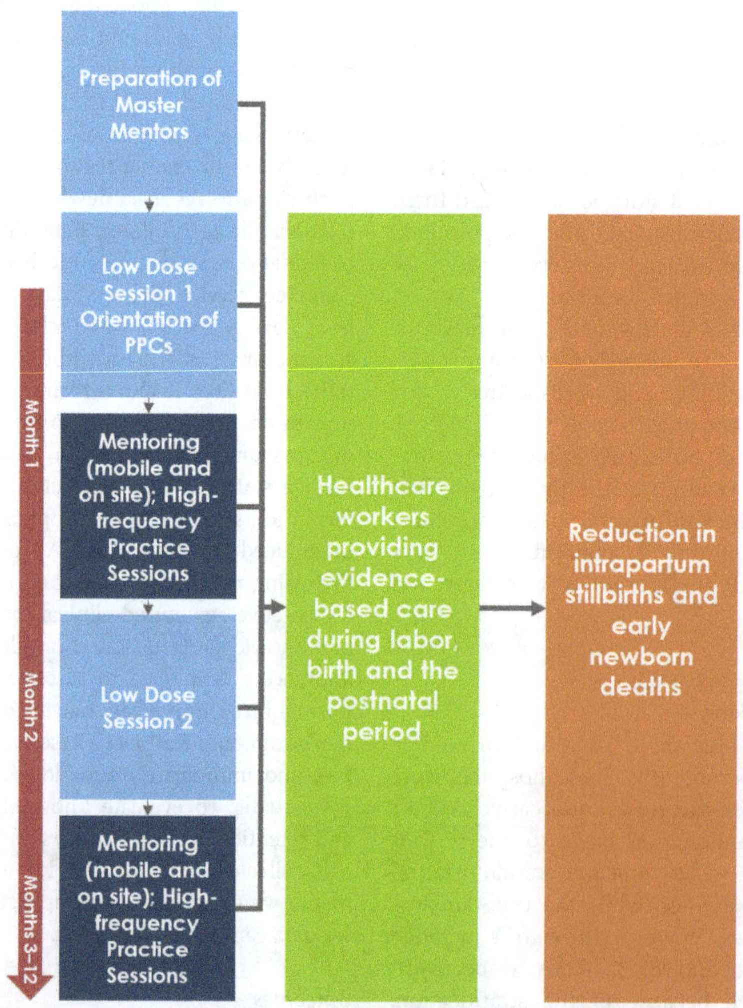

Fig. 2 Low-dose, high-frequency training approach to reduce newborn mortality and intrapartum stillbirths in Ghana. Describes the inputs, outcomes and impact of the project

who breathed at birth. The institutional 24-h newborn mortality rate was defined as deaths in the first 24 h per 1000 facility live births. Intrapartum stillbirth was defined as the death of a baby who had heart tones present at the time of the mother's admission to the facility, was born with no signs of maceration, and did not breathe at birth, and on whom resuscitation attempts were unsuccessful. The institutional intrapartum stillbirth rate was defined as the proportion of all facility births that resulted in intrapartum stillbirth. Training results were the proportion of total test items (knowledge questions or skill steps) performed correctly.

Statistical analysis

We ran a simulation to assess statistical power to detect a reduction in the primary outcome, 24-h newborn mortality, in the original 42 study sites. In each simulation run, the study design was replicated, with four study entry time points (i.e., strata) for 42 facilities. A random effect Poisson model was fit to each study replicate to estimate the intervention effect on the number of newborn deaths, adjusting for the stratum, with the number of deliveries per facility as the offset term. Across the multiple iterations of the study, we calculated the empirical statistical power as the proportion of the simulation runs in which the p-value was less than 0·05 level of significance, indicating that the null hypothesis of no post-intervention difference in the number of deaths is rejected. Results indicated that we had 99% power to detect a 25% decrease in the number of newborn deaths after the intervention.

We assessed institutional mortality rates and SBA competency at all facilities post-implementation compared to pre-implementation and assessed differences between institutional mortality rates at a subset of intervention and non-intervention (i.e., control) facilities during three 6-month time intervals. The entire study period (March 2014 to February 2017) was subdivided into four intervention waves, based on the start date of the intervention, and six calendar periods. For each facility the following variables were defined: intervention stage (coded as 0 for baseline, 1 for months 1–6 after Low-Dose 1, and 2 for months 7–12 after Low-Dose 1), wave (from 1 to 4, depending on the start of the intervention), and calendar period (from 1 to 6). Exploratory analyses included comparison of the observed intrapartum stillbirth or newborn death rates by intervention stage, wave, calendar period, and region. Outcome rate trajectories were plotted over the calendar period by wave to assess for within-group trends. Baseline mortality rates were calculated as a facility-weighted *(births or live births)* average over the 6-month baseline period. Comparability of mortality rates at baseline was assessed using analysis of variance (ANOVA).

To estimate the effect of the intervention, we fit a series of generalized population-average linear models with negative binomial distribution and a log-link with exchangeable working correlation structure. The models were estimated using generalized estimating equations with robust variance estimates and a negative binomial distribution.

The base model included two indicator variables for intervention (months 1–6 and months 7–12) and adjustment for the region and level of the health facility (regional hospital or district hospital/polyclinic). Exponentiated beta coefficients for the two intervention variables were interpreted as the relative risk (RR) of the outcome post-intervention compared to the historical control (baseline) period.

To assess whether the effect of the intervention varied significantly by wave or region, the base model was modified to include the appropriate interaction terms. Secondary analyses were conducted using time as a continuous variable in a similar model to assess the monthly change in mortality rates prior to and after intervention. In addition, we used interaction terms in a modified model to assess the effect of the intervention comparing intervention and control facilities in the same calendar period, adjusting for effect of facility level on the outcome measures.

OSCE and knowledge test scores were calculated based on the number of steps correct in the OSCE or number of items correct on the knowledge test out of the total possible correct on each test. Scores were analyzed using ordinary least-squares linear regression that tested for a difference in individuals' pre- and post-test assessment scores, and pre-test and 1-year assessment scores, adjusting for clustering of SBAs within the facility.

Data were analyzed using Stata Version 14 (StataCorp LLC, College Station, TX, USA).

Results

In the 40 facilities, 403 SBAs consented and were enrolled in the study. Two hundred and one SBAs (50%) were available for OSCE and knowledge assessment at 1 year after the intervention due to SBA rotation to other facilities, further education, and annual leave (Fig. 3).

The pre-intervention period included 38,192 births (Table 3). Months 1–6 and months 7–12 included 36,160 and 31,498 births, respectively. The total numbers of 24-h newborn deaths and intrapartum stillbirths in the 40 sites, including baseline and the intervention periods, were 528 and 799, respectively.

Delivery caseloads, intrapartum stillbirth rates, and 24-h newborn mortality rates prior to intervention were comparable across waves (ANOVA $p = 0{\cdot}818$ and $p = 0{\cdot}527$, respectively) (Table 4).

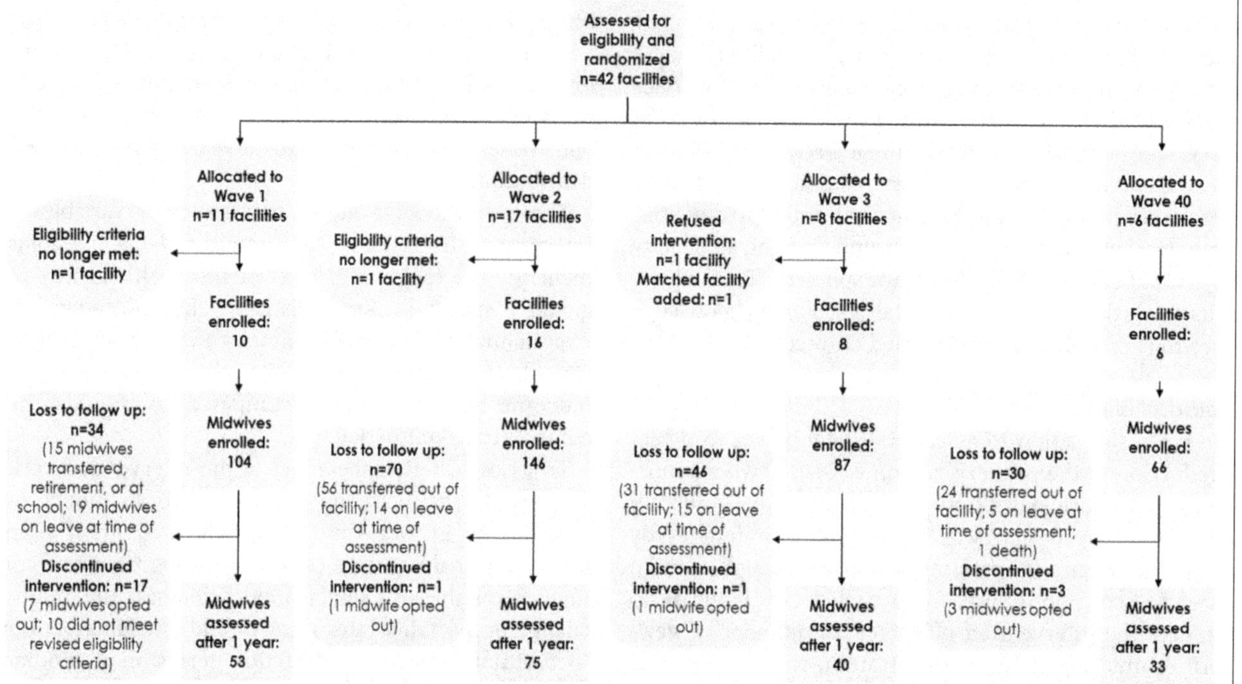

Fig. 3 Trial profile. Describes the allocation of trial facilities into the four waves, the number of midwives enrolled in the trial and the number assessed after 1 year of implementation

Implementation of the LDHF package resulted in a 55% reduction in risk of newborn mortality within 24 h of birth in the 6 months after LD1 (unadjusted RR 0·45, 95% CI 0·35–0·58; $p < 0·001$) and a 65% reduction in risk in the next 6-month follow-up period (unadjusted RR 0·35, 95% CI 0·24–0·50; $p < 0·001$). After adjusting for region and facility level, the reduction in risk increased to 59% and 70%, respectively (adjusted RRs 0·41, 95% CI 0·32–0·51 and 0·30, 95% CI 0.21–0.43, in months 1–6 and months 7–12, respectively). Regional-level facilities had a significantly greater risk of 24-h newborn mortality compared to district-level facilities and polyclinics (RR 5·11, 95% CI 3·55–7·36; $p < 0·001$).

The intervention resulted in a 35% reduction (RR 0·65, 95% CI 0·54–0·78; $p < 0001$) in the risk of intrapartum stillbirth (unadjusted analysis) comparing months 1–6 to the pre-intervention period, and a 51% reduction in risk (RR 0·49, 95% CI 0·36–0·65; $p < 0·001$) in months 7–12 (Table 5). Results in a model adjusting for level of facility (regional vs. district level or polyclinic) and region did not substantially differ compared to the unadjusted model. Regional-level facilities had a significantly greater risk of intrapartum stillbirth compared to district-level facilities and polyclinics (RR 1·33, 95% CI 1·03–1·70; $p = 0·027$).

Pre-test scores on the low-dose session 1 (LD1) knowledge test and OSCE were 76% and 44%, respectively (Table 6). Low-dose session 2 (LD2) pre-test scores were slightly higher at 91% and 52%, respectively. Post-test scores increased by 11% (95% confidence interval [CI] 9–12; $p < 0·001$) and 4% (95% CI 2–6; $p = 0·001$) on LD1 and LD2 knowledge tests,

Table 3 Outcomes of interest during pre- and post-intervention periods

	Pre-intervention	Post-intervention	
	Baseline	Months 1–6	Months 7–12
Number of births	38,192	36,160	31,498
Number of live births	37,204	35,352	30,940
Number of intrapartum stillbirths	392	242	165
Number of newborn deaths within 24 h of birth	284	140	104
Intrapartum stillbirth rate (per 1000 births)	10·3	6·7	5·2
24-h newborn mortality rate (per 1000 live births)	7·6	4·0	3·4

Table 4 Baseline facility characteristics

	Wave				ANOVA *p*-value
	1	2	3	4	
	Mean (+/– SD)	Mean (+/– SD)	Mean (+/– SD)	Mean (+/– SD)	
Number of births per month	194 (99)	117 (70)	136 (58)	110 (42)	0·0628
Births per month per participant trained	25 (18)	13 (8)	13 (7)	10 (4)	0·0336
Intrapartum stillbirth rate	9·0 (6·0)	10·7 (6·3)	12·0 (9·7)	12·0 (9·1)	0·818
24-h newborn mortality rate	11·7 (10·4)	8·2 (8·3)	5·9 (6·4)	7·0 (7·4)	0·527

respectively, and 44% (95% CI 40–48; $p < 0{\cdot}001$) and 40% (95% CI 37–43; $p < 0{\cdot}001$) on the LD1 and LD2 OSCEs, respectively. After 1 year, participants retained most knowledge and skills gains. Participants scored 31% and 28% higher on OSCE content from LD1 and LD2 at 1 year, respectively, compared to pre-test scores (LD1 95% CI 27–36; $p < 0{\cdot}001$; LD2 95% CI 25–32; $p < 0{\cdot}001$), and 8% and 2% higher, respectively, on knowledge content from LD1 and LD2 at 1 year, compared to pre-test scores (LD1 95% CI 6–10; $p < 0{\cdot}001$; LD2 95% CI 0–4; $p = 0{\cdot}025$).

There was no evidence of a temporal trend in intrapartum stillbirth or 24-h newborn mortality rates in study sites before the intervention. Therefore, the model did not adjust for calendar time. Once the intervention began, newborn mortality declined significantly from 1 month to the next over the one-year intervention period. Intrapartum stillbirth rates did not change significantly on a monthly basis; from this, we infer that the reduction in stillbirth rate was more drastic and immediate following the start of the intervention, and remained low for the remainder of the one-year follow-up period. Wave 3 facilities showed a greater reduction in risk of 24-h newborn mortality during months 7–12 post-intervention compared to facilities in the other three waves. Risk of intrapartum stillbirth decreased more dramatically in wave 2 facilities compared to other facilities (Additional files 1 and 2: Tables S1 and S2). We found no significant difference in the mortality rates as a result of a master mentor being present at a study site.

We tested to see if there is a difference in the mortality rates between cohorts of facilities in the intervention phase and the baseline phase during the same calendar period. In all three time periods analyzed, newborn mortality rates were significantly lower in facilities in the intervention phase compared to those in the baseline phase; intrapartum stillbirth rates were also lower but only statistically significant in two of the three analyzed calendar periods. This analysis was conducted for a subset of the total study time and outcome observations, as the study was not designed or resourced to conduct a full randomization with comparison sites throughout the study duration.

Discussion

The primary aim of the study was to assess newborn outcomes. Results showed significant reduction in intrapartum stillbirth and newborn death within 24 h. This could indicate that the quality of care during labor was sufficient to maintain maternal and fetal well-being. In addition, since resuscitation was attempted for all non-macerated newborns not breathing at birth, many babies who would otherwise have been declared intrapartum stillbirths but actually had intrapartum-related asphyxia, were successfully resuscitated [11] corroborating the assertion by Wall et al. that training SBAs in newborn resuscitation could prevent up to 30% of mortality in full-term babies due to intrapartum-related events [12]. Reduction in newborn deaths within 24 h may be

Table 5 Mortality outcomes in 40 sites

	Unadjusted risk ratio	95% CI	*p*-value	Adjusted risk ratio[a]	95% CI	*p*-value
Pre-intervention (6 months prior to intervention)	REF	REF	REF	REF	REF	REF
Newborn death within 24 h						
Months 1–6	0·45	0.35–0.58	< 0·001	0·41	0·32–0·51	< 0·001
Months 7–12	0·35	0.24–0.50	< 0·001	0·30	0·21–0·43	< 0·001
Intrapartum stillbirth						
Months 1–6	0·65	0·54–0·78	< 0·001	0·64	0·53–0·77	< 0·001
Months 7–12	0·49	0·36–0·65	< 0·001	0·48	0·36–0·63	< 0·001

OSCE objective structured clinical examination
[a]Adjusted for region and facility level (polyclinic or district hospital vs. regional hospital)

Table 6 Skilled birth attendant retention of key knowledge and skills

	Pre-test (%)	Post-test (%)	Difference (%) (post–/pre-)	*p*-value	1-year assessment (%)	Difference (%) (1-yr/pre-)	*p*-value
	Mean (+/– SD)	Mean (+/– SD)	Mean (95% CI)		Mean (+/– SD)	Mean (95% CI)	
Low-dose session 1							
Knowledge assessment	76 (9)	87 (7)	11 (9–12)	< 0·001	85 (8)	8 (6–10)	< 0·001
OSCE	44 (13)	88 (9)	44 (40–48)	< 0·001	76 (14)	31 (27–36)	< 0·001
Low-dose session 2							
Knowledge assessment	91 (10)	95 (6)	4 (2–6)	0·001	94 (10)	2 (0–4)	0·025
OSCE	52 (14)	92 (7)	40 (37–43)	< 0·001	81 (12)	28 (25–32)	< 0·001

attributed to the use of newborn care interventions for every baby (immediate drying and warming, skin-to-skin-contact, and immediate and exclusive breastfeeding) as well as rapid recognition and appropriate management of intrapartum-related asphyxia.

A second aim of the study was to assess the effect of the LDHF package on retention of key knowledge and skills after 1 year. We found that SBAs retained most knowledge and skills gained during low-dose sessions, which contributed to their ability to apply appropriate clinical interventions for improved newborn outcomes. The expectation after the low-dose sessions was that SBAs' skills should not be lost after training, but maintained or even improved. The lowest 1-year OSCE score occurred in relation to LD1, which dealt with care during normal labor and birth and newborn resuscitation. This implies that although SBAs attended many births, their practices did not reflect the evidence-based approaches presented during the first low-dose session. Thus, they might have needed more practice in simulated and clinical settings in the updated skills and/or reinforcement by PPCs or master mentors. Similarly, the skills for newborn resuscitation were new for most SBAs, and since resuscitation is a comparatively rare event, there may have been a need for reinforcement over time to maintain them. This is consistent with evaluations of maintenance of newborn resuscitation skills during which SBAs had the opportunity to review and practice skills on a regular basis after training [13].

In addition, our results demonstrate the impact and importance of an integrated package of evidence-based, clinical interventions that considers the continuum of care for the mother and baby on the day of birth. The components of the LDHF approach were chosen to target the major global causes of intrapartum-related events that are associated with up to 42% of maternal mortality, 32% of stillbirths, and 23% of newborn mortality [14]. They included cross-cutting elements of care that can improve maternal and newborn outcomes, such as respectful maternity care, which includes encouragement of continuous support during labor, ambulation, and positions of choice for labor and birth. These have been shown to decrease the duration of labor and the use of cesarean or assisted delivery [15, 16]. Key evidence-based infection prevention practices were introduced during LD1 to decrease the risk of maternal and newborn sepsis. Hand hygiene, [17] instrument processing, [18] reduction of vaginal exams during labor, [19] avoiding routine rupture of membranes, [20] and prompt management of maternal fever and newborn sepsis were emphasized [21]. Severe pre-eclampsia and eclampsia are implicated globally in up to 4·7% of stillbirths, with the highest burden in south Asia and sub-Saharan Africa. Improved management of these disorders during labor could avert these deaths [22, 23]. Respectful maternity care and infection prevention were part of all OSCEs and skills checklists used by providers during training and high-frequency practice sessions.

The study emphasized correct use of the partograph to monitor labor and support clinical decision-making, which has been shown to improve identification of prolonged labor, a major contributor to perinatal mortality [24]. Best practices for immediate newborn care included immediate drying and skin-to-skin contact, [25, 26] delayed cord clamping, [27] and breastfeeding in the hour following birth [25].

Leading causes of maternal mortality in sub-Saharan Africa include hemorrhage (25%), hypertension (16%), and sepsis (10%) [5]. Data for Ghana indicate that hemorrhage causes 24·3% of maternal mortality, hypertension accounts for 8·5%, and sepsis is the cause of 6·7% of deaths [28]. Thus, the LDHF approach targeted management of severe pre-eclampsia/eclampsia, using magnesium sulfate and antihypertensive medications, [29] and prevention and treatment of postpartum hemorrhage [30].

One of the factors contributing to effective implementation of the LDHF approach was close collaboration with all levels of the Ghana Health Service. National-level support was obtained at the outset, and regional health directors agreed to implementation in their regions. They also selected the MMs who carried out study activities as part of their normal duties; no MMs or SBAs were hired for the study. The investment in the development of a cadre of ten MMs in each region enabled close local follow-up of PPCs and SBAs in study facilities, both face-to-face and via mMentoring.

This study provides evidence that can guide strategies for health worker capacity-building at scale. Our results show a plausible causative association between use of an LDHF approach for facility-based in-service training and significant reductions in intrapartum stillbirths and newborn deaths in health facilities in low-resource settings. Health facilities did not undergo structural changes or receive additional equipment beyond delivery sets and resuscitation equipment. The LDHF approach built SBAs' competency in essential maternal and newborn health care practices. In each facility, all SBAs providing intrapartum and immediate postpartum care participated in this approach, resulting in facility-wide improvement in service quality, while minimizing the amount of time the SBAs spent outside of their facilities. It also enabled nearly all SBAs in each facility to receive the same training and follow-up support, which may have enhanced consistency of knowledge and skill transfer to the clinical setting. The critical mass of trained SBAs at each facility reinforces learning and builds a system of checks and balances throughout the health facility, likely rendering the change more sustainable. Coupled with ongoing practice and mentorship, improved practices are sustained and health outcomes continue to improve over time, even with staff attrition and turnover, as new SBAs are taught the skills by existing staff and can practice them on the simulators. Moreover, a pool of highly competent MMs enables continued application of the package after the study ends.

There are methodological limitations to consider in assessing the study implications. Because the study was embedded in program implementation, facility staff were aware of the outcome of interest, which could have affected their actions and performance. The presence of MMs at some facilities before intervention start-up could also have affected baseline outcome measurement rates. However, our analysis shows that mortality rates in all waves were comparable at baseline, and therefore we do not believe this has an effect on the results achieved. In addition, our study was not designed to be able to conduct a full time-series or randomized control trial analysis, due to resource limitations on baseline and control site data collection. Multiple analyses conducted using available data demonstrate qualitatively the same result. Other sources of potential bias include lack of concealment in group (i.e., wave) assignment and information bias such that data quality may have improved after the intervention started. In all likelihood, improved data quality following the intervention would result in more deaths being reported, rather than fewer, resulting in a smaller observed effect.

Although the regions for study implementation were chosen specifically to avoid overlap with other interventions conducted by the GHS and nongovernmental organizations, some SBAs from study facilities were invited to attend training on content related to BEmONC and/or newborn resuscitation, but none of the training was similar to the LDHF approach. However, the influence of these activities on our outcomes cannot be ruled out.

Finally, while the technical approach demonstrates results, other factors such as cost and human resource availability (for trainers and mentors) must be considered. A nested costing study showed that the LDHF package was less expensive per participant compared to the traditional approach [31].

Conclusions

Implementation of an LDHF approach to train SBAs in key evidence-based intrapartum and immediate newborn care practices is associated with a significant reduction in the risks of intrapartum stillbirth and newborn mortality within 24 h of birth. The components of the approach were chosen specifically to address the most common causes of intrapartum stillbirth and early newborn death in Ghana and were reinforced in multiple ways: classroom learning and practice with simulators during and between low-dose sessions; peer-led practice and feedback between and after low-dose sessions; follow-up via targeted SMS messaging and support by a master mentor; and robust data collection and reporting. In addition, all training was done onsite and involved nearly all maternity ward SBAs at each site. These elements contributed to transfer of knowledge and skills to the clinical setting and thus to improved outcomes. The adoption of the LDHF approach in Ghana and other low-resource countries has the potential to contribute to the acceleration of newborn survival and the achievement of Sustainable Development Goal 3 (reduction of neonatal mortality to at least as low as 12 per 1000 by 2030).

Policymakers and health partners should review current approaches to improving service delivery in maternal and newborn health, and consider investing in and adopting this approach as an innovative and effective method of training health care workers. While further research is necessary, we believe this approach should be considered for the improvement of clinical services in other technical areas that mandate acquisition and retention of skills to improve health outcomes.

Endnotes

[1]UN Sustainable Development Goals (http://www.un.org/sustainabledevelopment/health/page/2/0; accessed 26 January 2017)

[2]A skilled attendant is an accredited health professional such as a midwife, doctor, or nurse who has been

educated and trained to proficiency in the skills needed to manage normal (uncomplicated) pregnancies, childbirth, and the immediate postnatal period, and in the identification, management, and referral of complications in women and newborns. (WHO, ICM and FIGO. *Making pregnancy safer: the critical role of the skilled attendant. A joint statement by WHO, ICM and FIGO.* Geneva, 2004.)

[3]Project Fives Alive! is implemented by the Institute for Healthcare Improvement and the National Catholic Health Service in collaboration with the Ghana Health Service.

Additional files

Additional file 1: Table S1. Newborn mortality risk ratio by wave. Describes the effect of the intervention on newborn mortality by intervention wave.

Additional file : Table S2. Intrapartum stillbirth risk ratio by wave. Describes the effect of the intervention on intrapartum stillbirth by intervention wave.

Abbreviations
ANOVA: Analysis of variance; BEmONC: Basic emergency obstetric and newborn care; CI: Confidence interval; GHS: Ghana Health Service; LD1: Low dose session 1; LD2: Low dose session 2; LDHF: Low dose, high frequency; MM: Master mentor; OSCE: Objective structured clinical examination; PPC: Peer practice coordinator; RR: Relative risk; SBA: Skilled birth attendant; SMS: Short message service; U5: Under 5

Acknowledgements
The authors thank The Bill & Melinda Gates Foundation for their support of this work. They also thank the Institute for Healthcare Improvement and the director of its Project Fives Alive! initiative in Ghana, Dr. Sodzi Sodzi-Tetteh, for their fruitful collaboration during this study. We also extend great appreciation to the Ghana Health Service and the National Catholic Health Service for allowing us to carry out our work in their facilities. We especially recognize and are grateful to Mary Drake, Jhpiego Tanzania, for her contribution to the initial design of this study, and Gayane Yenokyan, Johns Hopkins Bloomberg School of Public Health, for her support in data analysis. We are indebted to Heather Harrison, Jhpiego Baltimore, who provided unfaltering program support and guidance throughout the study. The entire Ghana-based study team's rigorous fieldwork was inspiring and we congratulate them. Not least, we would like to thank the midwives and doctors who so enthusiastically participated in this study and made their constant priority the improvement of maternal and newborn care in their workplaces.

Funding
This research was funded by the Bill & Melinda Gates Foundation. The funders had no role in data collection, data analysis, data interpretation, or manuscript development. The contents of this publication are the responsibility of the authors and do not necessarily reflect the views of the funder.

Authors' contributions
PG, MA and CA contributed to the study design and AA, EA, DA, MA, CA, PD, JD, FE, and AN to study implementation and data collection. AN, AA and HT performed data analysis. All authors (PG, AN, AA, EA, DA, CA, MA, CB, PD, JD, FE, HT contributed to interpretation of findings, drafted the manuscript and contributed to manuscript revision. All authors read and approved the final manuscript.

Authors' information
N/A

Competing interests
The authors declare that they have no competing interests.

Author details
[1]Jhpiego/Baltimore, 1615 Thames Street, Baltimore, MD 21232, USA. [2]Jhpiego/Liberia, UN Drive, OPP Rock Compound, Mamba Point, Monrovia, Liberia. [3]Jhpiego Ghana, 14 Ollenu Street, East Legon, Accra, Ghana. [4]Ghana Health Service, Private Mail Bag, Ministries, Accra, Ghana.

References

1. World Health Organization. Children: reducing mortality. WHO fact sheet, updated September 2016. http://www.who.int/mediacentre/factsheets/fs178/en/. Accessed 23 Jan 2017.
2. Liu L, Oza S, Hogan D, et al. Global, regional, and national causes of under-5 mortality in 2000–15: an updated systematic analysis with implications for the sustainable development goals. Lancet. 2016;388:3027–35.
3. Lawn J, Blencowe H, Waiswa P, et al. Stillbirths: rates, risk factors, and acceleration towards 2030. Lancet. 2016;387:587–603.
4. Ghana Statistical Service (GSS), Ghana Health Service (GHS), and ICF International. Ghana demographic and health survey 2014. Rockville: GSS, GHS, and ICF International; 2015.
5. UNICEF and the World Health Organization. A decade of tracking progress for maternal, newborn and child survival: the 2015 report. Geneva: UNICEF and WHO; 2015.
6. Ghana Ministry of Health. Ghana national newborn health strategy and action plan 2014–2018. Accra: Ghana Ministry of Health; 2014.
7. Ameh CA, van den Broek N. Making it happen: training health-care providers in emergency obstetric and newborn care. Best Pract Res Clin Obstet Gynaecol. 2015;29(215):1077–91.
8. Bluestone J, Johnson P, Fullerton J, Carr C, Alderman J, Bon Tempo J. Effective in-service training design and delivery: evidence from an integrative literature review. Hum Resour Health. 2013;11(1):Article 51.
9. Sutton RM, Niles D, Meaney PA, et al. Low-dose, high-frequency CPR training improves skill retention of in-hospital paediatric providers. Paediatr. 2011;128(1):e145–51.
10. Anderson JM, Warren JB. Using simulation to enhance the acquisition and retention of clinical skills in neonatology. Semin Perinatol. 2011;35:59–67.
11. Goldenberg RL, McClure EM, Jobe AH, Kamath-Rayne BD, Gravette MG, Rubens CE. Stillbirths and neonatal mortality as outcomes. Int J Gynecol Obstet. 2013;123:252–3.
12. Wall SN, Lee ACC, Niermeyer S, et al. Neonatal resuscitation in low-resource settings: what, who, and how to overcome challenges to scale up? Int J Gynecol Obstet. 2009;107:S47–64.
13. Ashish KC, Wrammert J, Nelin V, et al. Evaluation of Helping Babies Breathe Quality Improvement Cycle (HBB-QIC) on retention of neonatal resuscitation skills six months after training in Nepal. BMC Pediatr. 2017;17:103.
14. Lawn JE, Kinney M, Lee AC, et al. Reducing intrapartum-related deaths and disability: can the health system deliver? Int J Gynecol Obstet. 2009; 107(Suppl 1):S123–40.
15. Lawrence A, Lewis L, Hofmeyr GJ, Dowswell T, Styles C. Maternal positions and mobility during first stage labor (Review). Cochrane Database Syst Rev. 2013;(8). https://doi.org/10.1002/14651858.CD003934.pub3.
16. Hodnett ED, Gates S, Hofmeyr GJ, Sakala C, Weston J. Continuous support for women during childbirth (Review). Cochrane Database Syst Rev. 2017;(7). https://doi.org/10.1002/14651858.CD003766.pub6
17. World Health Organization. WHO guidelines on hand hygiene in health care. Geneva: WHO; 2009.
18. World Health Organization (WHO) and Pan American Health Organization (PAHO). Decontamination and reprocessing of medical devices for health-care facilities. Geneva: WHO and PAHO; 2016.
19. Downe S, Gyte GM, Dahlen HG, Singata M. Routine vaginal examinations for assessing progress of labour to improve outcomes for women and babies at term (Review). Cochrane Database Syst Rev. 2013;7:CD010088.
20. Smyth RMD, Markham C, Dowswell T. Amniotomy for shortening

spontaneous labor (Review). Cochrane Database Syst Rev. 2013;(6). https://doi.org/10.1002/14651858.CD006167.pub4.

21. World Health Organization. WHO recommendations for prevention and treatment of maternal peripartum infections. Geneva: WHO; 2015.
22. World Health Organization. WHO recommendations for management of common childhood conditions: evidence for technical update of pocket book recommendations. Geneva: WHO; 2012.
23. von Dadelszen P, Firoz T, Donnay F, et al. Preeclampsia in low and middle income countries—health services lessons learned from the PRE-EMPT (PRE-eclampsia–eclampsia monitoring, prevention & treatment) project. J Obstet Gynaecol Can. 2012;34(10):917–26.
24. Hofmeyr GJ, Haws RA, Bergström S, et al. Obstetric care in low-resource settings: what, who, and how to overcome challenges to scale up? Int J Gynecol Obstet. 2009;107:S21–45.
25. American Academy of Pediatrics (AAP). Helping babies breathe provider guide. 2nd ed. AAP: Elk Grove Village; 2016.
26. Moore ER, Bergman N, Anderson GC, Medley N. Early skin-to-skin contact for mothers and their healthy newborn infants (Review). Cochrane Database Syst Rev. 2016;(11). https://doi.org/10.1002/14651858.CD003519.pub4.
27. World Health Organization. Guideline: delayed umbilical cord clamping for improved maternal and infant health and nutrition outcomes. Geneva: WHO; 2014.
28. Ghana Statistical Service (GSS), Ghana Health Service (GHS), and Macro International. Ghana maternal health survey 2007. Calverton: GSS, GHS, and Macro International; 2009.
29. World Health Organization. WHO recommendations for prevention and treatment of pre-eclampsia and eclampsia. Geneva: WHO; 2011.
30. World Health Organization. WHO recommendations for the prevention and treatment of postpartum haemorrhage. Geneva: WHO; 2012.
31. Willcox M, Harrison H, Asiedu A, Nelson A, Gomez P, LeFevre A. Incremental cost and cost-effectiveness of low-dose, high-frequency training in basic emergency obstetric and newborn care as compared to status quo: part of a cluster randomized training intervention evaluation in Ghana. Glob Health. 2017;13:88. https://doi.org/10.1186/s12992-017-0313-x. Published online 6 Dec 2017

21

A rare case of spontaneous hepatic rupture in a pregnant woman

Xiao Zhou, Meng Zhang, Zhuang Liu, Meili Duan and Lei Dong*

Abstract

Background: Spontaneous hepatic rupture in pregnancy is a rare and life-threatening event during the perinatal period.

Case presentation: We report a case of a 33-year-old woman with 36 + 6 weeks' gestation that present with elevated blood pressure before delivery, who was admitted to our hospital due to irregular abdominal pain. Diagnosed with abdominal paracentesis, the emergent caesarean section and laparotomy were performed. Postoperatively, the patient experienced 22-day intensive therapy in ICU and was transferred to the General Surgery Department in good physical condition without post-operative complications.

Conclusions: This case indicates that making an accurate and timely diagnosis and taking multidisciplinary approach contribute to a successful clinical outcome.

Keywords: Perinatal mortality, Pregnancy complications, Rupture, Spontaneous, Fatty liver

Background

Spontaneous hepatic rupture in pregnancy is a rare condition and carries a high maternal and perinatal mortality [1]. It is usually associated with hepatic hemangiomata, hepatic metastases from choriocarcinoma, or some unknown causes. Its sudden appearance and potentially fatal outcome make it an important diagnostic and therapeutic challenge.

We reported a successfully treated case of spontaneous hepatic rupture in a pregnant woman. It emphasizes the need for the early diagnosis as well as the timely surgical management and the postoperative monitoring of patients in the intensive care unit. The relevant literature is also reviewed.

Case presentation

A 33-year-old primigravida woman, a body mass index of 31 kg/cm2, was admitted to the emergency department at36 + 6 weeks gestation with abdominal pain that had lasted for 6 h. She did not have a history of trauma. Her antenatal period had been uneventful except for one episode of hypertension (141/84 mmHg). Physical examination revealed a blood pressure of 102/62 mm/Hg, a heart rate of 80 beats/min and a temperature of 36.6 °C. Blood tests showed hemoglobin of 95 g/L,Hematocrit of 28.9%, platelet count of 111×10^9/L(reference range, 110-300 × 10^9/L), reticulocyte count of 0.0525×10^{12}/L(reference range, 0.014-0.09 × 10^{12}/L), liver enzymes with an alanine aminotransferase of 281 U/L, aspartate aminotransferase of 392 U/L, lactate dehydrogenase of 525 U/L, total bilirubin levels of 19 μmol/L(reference range, 3.42-17.1umol/L), and normal alpha fetoprotein. Serological markers of hepatitis B and hepatitis C virus were negative. Ultrasound scan showed that fetal heart beats could not be found and free abdominal fluid was present. There were no images suggesting placental abruption. Ultrasound-guided intra-abdominal puncture revealed active intraperitoneal bleeding.

In less than 3 h of admission, an emergency laparotomy was performed and a dead fetus was delivered by cesarean section. No evidence of placental abruption or active intrauterine bleeding was detected. Exploration of the ovarian tubes and ovaries revealed no bleeding or neoplasm. Two liters of hemoperitoneum was removed from abdominal cavity. Active hemorrhage came from rupture of the right lobe of the liver which appeared fatty liver. Direct hemostasis was not achievable because the liver was edematous and was ruptured during the performance of sutures. Thus perihepatic packing was done by seven large gauze packs and hemostatic sponges were used to compress the bleeding

* Correspondence: 18618334341@163.com
Department of Intensive Care Unit, Beijing Friendship Hospital, Capital Medical University, No. 95 Yong-An Road, Xi Cheng District, Beijing 100050, China

lesions. Throughout the laparotomy, intraoperative bleeding was 2000 mL and the patient received 8 units of RBC and 1200 ml of plasma.

The patient was transferred to the ICU after surgery to continue resuscitation with intravenous fluids and vasoactive support. The following day in ICU, she had high fever and developed the acute kidney injury and severe acute respiratory distress syndrome. She was managed by massive blood transfusion, mechanical ventilation, renal replacement therapy and antibiotic treatment. Intra-abdominal pressure was maintained between 7.5 and 11.3 mmHg (1–1.5 KPa) by abdominal binder.

A second laparotomy was performed on the 6th postoperative day. A large hematoma and rupture of the right liver lobe were visible after removing the gauze packs (Fig. 1a), which was still bleeding (Fig. 1b). The patient was treated with argon laser to stop bleeding (Fig. 1c). Moreover, one drain was left in the abdomen. Postoperatively, ultrasound showed perihepatic and pelvic free fluid that required percutaneous drainage. Abdominal computed tomography (CT) scan (Fig. 2) revealed perihepatic effusion with laceration of the right liver lobe and hypo-density of fluid in the peritoneal cavity. Decreasing in volume of the perihepatic effusion was observed by subsequent CT scan (Fig. 2). After 22 days of recovery in ICU, the patient was transferred to the surgical department where she remained for further 3 weeks with regular post-operative course. She was discharged in normal physical condition after 45 days.

Discussion and conclusions

Spontaneous hepatic rupture in pregnancy, which was first described by Abercrombie in 1984, is a rare condition associated with high maternal and perinatal mortality [1], with its incidence ranging from 1 in 45,000 tol in 225,000 deliveries [2]. A recent literature review of hepatic rupture revealed a maternal mortality rate of 39% [3] and a perinatal mortality rate of 42% [4]. Spontaneous hepatic rupture is commonly caused by hepatic hemangiomata, hepatocellular carcinoma, hepatic adenoma, of which were reported to be pregnancy-related but rare [5]. Other causes arehepatic metastases from choriocarcinoma, focal nodular hyperplasia, peliosishepatis, trauma, infection (malaria, syphilis, amoebic abscess), aneurysms; granulomas, the use of cocaine during pregnancy, anabolic steroid therapy, systemic amyloidosis [6] and unknowns [7, 8]. Hepatic rupture in pregnancy usually is associated with pre-eclampsia, eclampsia, or Hemolysis Elevated Liver enzymes and Low Platelet count (HELLP) syndrome [9]. Spontaneous hepatic rupture in uncomplicated pregnancy also has been reported but is extremely rare [10]. The presenting symptoms and signs of liver bleeding are subtle and non-specific, the most common are abdominal pain, shoulder pain and vomiting. Thus, a high index of clinical suspicion is necessary and emergency ultrasonography, CT, or magnetic resonance imaging should be considered to reach the diagnosis of spontaneous hepatic rupture in a timely manner. As a pregnant woman presents with a sudden onset of unexplained, severe abdominal pain, spontaneous rupture of the liver should be suspected.

Hepatic rupture requires immediate laparotomy to stop bleeding, therapeutic options involves perihepatic packing, placement of sponges or absorbable mesh, fibrin glue, argon laser coagulation and hepatic artery ligation. Partial liver resection or even liver transplantation has been described in the literatures. The outcome of patients with spontaneous hepatic rupturegreatly depends on the etiology and severity of the hemorrhage [11, 12].

In this case, the patient had no history of trauma, excessive alcohol consumption, or use of hepatotoxic

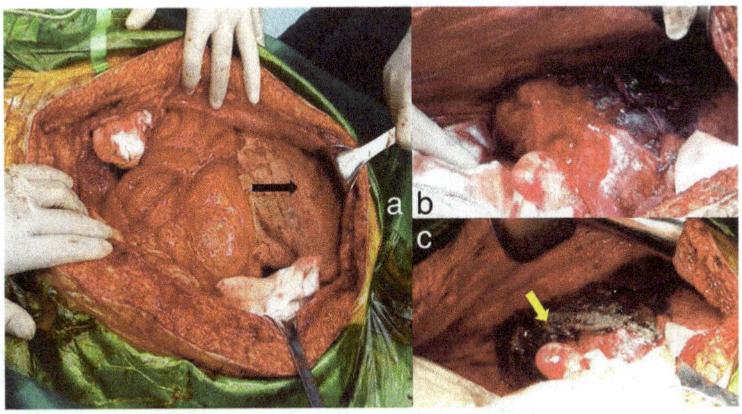

Fig. 1 The 2nd operation findings. **a** liver packing (black arrow shows gauzes). **b** liver hemotoma. **c** Argon laser to stop bleeding (yellow arrow shows laser-coagulation)

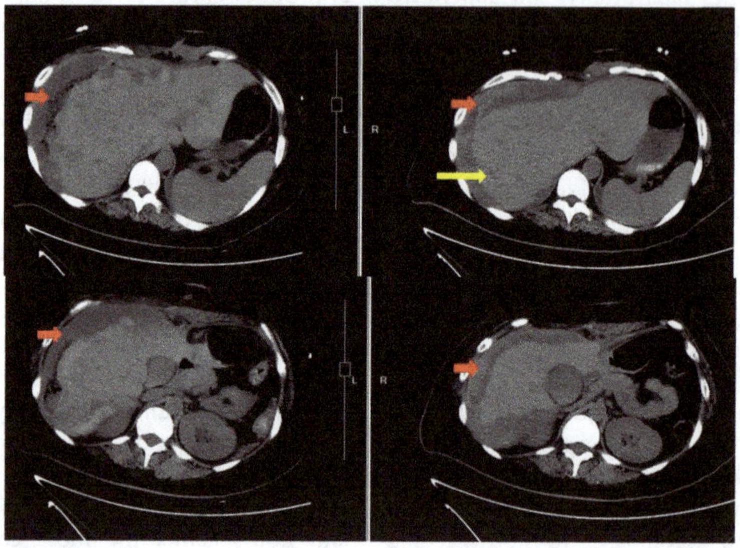

Fig. 2 Abdominal CT scans on the 3rd day (left) and 13th day (right) post the second surgery. Red arrows (hypodense collection) show perihepatic effusion. Yellow arrow shows the ruptures of the liver

medications, moreover, she did not have pre-eclampsia or eclampsia during this pregnancy, tumor biomarkers as well as clinical tests of hepatitis B and C virus infection were negative. Liver lesions were not visible at operation or with imaging. There was insufficient evidence for the diagnosis of HELLP syndrome: the platelet count was marginally low even with massive hemorrhage, tests of hemolysis were negative (serum indirect bilirubin, reticulocyte count, Coombs test, and Ham's test), and liver enzymes before acute hemorrhage were mildly elevated. Nevertheless, HELLP syndrome cannot be totally excluded due to the presence of hypertension. HELLP syndrome is considered as a risk factor for hepatic rupture in pregnancy. Vigil-De et al. reported that it was present in 92.8% of cases in their series during the past two decades [12]. With this case of a high BMI, fatty liver was suspected during laparotomy but no evidence from the biopsy yet. A few cases of fatty liver disease associated with hepatic rupture have been reported, the incidence was about 1 in 13,000 pregnancies [13].

A large hematoma was on the right lobe of the liver in this patient. Perihepatic packing was carried out to control the bleeding in this case, however, she remained at risk for complications, such as intraperitoneal infection. For patient with continued bleeding after the first surgical operation, ICU assistance played a valuable role on the recovery during the post-operative course. The right hepatic lobectomy was another choice for the surgeon when hemorrhage remained uncontrolled, which probably led to postoperative liver dysfunction. Hence, an effort should be made to gain hemostatic control while avoiding large resections as much as possible.

In conclusion, spontaneous hepatic rupture in pregnancy is rare but life-threatening. A high level of alertness for the diagnosis aided by timely ultrasonography and CT scan is critical to prompt intervention, which requires multidisciplinary approach to achieve a successful outcome.

Abbreviations

CT: Computer tomography; HELLP: Syndromehemolysis elevated liver enzymes and low platelet syndrome; ICU: Intensive care unit

Acknowledgements

The authors give special thanks to Professor Jingfeng Liu who guided this work.

Funding

Not applicable.

Authors' contributions

LD and MLD made the treatment strategies to the patient. XZ, MZ and ZhL underwent treatments and read the literature. XZ was a major contributor in writing the manuscript. All authors read and approved the final manuscript.

Competing interests

The authors declare that they have no competing interests.

References

1. Poo JL, Gongora J. Hepatic hematoma and hepatic rupture in pregnancy. Ann Hepatol. 2006;5(3):224–6.
2. Wicke C, Pereira PL, Neeser E, et al. Subcapsular liver hematoma in HELLP syndrome: evaluation of diagnostic and therapeutic options—a unicenter study. Am J Obstet Gynecol. 2004;190(1):106–12.

3. Reck T, Bussenius-Kammerer M, Ott R, et al. Surgical treatment of HELLP syndrome-associated liver rupture-an update. Eur J Obster Gynecol Reprod Biol. 2001;99(1):57–65.
4. Marsh FA, Kaufmann SJ, Bhabra K. Surviving hepatic rupture in pregnancy-a literature review with an illustrative case report. J Obstet Gynecol. 2003; 23(2):109–13.
5. Srinivasa S, Lee WG, Aldameh A, et al. Spontaneous hepatic haemorrhage: a review of pathogenesis, aetiology and treatment. Int Hepato-Pancreato-Biliary Assoc. 2015;17:872–80.
6. Suda T, Oguri HA. Case of primary amyloidosis with spontaneous hepatic rupture. Nihon Shokakibyo Gakkai Zasshi. 2017;114(6):1039–45.
7. Sommacale D, Palladino E, Tambya EL, et al. Spontaneous hepatic rupture in a patient with peliosishepatis: a report of one case. Int J Surg Case Rep. 2013;4(5):508–10.
8. Sommacale D, Palladino E, Esther L, et al. Spontaneous hepatic rupture in a patient with peliosishepatis: a report of one case. Int J Surg Case Rep. 2013;4(5):508–10.
9. Kjell Haram, Einar Svendsen, Ulrich Abildgaard. A Review. Am J Forensic Med Pathol. BMC Pregnancy Childbirth 2009; 9: 8.
10. Abdi S, Cameron IC, Nakielny RA, et al. Spontaneous hepatic rupture and maternal death following an uncomplicated pregnancy and delivery. BJOG. 2001;108(4):431–3.
11. Miguelote RF, Costa V, Vivas J, et al. Postpartum spontaneous rupture of a liver hematoma associated with preeclampsia and HELLP syndrome. Arch Gynecol Obstet. 2009;279(6):923–6.
12. Vigil-De Gracia P, Ortega-Paz L. Pre-eclampsia/eclampsia and hepatic rupture. Int J Gynaecol Obstet. 2012;118(3):186–9.
13. Pereira SP, O'Donohue J, Wendon J, et al. Maternal and perinatal outcome in severe pregnancy-related liver disease. Hepatology. 1997;26:1258–62.

22

Task shifting in active management of the third stage of labor

Tessa M. Raams[1*], Joyce L. Browne[1], Verena J. M. M. Festen-Schrier[1], Kerstin Klipstein-Grobusch[1,2] and Marcus J. Rijken[1,3]

Abstract

Background: Active management of the third stage of labor (AMTSL) describes interventions with the common goal to prevent postpartum hemorrhage (PPH). In low- and middle-income countries, implementation of AMTSL is hampered by shortage of skilled birth attendants and a high percentage of home deliveries. Task shifting of specific AMTSL components to unskilled birth attendants or self-administration could be a strategy to increase access to potentially life-saving interventions. This study was designed to evaluate the effect, acceptance and safety of task shifting of specific aspects of AMTSL to unskilled birth attendants.

Methods: A systematic search was conducted in five databases in September 2015 to identify intervention studies of AMTSL implemented by unskilled birth attendants or pregnant women themselves. Quality of studies was evaluated with an adapted Cochrane Collaboration assessment tool.

Results: Of 2469 studies screened, 21 were included. All studies assessed implementation of uterotonics (misoprostol tablets or oxytocin injections), administered by community health workers (CHWs), auxiliary midwives, traditional birth attendants (TBAs) or self-administration at antenatal (home) visits or delivery. Task shifting for none of the other AMTSL components was reported. Task shifting of provision of uterotonics reduced the risk of PPH (RR 0.16 to 1) compared to standard care (13 studies, $n = 15.197$). The correct dose and timing was reported for 83.4 to 99.8% (5 studies, $n = 6083$) and 63 to 100% (9 studies, $n = 8378$) women respectively. Uterotonics were recommended to others by 80 to 99.7% (7 studies, $n = 6445$); 80 to 99.4% (5 studies, $n = 2677$) would use the drug at next delivery. Willingness to pay for uterotonics varied from 54.6 to 100% (7 studies, $n = 6090$).

Conclusion: Task shifting of AMTSL has thus far been evaluated for administration of uterotonics (misoprostol tablets and oxytocin injected by CHWs and auxiliary midwives) and resulted in reduction of PPH, high rates of appropriate use and satisfaction among users.

In order to increase AMTSL coverage in low-staffed health facilities, task shifting of uterine massage or postpartum tonus assessment to unskilled attendants or delivered women could be considered. Task shifting of controlled cord traction is currently not recommended.

Keywords: Active management of the third stage of labor, Community health workers, Low- and middle-income countries, Postpartum hemorrhage, Self-administration, Task shifting, Traditional birth attendants

* Correspondence: tessa.raams@gmail.com
[1]Julius Global Health, Julius Center for Health Sciences and Primary Care, University Medical Center Utrecht, Heidelberglaan 100, 3584 Utrecht, The Netherlands
Full list of author information is available at the end of the article

Background

Postpartum hemorrhage (PPH) is the leading cause of maternal mortality worldwide and accounts for 34% of maternal deaths in low- and middle-income countries (LMIC) [1]. PPH is defined as blood loss of 500 ml or more within 24 h after delivery and most frequently occurs during the third or fourth stages of labor, the period from delivery of the infant until placental delivery and 2 h postpartum [2]. Active management of the third stage of labor (AMTSL) describes a set of interventions aimed at the prevention of PPH [3, 4]. AMTSL includes the administration of uterotonics (for example oxytocin or misoprostol) preferably within 1 min after delivery to all women, controlled cord traction (CCT) to stimulate placental delivery, uterine massage to activate uterine contraction and assessment of uterine tonus every 15 min during 2 h postpartum to early identify uterine atony [1, 4–6]. The World Health Organization (WHO) recommends AMTSL to be performed by skilled birth attendants and health workers trained in the management of pregnancy and delivery [4]. WHO recommendations regarding implementation are component-dependent: uterotonics are recommended for all delivered women. CCT is considered optional in settings with skilled birth attendants, continuous uterine massage is not recommended if prophylactic oxytocin is provided and uterine tonus surveillance is recommended for all delivered women [4, 7–9].

Almost 60% of births in low- and middle-income countries occur in rural areas outside health facilities and are assisted by traditional birth attendants or family members not (formally) trained in obstetric care. Despite attempts to increase skilled attendance at (home) deliveries, this remains challenging due to a shortage of skilled birth attendants and significant travel distances in rural areas [10, 11]. As a consequence, the implementation of AMTSL is limited despite its paramount importance, especially in areas with low access to emergency obstetric care [5, 11–13].

In 2012, the WHO published recommendations on task shifting in maternal and newborn health care in an attempt to optimize the potential of the existing health workforce [14]. These recommendations include for example the administration of misoprostol by lay health workers to prevent postpartum hemorrhage, but don't address all components of AMTSL. The effects of task shifting of individual components of AMTSL have never been reviewed [14].

Of the AMTSL interventions, uterotonics are the most effective in terms of prevention of PPH, although the relative contribution of each of AMTSL components has not been well-studied [4, 15]. Oxytocin is the preferred uterotonic drug and recommended by the WHO if skilled birth attendants are available. However, as oxytocin is thermo-unstable it requires cold-chain handling which increases costs. Additionally it should be injected intramuscularly or intravenously by skilled birth attendants. Misoprostol is considered a safe, cheap and only slightly less effective alternative [16–19]. The WHO recommends the provision of misoprostol by community health workers for PPH prevention in rural areas and homebirths in absence of skilled attendance [4]. Community distribution of misoprostol to pregnant women for self-administration is also widely explored as an option, but currently not recommended [20–22].

The aim of this systematic review is to evaluate the evidence on the effect, women's acceptance and safety of task shifting of different components of AMTSL to unskilled birth attendants or self-administration.

Methods

Protocol

This review was designed in accordance with the PRISMA guidelines [23].

Eligibility criteria

Type of study

Randomized controlled trials (RCTs) or quasi-experimental trials evaluating the effect of implementation of components of AMTSL to unskilled birth attendants or delivering women on the incidence of PPH compared to the current situation, which is mostly no implementation of components of AMTSL at all. No restrictions on language and publication date were applied. Case reports, reviews and proceedings were excluded.

Type of participants

Women delivering in a community setting or health facility center in LMIC without skilled birth attendants present. Skilled birth attendants are defined as accredited health professionals (midwife, nurse) who are trained to assist pregnancies and postpartum care. Unskilled birth attendants are nonprofessionals, educated in a specific task of pregnancy care and postpartum care [24].

Type of intervention

Trials evaluating the effect on outcome measures of implementation of administration of uterotonics (oxytocin or misoprostol), controlled cord traction, uterine massage, assessment of uterine tonus during 2 hpostpartum to unskilled birth attendants in areas without standardized postpartum care according to AMTSL. By evaluating the effect and safety of AMTSL performed by unskilled birth attendants, effect and safety of task shifting is indirectly measured. Task shifting is defined as a process in which tasks are moved from skilled to less skilled health workers [14].

Type of outcome measures

The primary outcome measure was the incidence of postpartum hemorrhage, defined as blood loss of 500 ml or more in the first 24 h postpartum. Secondary outcomes were women's acceptance and safety. The first defined as recommending the care to friends or family, willingness to receive the same care at their next delivery and willingness to pay for uterotonics at the next delivery. The latter defined as receiving the care at the correct time during third stage of labor and using correct methods as described in the WHO guidelines [4]. Safety also included adverse effects of interventions.

Information sources

The search was performed in the following electronic databases: The Cochrane Library (Cochrane Database of Systematic Reviews), EMBASE, Global Health Library, POPLINE and PubMed for all publications up to September 2015. Full texts were available for all included studies. In addition, included studies were screened for additional relevant studies through their reference lists and cross-referenced in Web of Science.

Search

Synonyms for 'Active Management of the Third Stage of Labor' and its components, i.e. 'uterotonics', 'cord traction', 'uterine massage' and 'uterine tonus' combined with synonyms for 'task shifting' and correlating Mesh terms were used as search strategy. The full search strategy including a list of synonyms is available in the Additional file 1.

Study selection

After removal of duplicates, the title and abstract of retrieved studies were screened by two independent reviewers (TR, VS) using predefined inclusion and exclusion criteria. Any discrepancies between the two reviewers in this process were discussed and full text accessed if necessary for further clarification. If results were published multiple times, data were used only once from the most complete article.

Data collection process and data items

Data were extracted from each individual article using a standardized extraction form and included: study design, study setting and location, number of delivered women and population characteristics including age, parity and educational level, intervention as part of AMTSL, by whom this was performed and educational level or training received, incidence of PPH and relative risks with corresponding 95% confidence interval, women's acceptance including willingness to pay for uterotonics, recommendations to friends and family and wish to receive same care or drugs at next delivery, safety including correct dose, correct time and duration of intervention and reported side effects. The extraction was performed by one reviewer (TR) and a second reviewer was available for discussion or clarification processes. Corresponding authors were contacted in case further information was required.

Quality assessment

Quality of studies was assessed at study level using an adapted version of the Cochrane Collaboration's tool for assessing risk of bias for systematic reviews of interventions [25]. Studies were scored for detection bias, evaluating blinding of participants for outcome measurements; attrition bias, evaluating completeness and origin of data; reporting bias, evaluating origin of data, definition and assessment of outcome measurements; and possible confounders. Risk of bias was assigned as low, high or unclear risk, according to the quality assessment tool, attached as a Additional file 2. Any disagreements were discussed until consensus was achieved.

Summary measures

Incidence of PPH was reported in relative risks (RR) and 95% confidence interval (CI). If these were not reported, they were calculated using SPSS v20.0 software [26]. Women's acceptance and safety were reported in percentages.

Synthesis of results

Results were narratively described because the heterogeneity of the interventions and settings did not allow for a meaningful meta-analysis.

Results

Study selection

The systematic search identified 2469 studies after removal of duplicates, of which 60 studies remained after title and abstract screening [Fig. 1]. Of these studies, 21 met the inclusion criteria. No additional studies were obtained through snowballing. All studies aimed to evaluate effect and safety of implementation of AMTSL to unskilled attendants compared to standard of care (mostly no standardized care). No studies were found reporting on task shifting of components of AMTSL from skilled to unskilled birth attendants.

Study characteristics

Study characteristics are presented in Tables 1 and 2. Five studies were RCTs [11, 17, 27–29] and sixteen were quasi-experimental trials [5, 10, 12, 13, 22, 30–40]. Studies were published between 2005 and 2014 and reported on 236 to 77.337 included pregnant women in community centers or at home births in LMIC in Africa (48%, $n = 10$) Asia (43%, $n = 9$) and Central America (2%,

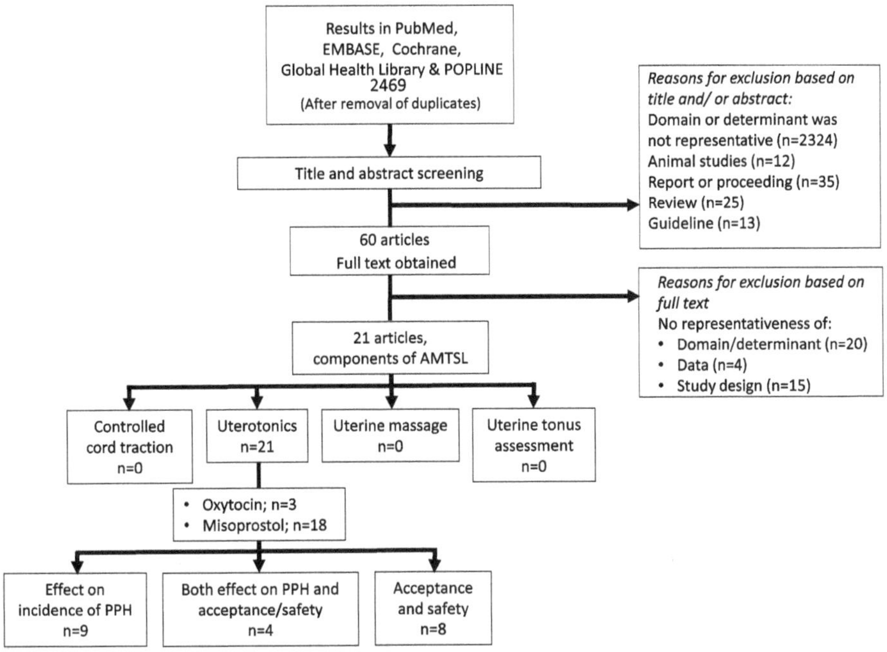

Fig. 1 Flowchart of literature search and selection process. PPH: postpartum haemorrhage

n = 2). Tasks were shifted to community health workers (19%, *n* = 4), auxiliary midwives (19%, n = 4), traditional birth attendants (38%, *n* = 8) or self-administered by delivered women (48%, n = 10).

All studies assessed the administration of uterotonics; misoprostol tablets or oxytocin injections. Misoprostol tablets for self-administration were distributed at antenatal (home) visits (*n* = 5), at delivery (*n* = 12) or both (*n* = 4). Controlled cord traction, uterine massage and uterine tone assessment and their effect on reduction of PPH were not reported in any of the studies. Therefore the main focus of the remainder of this article will be on task shifting of uterotonic admission.

Risk of bias within studies

The overall risk assessment is summarized in Fig. 2, the individual study risk of bias assessment is available as a Additional file 2.

Detection bias

In 14% (*n* = 3) of 21 studies both delivered women as participants were blinded for intervention and outcome. In one study the outcome was measured by workers who were not involved in the distribution process. In the remaining studies participants performing the intervention were also involved in the measurement of outcomes. In none of the articles a bias effect is mentioned and because of possible influence on outcomes, risk of bias was scored as unclear.

Attrition bias

Data on baseline characteristics were obtained at antenatal care visits in facility centers or during home visits. Data on intervention and outcome measures were obtained at delivery by auxiliary midwives, community health workers or traditional birth attendants by interviewing women postpartum. All health workers received training on how to collect data and therefore low risk of bias for origin of data was scored. In 81% (*n* = 17) of studies were less than 10% missing data of outcome measures or loss to follow up and therefore low risk of bias on completeness of data was scored. One article had more than 10% missing data [22].

Reporting bias

In 86% (*n* = 18) of articles the definition of PPH was clear. In the other articles PPH was defined as 'need for referral' or 'heavy bleeding'. Blood loss was objectively measured in 62% (*n* = 8) of studies with a calibrated scale. In 38% (*n* = 5) of studies blood loss was visually estimated by health workers or blood loss was subjectively estimated by delivered women and was therefore scored as a high risk of bias. PPH was not measured in eight articles and scored as 'not applicable'.

Possible confounders

Confounders were scored as low risk of bias in randomized controlled trials without differences in baseline characteristics. In 71% (*n* = 15) of studies possible confounders were not reported and therefore risk of bias was scored 'unclear'.

Table 1 Administration of uterotonics. Self-administered, by TBAs, auxiliary midwives or community health workers: RR (95% CI) for PPH ($n = 13$)

Study (first author, year of publication)	Design	Location	Deliveries (N per group)	Population (age, parity, education)[a]	PPH (%)	RR (95% CI)
Misoprostol[b], self- administered						
Geller et al., 2013 [22]	Quasi exp. trial	30 communities in Ghana	102 (82) misoprostol, 107 (92) control	Age: 26.6 ± 6.7 Parity(2–4): 46% Education: n/a	Misoprostol 1.2% (1/82), Control 3.3% (3/92)	0.38 (0.04–3.57)
Mir et al., 2012 [31]	Quasi exp. trial	Districts of Dadu and Khanewal, India	678 (678) misoprostol, 720 (720) control	Age: 28 ± 5.7 Parity: n/a No education: 73%	Misoprostol (3/678) 0.4%, Control ($n = 5/720$) 0.6%	0.42 (0.08–2.18)
Misoprostol, TBAs						
Mobeen et al., 2010 [17]	RCT	46 villages in Chitral, Pakistan	533 (514) misoprostol, 583 (558) control	Age: 28 ± 5 Parity (3–5): 42.4% No education: 72.7%	Misoprostol 16.5% (85/514), Control 21.9% (122/558)	0.76 (0.59–0.97)
Prata et al., 2009 [32]	Quasi exp. trial	Rural villages of Tigray, Ethiopia	485 (485) misoprostol, 481 (481) control	Age: 27.7 ± 6.7 Parity: 3.4 ± 2.0 No education: 80.2%	Misoprostol 8.9% (43/485), Control 18.9% (91/481)	0.47 (0.33–0.66)
Walraven et al., 2005 [11]	RCT	26 villages of the North Bank East Health Division, The Gambia	629 (629) misoprostol + 4 placebo tablets, 599 (599) ergometrine[c] + 3× placebo	Age: 25.9 ± 5.3 Parity(≥6): 18.6% No education: 95.2%	Misoprostol 11.0% (69/629), Ergometrine 12.0% (72/599)	0.91 (0.67–1.25)
Misoprostol, TBAs or self-administered						
Ejembi et al., 2014 [30]	Quasi exp. trial	5 communities in North-West Nigeria	1239 (1239) misoprostol, 231 (231) control	Age, parity, education: n/a	Misoprostol 8.1% (100/1239), Nothing 9.5% (22/231)	0.84 (0.54–1.30)
Prata et al., 2012a [33]	Quasi exp. trial	5 communities in North-West Nigeria	1421 (1421) misoprostol, 303 (303) control	Age, parity, education: n/a	Misoprostol 1.2% (17/1421) Nothing 7.6% (23/303)	0.16 (0.09–0.31)
Misoprostol, auxiliary midwives						
Chandhiok et al., 2005 [27]	Cluster-RCT	30 PHCs from 5 states in India	600 (600) misoprostol, 600 (600) standard (methergine[d]/ nothing)	Age:24.3 ± 3.6, Gravida (2–3): 56.3%, Literate: 62%	Misoprostol 0.7% (4/600), Control 0.8% (5/600)	0.80 (0.22–2.96)
Derman et al., 2006 [28]	RCT	4 PHCs of Belgaum district, India	812 (809) misoprostol, 808 (807) placebo	Age:23.3 ± 3.3 Parity (1–2): 58.1% Literacy: 62.9%	Misoprostol 6.4% (52/809), Control 12.0% (97/807)	0.53 (0.39–0.74)
Oxytocin[e], auxiliary midwives						
Low et al., 2008 [34]	Quasi exp. trial	Public birth center in Morazan, Honduras	146 (146) oxytocin, 83 (83) control	Age:23.5 Parity (1–4): 49.2% Education: n/a	Oxytocin 12.3% (18/146), No oxytocin 19.3% (16/83)	0.64 (0.35–1.19)
Low et al., 2012 [35]	Quasi exp. trial	Public birth center in Morazan, Honduras	339 (339) intervention, 229 (229) pre-intervention	Age: 23.1 ± 6.5, Parity: 1.5 ± 2.1 Education: n/a	Intervention 5.9% (20/339), Pre-intervention 14.8% (34/229)	0.40 (0.23–0.67)
Misoprostol 2x200mcg, community health worker						
Nasreen et al., 2011 [36]	Quasi exp. trial	2 districts, northern Bangladesh	884 (884) misoprostol, 1008 (1008) control	Age:23.0 ± 4.8 Gravida: 2.6 ± 1.4 vs 2.1 ± 1.2	Misoprostol 1.6% (14/884), Control 6.4% (65/1008)	0.25 (0.14–0.43)

Table 1 Administration of uterotonics. Self-administered, by TBAs, auxiliary midwives or community health workers: RR (95% CI) for PPH ($n = 13$) *(Continued)*

Study (first author, year of publication)	Design	Location	Deliveries (N per group)	Population (age, parity, education)[a]	PPH (%)	RR (95% CI)
				No education: 36.1% vs 21.2%		
Oxytocin uniject device, community health worker						
Stanton et al., 2013 [29]	Cluster RCT	4 rural districts in Brong-Ahafo region, Ghana	689 (682) oxytocin 888 (888) control	Age: 27.5 ± 6.6. Parity(2–4): 43.3% No education: 48%	PPH-1:[f] 2.6% (18/682) vs 5.5% (49/887) PPH-2: 3.8% (26/682) vs 10.8% (96/887) PPH-3: 4.1% (28/682) vs 11.1% (99/888) Severe PPH 0.1% (1/682) vs 0.9% (8/887)	PPH-1: 0.49 (0.27–0.88) PPH-2: 0.34 (0.18–0.63) PPH-3: 0.36 (0.20–0.66) Severe PPH: 1 (0.013–1.7)

CCT controlled cord traction, *CHW/O* community health worker/officer, *CI* confidence interval, *IU* international unit; mcg: microgram, *Ml* milliliters, *n/a* not available, *PHC* public health center, *PPH* postpartum hemorrhage, *RR* relative risk, *RCT* randomized controlled trial, *Quasi exp.* quasi experimental, *TBA* traditional birth attendant

[a]Population characteristics of intervention group if no statistical differences, reported in mean and standard deviation or percentage

[b]Tablets of misoprostol of 3x200micrograms if not otherwise described

[c]Ergometrine given as four tablets of 0.5 mg, as standard treatment at location of research

[d]Methergine given as intramuscular injections in a dose of 0.2 mg or 0.125 mg

[e]Oxytocin 10 international units, intramuscular injection

[f]PPH-1: blood loss ≥500 ml, PPH-2: PPH-1 plus any woman receiving early treatment for PPH, PPH-3: any woman without a quantitative blood loss measure who is referred to higher care for PPH

Table 2 Safety and acceptance of task shifting intervention in included studies ($n = 12$)

Study (first author, year of publication)	Study Design	Location	Population (age, parity, education)[a]	Training of intervention	Intervention – what/who[b]	Distribution complete - % of deliveries	Intervention – correct dose and/or timing (%)	Intervention – acceptance (%)
Diadhiou et al., 2011 [37]	Quasi-exp. trial	health center/post and maternity huts in 2 districts, Senegal	Age: 26.4 ± 5.5 Parity: 2.9 ± 2.2 No education: 43%	6 days course including 5 days on EoC and 1 day on misoprostol administration[c]	Misoprostol *auxiliary midwives*	16.1% (41/255) in Thies, 4.2% (9/214) in Kaolack, both percentages refer to distribution in maternity huts	Correct dose and timing: 100% (245/245) in HC/HP and MH	Recommended to friends: n/a Use at next delivery: n/a Willing to pay: 85.6% (160/187) in HC, 100% (8/8) in HP, 100% (50/50) in MH
Ejembi et al., 2014 [30]	Quasi-exp. trial	5 communities North-West Nigeria	Age, parity, education: n/a	TBAs: 6 days course on home-based EoC and misoprostol administration. Women: educated on misoprostol use at home visits of TBAs.	Misoprostol, distribution by drug keeper to *TBA, self-administration, friend/relative, doctor/midwife*	80.2% (1265/1577), total group - *TBA*:88.1% (919/1043) - *Self-administered:* 66.3% (106/160) - *Friend:* 67.1% (147/219) - *Midwife*:46.1% (47/102) - Attendant unknown for 53 deliveries	- *Total group:* dose 93.2% (1179/1265), time 87.3% (1104/1265) - *TBA:* dose 96.2% (884/919), time 88.9% (817/919) - *Self-administered:* dose 96.2% (102/106), time 77.4% (82/106) - *Friend:* dose 95.9% (141/147), time 85% (125/147) - *Midwife:* dose 93.6% (44/47), time 78.7% (37/47)	Recommended to friends: 99.7% (1260/1264) Use at next delivery: 99.4% (1256/1264) Willing to pay: 99.1% (1253/1264) Post-delivery data for this topic is missing for $n = 1$ delivery
Geller et al., 2014 [22]	Quasi-exp. trial	30 communities in rural Ghana	Age: 24.4 ± 6.56 Parity: 2.5 ± 2.05 Education: n/a	Training of midwives and CHWs on misoprostol administration. Use of pictorial charts for women.	Misoprostol, *self-administered*	65% (654/999) of misoprostol tablets distributed by midwives at antenatal care visits. $N = 105$ (96 at home, 9 institutional) women take misoprostol	Correct dose: n/a Correct timing: 98.9% (92/93) No data collected for institutional deliveries	Recommended to friends: 98.6% (71/72) Use at next delivery: 98.6% (71/72) Willing to pay: n/a Post-delivery data for this topic is missing for $n = 21$ deliveries
Mir et al.,2012 [31]	Quasi-exp trial	Dadu and Khanewal districts, India	Age 28 ± 5.7 Parity: n/a No education: 73%	Creating of community awareness & family education regarding use of misoprostol. 1 month before delivery women were assessed retention of knowledge. 15 days before delivery again briefed on information	Misoprostol, *self-administered*	88% (678/770) of women that delivered at home took misoprostol	Correct dose and timing: 95% (647/678)	Recommended to friends: 80% (616/770) Use at next delivery: 80% (616/770) Willing to pay: 74% (570/770)
Prata et al., 2012a [33]	Quasi-exp trial	5 rural communities North-West Nigeria.	Age, parity, education: n/a	TBAs were trained to counsel pregnant women about bleeding after delivery, the importance of delivery at a health facility, and the role of misoprostol and its administration.	Misoprostol, *TBA or self-administration*	79% (1421/1800) of women that were interviewed postpartum took misoprostol	Correct dose: 98% (1393/1421) Correct time: 88% (1250/1421)	Recommendations, use at next delivery, willing to pay: n/a
Prata et al., 2012b [38]	Quasi-exp trial	6 rural districts in Bangladesh	Age, parity, education: n/a	Training concerning various aspects of misoprostol and	Misoprostol, *RDRS trained and non-RDRS*	RDRS-trained TBA: 81.3% (1041/1280)	Correct dose: n/a	Recommended to friends: 98.6% (1903/1930)

Table 2 Safety and acceptance of task shifting intervention in included studies ($n = 12$) *(Continued)*

Study (first author, year of publication)	Study Design	Location	Population (age, parity, education)[a]	Training of intervention	Intervention – what/*who*[b]	Distribution complete - % of deliveries	Intervention – correct dose and/or timing (%)	Intervention – acceptance (%)
				the usage of a delivery mat to measure blood loss.	*TBAs, self-administration, relative, nurse/ doctor*	Non-RDRS TBA: 69.9% (533/762) Relative 64.8% (250/386) Alone 67.7% (44/65) Doctor 7.6% (18/236) Nurse 67.7% (44/65)	*-TBA (trained/untrained):* time 99.9% (1572/1574) - *other groups:* time 99.7% (355/356)	Use at next delivery: n/a Willing to pay: 84.6% (1633/1930) All women that were offered misoprostol, independent of birth attendant
Prata et al., 2014 [12]	Quasi-exp. trial	6 rural districts of Rangpur Division, Bangladesh	Age (15–29): 89.3% No education: 63% Gravidity (2+): 67.6%	RDRS trained TBAs received 2 days training on administration of misoprostol.	Misoprostol, *RDRS trained TBA, non-RDRS TBA, lay person*	67.4% (64.413/66489) RDRS trained TBA: 71% non-RDRS TBA 48% lay person 54%	Correct dose: n/a Correct time: n/a	Recommendations, use at next delivery, willing to pay: n/a
Rajbhandariet al., 2010 [39]	Quasi-exp. trial	30 clusters in 1 district in India, rural area.	Age: 25 yrs. Mean parity: 3; literate respondents: average 33%	Prenatal health education by female community health volunteers at home visits in 3–4 sessions. Other family members were involved. Advice on seeking prenatal care, planning institutional delivery, misoprostol, timely response to danger symptoms.	Misoprostol, *self-administered*	In study period (2006–2008) 74.5% (13969/18761) women took misoprostol. At end line of study 74% (604/816) of vaginal deliveries received misoprostol. 74% (447/604) of these women took misoprostol.	Correct dose: 98.2%(439/447) Correct time: 100% (447/447)	Recommendations, use at next delivery, willing to pay: n/a
Sanghvi et al., 2010 [10]	Quasi-exp. trial	8 districts in Afghanistan	Age: n/a Gravida > 1: 84.4% Education: n/a	Instructed by CHWs and SBAs during three home visits. Only received misoprostol when women were able to demonstrate understanding of the usage and risks.	Misoprostol, *self-administered*	99% (2021/2039) of pregnant women were offered misoprostol, 97.5% (1970/2021) accepted the drug. 70% (1421/2039) of all pregnant women, took the drug.	Correct dose: 99.8% (1418/1421) Correct time: 95.8% (1361/1421)	Recommended to friends: 92% (1876/ 2039) Use at next delivery: n/a Willing to pay: 88% (1794/2039)
Sibley et al., 2014 [5]	Quasi-exp. trial	3 districts in Amhara and Oromiya regions of Ethiopia	Age 20-34 yrs.: 76.5% No education: 71.9% Parity 2–4: 51%	Facility based Community Maternal and Neonatal Health Extension Program - training, no further specification.	Misoprostol, *health extension workers, CHWs, TBAs and self-administered*	58.9% (600/1019) of women received misoprostol. 97.5% (585/600) used it.	Correct dose and timing: 70.7% (412/585) Correct dose: 83.4% (483/585) Correct time: 84.1% (491/585)	Recommendations, use at next delivery, willing to pay: n/a
Smith et al., 2014a [13]	Quasi-exp. trial	2 districts in Grand Bassa county, Liberia	Age, parity, education: n/a	Explanation of misoprostol use to women at antenatal care visits or at home visits by district reproductive health supervisor.	Misoprostol, *self-administered*	53.7% (980/1826) of all women received misoprostol. Of a sample of 550 women who received misoprostol 302 delivered at home, 87.7% (265/302) of them took the drug.	Correct dose: n/a Correct time: 63% (167/265)	Recommended to friends: 99.6% (258/259) Use at next delivery: 98.1% (254/259) Willing to pay: 54.6% (142/260) For some questionnaires data were missing.

Table 2 Safety and acceptance of task shifting intervention in included studies ($n = 12$) *(Continued)*

Study (first author, year of publication)	Study Design	Location	Population (age, parity, education)[a]	Training of intervention	Intervention – what/*who*[b]	Distribution complete - % of deliveries	Intervention – correct dose and/or timing (%)	Intervention – acceptance (%)
								Data shown are independent of distributor of misoprostol
Smith et al., 2014b [40]	Quasi-exp. trial	Mundri East County and South Sudan, Sudan	Age, parity, education: n/a	Education of misoprostol use to women at pre-natal care visits or home visits by SBAs and maternal health workers	Misoprostol, *self-administered*	84.9% (787/927) of women received misoprostol during pregnancy. 98.9% (527/533) of women delivering at home received misoprostol. Postpartum data were gathered for 76.1% (599/787) of women of whom 81% (485/599) had home delivery with misoprostol.	Correct dose: n/a Correct time: 98.6% (478/485)	Recommended to friends: 95.1% (461/485) Use at next delivery: 99.0% (480/485) Willing to pay: 99.0% (480/485)

Articles sorted on alphabetical order. *n/a* not available, *CHW* community health worker, *EoC* emergency obstetric care, *HC* health centre, *HP* health post, *MH* maternity hut, *TBA* traditional birth attendant, *RDRS* Rangpur Dinajpur Rural Services, *SBA* skilled birth attendant

[a]Population characteristics of only intervention group if no statistical differences

[b]tablets of 3x200micrograms if not otherwise described

[c]misoprostol administration refers to misoprostol use as prevention for PPH and focuses on correct storage, dose, time and route of misoprostol administration, as well as side effect management

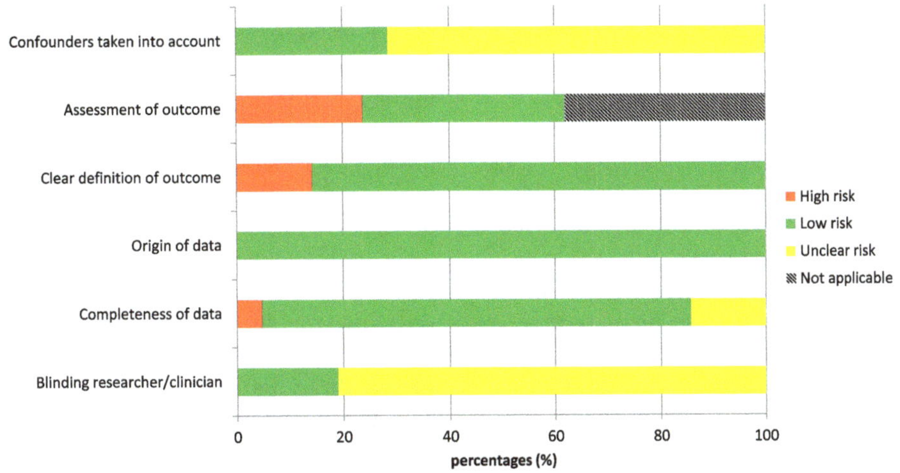

Fig. 2 Bar graph showing the risk distribution according to the different variables on which 21 articles were assessed. Blinding of researcher/clinician was only evaluated if intervention was compared to control group

Results of individual studies

Primary outcome: PPH incidence

In thirteen studies (15.197 women), the primary outcome assessed was the incidence of PPH when uterotonics were provided by unskilled birth attendants.

The incidence of PPH in delivered women who received misoprostol tablets ($n = 10$) was compared to the incidence in women treated by the standard care of no uterotonics ($n = 8$), ergometrine ($n = 1$) or methergine ($n = 1$). Intramuscular oxytocin injections (10 international units) were provided in three studies, in one of these a Uniject device, a disposable automatic syringe, was used. Oxytocin was administered by auxiliary midwives or community health workers. The relative risks of PPH incidence varied from 0.16 to 1 in favor of task shifting. For seven of thirteen articles relative risks were statistically significant [17, 28, 29, 32, 33, 35, 36].

In all studies, educational programs were organized before the start of the interventional trial. Most educational programs for community health workers, auxiliary midwives or traditional birth attendants included a multiple-day course on aspects of AMTSL, mainly focusing on administration of uterotonics. Pregnant women were educated on self-administration by nurses or health workers at antenatal care visits, both at home or in a clinic.

Secondary outcome: Acceptance and safety of task shifting

In twelve studies [5, 10, 12, 13, 22, 30, 31, 33, 37–40] the primary outcome assessed was women's acceptance and safety of community distribution of uterotonics [Table 2]. In all studies administration of uterotonics was evaluated.

Women's acceptance

Of delivered women who self-administered misoprostol tablets postpartum or received tablets from traditional birth attendants, 80% to 99.7% (7 studies, 6445 women) recommended taking misoprostol tablets at delivery to family or friends. Approximately the same percentage, 80% to 99.4% (5 studies, 2677 women), would use misoprostol at their next delivery and 54.6% to 100% (7 studies, 6090 women) were willing to pay for the tablets. Of delivered women who received tablets from auxiliary midwives, 85.6% to 100% (1 study, 218 women) were willing to pay for tablets. No data were available for women who received tablets from community health workers.

Safety of intervention

Of delivered women who self-administered misoprostol tablets or received tablets from traditional birth attendants 83.4% to 99.8% (5 studies, 4719 women) took misoprostol tablets at the correct dose and 63% to 100% (9 studies, 6757 women) took tablets at the correct time, after delivery of the baby and before placental delivery. Both correct dose and time was mentioned in two articles and achieved by 70.7% to 95% of women ($n = 1304$). Approximately the same percentages were observed for auxiliary midwives and community health workers, 83.4% (1 study, 483 women) took the correct dose, 84.1% (1 study, 491 women) at the correct time. Both correct dose and time was mentioned in two articles and achieved by 70.7% to 100% of women ($n = 657$). Incorrect use of misoprostol mostly included taking a lower dose or waiting too long for taking the tablets. Eight articles explicitly described that misoprostol was not taken before delivery of the baby, in one article less than

2 % of the pregnant women took misoprostol pre-infant delivery.

Adverse effects of uterotonics

Adverse effects of misoprostol or oxytocin in the community setting were mentioned in fourteen articles [10,11,13,17,22,27,28,30,31,32,36,37,39,40, Additional file 3]. Mild-to-moderate adverse effects of misoprostol included nausea, vomiting, shivering and/or fever. There were no significant differences in these adverse effects between intervention and control groups of no uterotonics, ergometrine (n = 1 study) or methergine (n = 1 study).

Discussion

This systematic review about task shifting within AMTSL interventions shows that only administration of uterotonics has been evaluated in community and health facility settings in low- and middle-income countries. No data are available for task shifting of controlled cord traction, uterine massage or uterine tone assessment and its effect on incidence of PPH.

Compared to no AMTSL, the administration of uterotonics by traditional birth attendants, auxiliary midwives, community health workers or the woman herself reduced the incidence of PPH. Task shifting of this part of AMTSL to unskilled birth attendants was generally accepted by women and care providers and was reported to be a safe intervention.

Community distribution of misoprostol and oxytocin by auxiliary midwives and lay health workers as a strategy to increase uterotonic coverage is currently included in WHO guidelines on the prevention of postpartum hemorrhage [4]. The results of this review confirm the safety and effectiveness of this strategy. Administration of misoprostol or oxytocin self-administered by delivered women is not yet recommended in WHO guidelines, and could be considered a strategy to further increase access to AMTSL.

A number of challenges in improving the implementation of AMTSL through task shifting have been suggested. First, misoprostol can be used as an abortifacient and mistimed administration could lead to premature deliveries [39]. Although misoprostol is recognized as an essential medicine by the WHO, worries of mistimed administration have prevented the registration in many countries [41]. While no data were available for number of abortions or preterm deliveries, this remains a potential serious side effect of mistimed administration of misoprostol. The results of this study show that the vast majority of women took or received tablets at the correct time and in the correct dose. In addition, programs that encourage return of misoprostol tablets in case it was not used (e.g. in facility delivery where oxytocin was available), had a near-complete recovery rate [22]. Our results are in line with a systematic review of Smith et al. [42], who described strategies and their safety when distributing misoprostol in the community. They identified 18 studies and showed that 0.06% (n = 7) of 12.615 women incorrectly used misoprostol. No significant differences were seen for the number of stillbirths or neonatal deaths in case uterotonics were provided.

Secondly, an emphasis on task shifting elements of AMTSL could send a mixed-message and may inadvertently stimulate pregnant women to deliver at home without skilled birth attendants. Therefore, the message should always be to promote facility based delivery and only use pragmatic rescue treatment if other options fail. As such, task shifting could be considered complementary in creating community awareness as an intermediate solution towards universal facility based deliveries. In fact, introducing misoprostol distribution programs and associated education training programs for implementation have been reported to increase awareness of the importance of medical care and referrals to Emergency Obstetric Care facilities [7, 31]. Prata et al. [38] observed that level of training is directly proportional to distribution rates of uterotonics, emphasizing the importance of education in creating community awareness. An additional advantage of an intense training program with task shifting of AMTSL to community health workers and traditional birth attendants may be to increase their awareness about referral indications and provide a bridge between community-based traditional care and facility-based obstetric care [7]. Task shifting of AMTSL may also provide an opportunity for facility-based obstetric care to improve quality of care in light of the continuing shortage of skilled birth attendants and to reduce workload for midwives. For example, a randomized controlled trial in a tertiary hospital in Ghana (clinicaltrials.gov, registration number: NCT02223806; [43]) suggested that the final step of postpartum assessment of the uterine tonus can be effectively conducted by patients, whilst regularly monitored by midwives (unpublished data). Recent evidence indicates that omission of CCT has little effect on the risk of severe hemorrhage and the WHO recommends not to include CCT in hemorrhage prevention programs for non-hospital settings [8, 9].

Strengths of this review include the broad focus to include multiple components of AMTSL. In contrast to earlier reviews, we did not only focus on the effect on PPH incidence and safety, but also included women's acceptance of the interventions [20, 42]. Limitations include our inability to conduct a meta-analysis due to heterogeneity of interventions, outcome measurements and contexts. Data were collected at antenatal care visits, during delivery or a few days or weeks postpartum by health workers or traditional birth attendants. Postpartum hemorrhage was measured using different methods varying from visual estimation to using a calibrated scale, possibly explaining the high differences in incidence of PPH between the included studies. Additional file 2 provides more detailed information on measurements of postpartum hemorrhage among the different studies. Educational programs differed between studies, varying from 1-day programs to 7-day programs which is likely to influence the level of skills. An additional limitation is that we only included peer-reviewed literature, which may have excluded intervention reports from the grey literature, for example from non-governmental organizations working in LMIC. All studies evaluating the safety of community distribution of misoprostol, compared reduction of PPH to standard care, which is (mostly) no use of uterotonics. No trials exist comparing the effect on PPH of uterotonics by unskilled birth attendants compared to administration by skilled attendants. However, by not only focusing on the effect of uterotonic administration itself but by also evaluating the effect and safety of task shifting in rural areas, this systematic review has also included safety and acceptance of community distribution.

This review supports the growing body of evidence that the potential of human resources should be maximized at all levels of the health-care system to reduce the burden of maternal morbidity and mortality. In line with this the Senegal Ministry of Health agreed in their national strategic plan for 2014–18 that misoprostol could be provided by auxiliary midwives in maternity huts [44]. In the prevention of PPH as major contributor to maternal mortality, the efficacy and safety of task shifting of all elements (except for controlled cord traction, which is discouraged by the WHO in case skilled birth attendants are absent) within AMSTL should be evaluated in future studies.

Conclusion

Task shifting of (parts of) AMSTL to community health workers, traditional birth attendants or self-administration has been explored in response to the shortages in skilled birth attendants and facility-based deliveries in low- and middle income countries. This systematic review showed that so far only task shifting in uterotonics (oxytocin and misoprostol) administration has been reported. The administration of misoprostol tablets by CHWs, traditional birth attendants or self-administered proved to be effective, safe and accepted in low resource settings. The administration of intramuscular oxytocin by CHWs and auxiliary midwives proved to be effective in reducing PPH. Educational programs are the key element for improvement of implementation of AMTSL and creating awareness of importance of timely referral for emergency obstetric care. As a comprehensive PPH-reduction-strategy based on the AMTSL requires implementation of all steps (except for controlled cord traction, which is discouraged by the WHO in case skilled birth attendants are absent) expanding task shifting to other relevant components of AMTSL will provide additional opportunities to prevent maternal morbidity and mortality due to PPH.

Additional files

Additional file 1: Full search strategy and list of synonyms.

Additional file 2: Individual study risk of bias assessment, according to quality assessment tool.

Additional file 3: Side effects of misoprostol during pregnancy / delivery ($n = 14$).

Abbreviations

AMTSL: Active management of the third stage of labor; CCT: Controlled cord traction; CHW: Community health worker; CI: Confidence interval; EOC: Emergency obstetric care; FIGO: International federation of gynecology and obstetrics; ICM: International confederation of midwives; LMIC: Low- and middle income country; Ml: Milliliters; PPH: Postpartum hemorrhage; RR: Relative risk; SBA: Skilled birth attendant; TBA: Traditional birth attendant; WHO: World Health Organization

Acknowledgements

No acknowledgements are added.

Funding

Not applicable

Authors' contributions

TMR conceived the research question, participated in search and selection of articles, and drafted the first version of the manuscript. JLB co-conceived the research question, was involved in the design and coordination of the study, drafting and revising the manuscript. VJMMS participated in selection of articles and revision of the manuscript. KKG co-conceived the research question and the study design, and revised the manuscript critically. MJR has been involved in coordination of the study process, drafting and revising the manuscript. All authors have approved the final version of the manuscript to be published.

Competing interests

Marcus J Rijken, one of the co-authors of this systematic review, is a member (associate editor) of the editorial board of BMC Pregnancy and Childbirth.

Author details
[1]Julius Global Health, Julius Center for Health Sciences and Primary Care, University Medical Center Utrecht, Heidelberglaan 100, 3584 Utrecht, The Netherlands. [2]Division of Epidemiology & Biostatistics, School of Public Health, Faculty of Health Sciences, University of the Witwatersrand, Johannesburg, South Africa. [3]Department of Obstetrics and Gynecology, University Medical Center Utrecht, Utrecht, The Netherlands.

References

1. Sheldon WR, Blum J, Vogel JP, Souza JP, Gülmezoglu AM, Winikoff B. Postpartum haemorrhage management, risks, and maternal outcomes: findings from the World Health Organization multicountry survey on maternal and newborn health. BJOG. 2014;121(Suppl):5–13.
2. Breu F, Guggenbichler S, Wollmann J. World health statistics 2013. Vasa. 2013;168
3. Lalonde A, Daviss BA, Acosta A, Herschderfer K. Postpartum hemorrhage today: ICM/FIGO initiative 2004-2006. Int J Gynaecol Obstet. 2006;94:243–53.
4. Dept. of Reproductive Health and Research. World Health Organization, dept. of reproductive health and research, World Health Organization. WHO recommendations for the prevention and treatment of postpartum haemorrhage. Geneva: World Health Organization Press; 2012.
5. Sibley LM, Spangler SA, Barry D, Tesfaye S, Desta BF, Gobezayehu AG. A regional comparison of distribution strategies and women's awareness, receipt, and use of misoprostol to prevent postpartum hemorrhage in rural Amhara and Oromiya regions of Ethiopia. J Midwifery Womens Health. 2014;59(Suppl 1):S73–82.
6. Lalonde A. Prevention and treatment of postpartum hemorrhage in low-resource settings. Int J Gynaecol Obstet. 2012;117:108–18.
7. Geller SE, Adams MG, Kelly PJ, Kodkany BS, Derman RJ. Postpartum hemorrhage in resource-poor settings. Int J Gynaecol Obstet. 2006;92:202–11.
8. Gülmezoglu AM, Lumbiganon P, Landoulsi S, Widmer M, Abdel-aleem H, Festin M, et al. Active management of the third stage of labour with and without controlled cord traction : a randomised, controlled, non-inferiority trial. Lancet Elsevier Ltd. 2007;379:1721–7.
9. Hofmeyr GJ, Mshweshwe NT, Gülmezoglu AM. Controlled cord traction for the third stage of labour (review). Cochrane Database Syst Rev 2015, issue 1. Art. no. : CD008020.
10. Sanghvi H, Ansari N, Prata NJV, Gibson H, Ehsan AT, Smith JM. Prevention of postpartum hemorrhage at home birth in Afghanistan. Int Fed Gynecol Obstet. 2010;108:276–81.
11. Walraven G, Blum J, Dampha Y, Sowe M, Morison L, Winikoff B, et al. Misoprostol in the management of the third stage of labour in the home delivery setting in rural Gambia: a randomised controlled trial. BJOG An Int. J. Obstet. Gynaecol. 2005;112:1277–83.
12. Prata N, Bell S, Holston M, Quaiyum MA. Is attendant at delivery associated with the use of interventions to prevent postpartum hemorrhage at home births? The case of Bangladesh. BMC Pregnancy Childbirth. 2014;14:24.
13. Smith JM, Baawo SD, Subah M, Sirtor-Gbassie V, Howe CJ, Ishola G, et al. Advance distribution of misoprostol for prevention of postpartum hemorrhage (PPH) at home births in two districts of Liberia. BMC Pregnancy Childbirth. 2014;14:189.
14. World Health Organization. Optimizing health worker roles to improve access to key maternal and newborn health interventions through task shifting. Geneva: World Health Organization; 2012.
15. Prata N, Bell S, Weidert K. Prevention of postpartum hemorrhage in low-resource settings: current perspectives. Int J Womens Health. 2013;5:737–52.
16. Miller S, Lester F, Hensleigh P. Prevention and treatment of postpartum hemorrhage: new advances for low-resource settings. J Midwifery Womens. Health. 2004;49:283–92.
17. Mobeen N, Durocher J, Zuberi N, Jahan N, Blum J, Wasim S, et al. Administration of misoprostol by trained traditional birth attendants to prevent postpartum haemorrhage in homebirths in Pakistan: a randomised placebo-controlled trial. BJOG. 2011;118:353–61.
18. Tunçalp Ö, Hofmeyr GJ, Gülmezoglu AM. Prostaglandins for preventing postpartum haemorrhage. Cochrane Database Syst Rev. 2012;8:CD000494.
19. Gulmezoglu AM, Villar J, Ngoc NT, Piaggio G, Carroli G, Adetoro L, et al. WHO multicentre randomised trial of misoprostol in the management of the third stage of labour. Lancet. 2001;358:689–95.
20. Oladapo OT, Fawole B, Blum J, Abalos E, Ot O, Fawole B, et al. Advance misoprostol distribution for preventing and treating postpartum haemorrhage (review). Cochrane Database Syst Rev. 2012;2:CD009336.
21. Prata N, Passano P, Bell S, Rowen T, Potts M. New hope: community-based misoprostol use to prevent postpartum haemorrhage. Health Policy Plan. 2013;28:339–46.
22. Geller S, Carnahan L, Akosah E, Asare G, Agyemang R, Dickson R, et al. Community-based distribution of misoprostol to prevent postpartum haemorrhage at home births : results from operations research in rural Ghana. BJOG An Int J Obstet Gynaecol. 2014;121:319–26.
23. Liberati A, Altman DG, Tetzlaff J, Mulrow C, Gøtzsche PC, Ioannidis JPA, et al. The PRISMA statement for reporting systematic reviews and meta-analyses of studies that evaluate health care interventions: explanation and elaboration. PLoS Med. 2009;6(7):e1000100.
24. World Health Organization. Making pregnancy safer : the critical role of the skilled attendant a joint statement by WHO, ICM and FIGO. Geneva: World Health Organization; 2004.
25. Higgins JPT, Green S (editors). Cochrane Handbook for Systematic Reviews of Interventions Version5.1.0 [updated March 2011]. The Cochrane Collaboration, 2011. Available from http://handbook.cochrane.org.
26. Field A. Discovering statistics using IBM SPSS statistics. Discov. Stat. Using IBM SPSS stat. hichester: Wiley; 2013. p. 297–321.
27. Chandhiok N, Dhillon BS, Datey S, Mathur A, Saxena NC. Oral misoprostol for prevention of postpartum hemorrhage by paramedical workers in India. Int J Gynecol Obstet. 2006;92:170–5.
28. Derman RJ, Kodkany BS, Goudar SS, Geller SE, Naik VA, Bellad MB, et al. Oral misoprostol in preventing postpartum haemorrhage in resource-poor communities: a randomised controlled trial. Lancet. 2006;368:1248–53.
29. Stanton CK, Newton S, Mullany LC, Cofie P, Tawiah Agyemang C, Adiibokah E, et al. Effect on postpartum hemorrhage of prophylactic Oxytocin (10 IU) by injection by community health officers in Ghana: a community-based. Cluster-Randomized Trial PLoS Med. 2013;10
30. Ejembi C, Shittu O, Moran M, Adiri F, Oguntunde O, Saadatu B, et al. Community-level distribution of Misoprostol to prevent postpartum hemorrhage at home births in northern Nigeria. Afr J Reprod Health. 2014;18:166–75.
31. Mir AM, Wajid A, Gull S. Helping rural women in Pakistan to prevent postpartum hemorrhage: a quasi experimental study. BMC Pregnancy Childbirth. 2012;12:120.
32. Prata N, Gessessew A, Abraha AK, Holston M, Potts M. Prevention of postpartum hemorrhage: options for home births in rural Ethiopia. Afr J Reprod Health. 2009;13:87–95.
33. Prata N, Ejembi C, Fraser A, Shittu O, Minkler M. Community mobilization to reduce postpartum hemorrhage in home births in northern Nigeria. Soc Sci Med Elsevier Ltd. 2012;74:1288–96.
34. Low LK, Bailey JM, Sacks E, Medina L, Piñeda HOL. Postpartum hemorrhage prevention: a case study in northern rural Honduras. J Midwifery Womens Health. 2008;53:e1–6.
35. Low LK, Bailey JM, Sacks E, Robles C, Medina L. Reduced postpartum hemorrhage after implementation of active management of the third stage of labor in rural Honduras. Int J Gynaecol Obstet. 2012;119:217–20.
36. Nasreen H-E, Nahar S, Al Mamun M, Afsana K, Byass P. Oral misoprostol for preventing postpartum haemorrhage in home births in rural Bangladesh: how effective is it? Glob Health Action. 2011;4:1–11.
37. Diadhiou M, Dieng T, Ortiz C, Mall I, Dione D, Sloan NL. Introduction of misoprostol for prevention of postpartum hemorrhage at the community level in Senegal. Int Fed Gynecol Obstet. 2011;115:251–5.
38. Prata N, Quaiyum MA, Passano P, Bell S, Bohl DD, Hossain S, et al. Training traditional birth attendants to use misoprostol and an absorbent delivery mat in home births. Soc Sci Med. 2012;75:2021–7.
39. Rajbhandari S, Hodgins S, Sanghvi H, McPherson R, Pradhan YV, Baqui AH. Expanding uterotonic protection following childbirth through community-based distribution of misoprostol: operations research study in Nepal. Int Fed Gynecol Obstet. 2010;108:282–8.
40. Smith JM, Dimiti A, Dwivedi V, Ochieng I, Dalaka M, Currie S, et al. Advance distribution of misoprostol for the prevention of postpartum hemorrhage in South Sudan. Int Fed Gynecol Obstet. 2014;127:183–8.
41. Smith HJ, Colvin CJ, Richards E, Roberson J, Sharma G, Thapa K, et al. Programmes for advance distribution of misoprostol to prevent post-

partum haemorrhage: a rapid literature review of factors affecting implementation. Health Policy Plan. 2015:1–12.
42. Smith JM, Gubin R, Holston MM, Fullerton J, Prata N. Misoprostol for postpartum hemorrhage prevention at home birth: an integrative review of global implementation experience to date. BMC Pregnancy Childbirth. 2013;13:44.
43. Browne JL, Damale NK, Raams TM, Van der Linden EL, Maya ET, Doe R, et al. Uterine tonus assessment by midwives versus patient self-assessment in the active management of the third stage of labor (UTAMP): study protocol for a randomized controlled trial. Trials. 2015:1–6.
44. Diop A, Daff B, Sow M, Blum J, Diagne M, Sloan NL, et al. Oxytocin via Uniject (a prefilled single-use injection) versus oral misoprostol for prevention of postpartum haemorrhage at the community level: a cluster-randomised controlled trial. Lancet Glob Health. 2016;4:e37–44. A

Permissions

All chapters in this book were first published in P&C, by BioMed Central; hereby published with permission under the Creative Commons Attribution License or equivalent. Every chapter published in this book has been scrutinized by our experts. Their significance has been extensively debated. The topics covered herein carry significant findings which will fuel the growth of the discipline. They may even be implemented as practical applications or may be referred to as a beginning point for another development.

The contributors of this book come from diverse backgrounds, making this book a truly international effort. This book will bring forth new frontiers with its revolutionizing research information and detailed analysis of the nascent developments around the world.

We would like to thank all the contributing authors for lending their expertise to make the book truly unique. They have played a crucial role in the development of this book. Without their invaluable contributions this book wouldn't have been possible. They have made vital efforts to compile up to date information on the varied aspects of this subject to make this book a valuable addition to the collection of many professionals and students.

This book was conceptualized with the vision of imparting up-to-date information and advanced data in this field. To ensure the same, a matchless editorial board was set up. Every individual on the board went through rigorous rounds of assessment to prove their worth. After which they invested a large part of their time researching and compiling the most relevant data for our readers.

The editorial board has been involved in producing this book since its inception. They have spent rigorous hours researching and exploring the diverse topics which have resulted in the successful publishing of this book. They have passed on their knowledge of decades through this book. To expedite this challenging task, the publisher supported the team at every step. A small team of assistant editors was also appointed to further simplify the editing procedure and attain best results for the readers.

Apart from the editorial board, the designing team has also invested a significant amount of their time in understanding the subject and creating the most relevant covers. They scrutinized every image to scout for the most suitable representation of the subject and create an appropriate cover for the book.

The publishing team has been an ardent support to the editorial, designing and production team. Their endless efforts to recruit the best for this project, has resulted in the accomplishment of this book. They are a veteran in the field of academics and their pool of knowledge is as vast as their experience in printing. Their expertise and guidance has proved useful at every step. Their uncompromising quality standards have made this book an exceptional effort. Their encouragement from time to time has been an inspiration for everyone.

The publisher and the editorial board hope that this book will prove to be a valuable piece of knowledge for researchers, students, practitioners and scholars across the globe.

List of Contributors

L. Lindroos, L. Ladfors and U.-B. Wennerholm
Department of Obstetrics and Gynecology, Institute of Clinical Sciences at Sahlgrenska Academy, Gothenburg University, Diagnosvägen 15, 416 85 Gothenburg, Sweden

A. Elfvin
Department of Pediatrics, Institute of Clinical Sciences at Sahlgrenska Academy, Gothenburg University, Gothenburg, Sweden

Patience Afulani and Dilys Walker
Obstetrics, Gynecology and Reproductive Sciences, UCSF, San Francisco, USA
Institute for Global Health Sciences, UCSF, San Francisco, USA

Caroline Kusi
Institute for Global Health Sciences, UCSF, San Francisco, USA

Leah Kirumbi
Kenya Medical Research Institute, Nairobi, Kenya

Brooke Thomson
School of Nursing, Midwifery and Paramedicine, Curtin University, Bentley, Perth, Western Australia 6102, Australia

Janice Butt, Chloe Western, Helen Overing, Corrinne Poletti and Jessica Priest
Department of Nursing and Midwifery Education and Research, King Edward Memorial Hospital, Subiaco, Western Australia 6008, Australia

Lucy Lewis and Yvonne L. Hauck
School of Nursing, Midwifery and Paramedicine, Curtin University, Bentley, Perth, Western Australia 6102, Australia
Department of Nursing and Midwifery Education and Research, King Edward Memorial Hospital, Subiaco, Western Australia 6008, Australia

Dawn Hudd
Family Birth Centre, Midwifery Group Practice and Community Midwifery Program, King Edward Memorial Hospital, Subiaco 6008, Western Australia, Australia

Maria S. Maputle
Department of Advanced Nursing, University of Venda, Thohoyandou 0950, South Africa

S. Connor
Department of Rural Nursing and Midwifery, La Trobe Rural Health School, Vic, Mildura 3500, Australia

K. Edvardsson
Judith Lumley Centre, School of Nursing and Midwifery, La Trobe University, Vic, Bundoora 3086, Australia
Department of Clinical Sciences, Obstetrics and Gynecology, Umeå University, 901 87 Umeå, SE, Sweden

E. Spelten
Department of Public Health, La Trobe Rural Health School, Mildura, Vic 3500, Australia

Birute Zilaitiene, Marius Dirzauskas, Rasa Verkauskiene and Rytas Ostrauskas
Institute of Endocrinology, Lithuanian University of Health Sciences, 50009 Kaunas, Lithuania

Joerg Gromoll and Eberhard Nieschlag
Center of Reproductive Medicine and Andrology, University of Münster, 48149 Münster, Münster, Germany

Yun Zhao, Mei Xiao and Wan Tang
Department of Obstetrics, Maternal and Child Health Hospital of Hubei Province, No 745 Wuluo Road, Wuhan City, People's Republic of China

Li Zou
Department of Obstetrics and Gynecology, Union Hospital of Tongji Medical College, Huazhong University of Science and Technology, Wuhan City, People's Republic of China

Hai-yi Niu and Fu-yuan Qiao
Department of Obstetrics and Gynecology, Tongji Hospital of Tongji Medical College, Huazhong University of Science and Technology, Wuhan City, People's Republic of China

Muhammad Zakria Zakar, Mudasir Mustafa and Aisha Jalil
Department of Sociology, Institute of Social and Cultural Studies, University of the Punjab, Lahore, Pakistan

Rubeena Zakar
Department of Public Health, Institute of Social and Cultural Studies, University of the Punjab, Lahore, Pakistan

Florian Fischer
Department of Public Health Medicine, School of Public Health, Bielefeld University, Bielefeld, Germany

Natnael Etsay Assefa, Hailemariam Berhe, Fiseha Girma, Kidanemariam Berhe, Yodit Zewdie Berhe, Gdiom Gebreheat, Weldu Mamu Werid, Almaz Berhe, Hagos B Rufae and Guesh Welu
Adigrat University College of Health Sciences, Adigart, Tigray, Ethiopia

Paola Colais, Katia Bontempi, Luigi Pinnarelli, Danilo Fusco and Marina Davoli
Department of Epidemiology, Lazio Regional Health Service, Via Cristoforo Colombo 112, 00142 Rome, Italy

Carlo Piscicelli and Ilenia Mappa
Cristo Re Hospital, Via delle Calasanziane, 25, 00167 Rome, Italy

Mali Abdollahian and Kaye Marion
School of Science (Mathematical and Geospatial Sciences), College of Science, Engineering, and Health, RMIT University, GPO Melbourne, VIC 3001, Australia

Dewi Anggraini
School of Science (Mathematical and Geospatial Sciences), College of Science, Engineering, and Health, RMIT University, GPO Melbourne, VIC 3001, Australia
Study Program of Statistics, Faculty of Mathematics and Natural Sciences, University of Lambung Mangkurat (ULM), Ahmad Yani Street, Km. 36, Banjarbaru, South Kalimantan 70714, Indonesia

Nia Holford
South Wales Clinical Psychology Doctorate Programme, Cardiff University, Cardiff, UK

Sue Channon
Centre for Trials Research, Cardiff University, Cardiff, UK

Jessica Heron
Action on Postpartum Psychosis, Department of Psychiatry, The Barberry National Centre for Mental Health, University of Birmingham, Birmingham, UK

Ian Jones
National Centre for Mental Health, Division of Psychological Medicine and Clinical Neurosciences, MRC Centre for Neuropsychiatric Genetics and Genomics, Cardiff University, Cardiff, UK

Bola Lukman Solanke and Semiu Adebayo Rahman
Department of Demography and Social Statistics, Faculty of Social Sciences, Obafemi Awolowo University, Ile-Ife, Nigeria

Chia-Hung Yu, Ying-Jen Chang and Chin-Chen Chu
Division of Women's and Children's Anesthesia, Department of Anesthesiology, Chi Mei Medical Center, 901 Zhonghua Road, Yongkang District, Tainan City 710, Taiwan

Yi-Chen Chen
Department of Medical Research, Chi Mei Medical Center, 901 Zhonghua Road, Yongkang District, Tainan City 710, Taiwan

Shih-Feng Weng
Department of Healthcare Administration and Medical Informatics, Kaohsiung Medical University, 100, Shih-Chuan 1st Road, Kaohsiung 807, Taiwan
Department of Medical Research, Chi Mei Medical Center, 901 Zhonghua Road, Yongkang District, Tainan City 710, Taiwan

Chung-Han Ho
Department of Medical Research, Chi Mei Medical Center, 901 Zhonghua Road, Yongkang District, Tainan City 710, Taiwan
Department of Pharmacy, Chia Nan University of Pharmacy and Science, Chi Mei Medical Center, 60, Sec. 1, Erren Rd., Rende Dist., Tainan City 717, Taiwan

Jen-Yin Chen
Division of Women's and Children's Anesthesia, Department of Anesthesiology, Chi Mei Medical Center, 901 Zhonghua Road, Yongkang District, Tainan City 710, Taiwan
Department of Senior Citizen Service Management, Chia Nan University of Pharmacy and Science, Chi Mei Medical Center, No.60, Sec. 1, Erren Rd., Rende Dist, Tainan City 717, Taiwan

Jhi-Joung Wang
Division of Women's and Children's Anesthesia, Department of Anesthesiology, Chi Mei Medical Center, 901 Zhonghua Road, Yongkang District, Tainan City 710, Taiwan
Department of Medical Research, Chi Mei Medical Center, 901 Zhonghua Road, Yongkang District, Tainan City 710, Taiwan

Ming-Ping Wu
Division of Urogynecology and Pelvic Floor Reconstruction, Department of Obstetrics and Gynecology, Chi Mei Medical Center, 901 Zhonghua Road, Yongkang District, Tainan City 710, Taiwan
Center of General Education, Chia Nan University of Pharmacy and Science, Chi Mei Medical Center, 60, Sec. 1, Erren Rd., Rende Dist.,, Tainan City 717, Taiwan

Wei Sun, Ying Zhang, Zeyu Yang, Ailu Cai, Yu Wang and Wenjia Lei
Department of Sonography, Shengjing Hospital of China Medical University, Shenyang, China

Shaowei Yin
Department of Obstetrics and Gynecology, Shengjing Hospital of China Medical University, Shenyang, China

Qiuju Wei
Department of Obstetrics and Gynecology, the University of Tennessee Health Science Center, Memphis, TN, USA

Nolwenn Lagadec, Magali Steinecker, Amar Kapassi, Anne Marie Magnier, Julie Chastang and Nadia Gaouaou
Department of Education and Research in General Medicine, Faculty of Medicine Pierre et Marie Curie, 27, rue Chaligny - 75571, cedex 12 Paris, France

Sarah Robert and Gladys Ibanez
Sorbonne Universités, UPMC Univ Paris 06, INSERM, Institut Pierre Louis d'épidémiologie et de Santé Publique (IPLESP UMRS 1136), F75012 Paris, France

Hans Järnbert-Pettersson
Karolinska Institutet - Department of Clinical Science and Education, Södersjukhuset, Stockholm, Sweden

Linda Vixner
Dalarna University- School of Education, Health and Social Studies, Falun, Sweden

Ahmed Kamel, Ayman A. Halim, Salwa AlFarra, Yahia El-faissal, Wafaa Ramadan and Ahmed M. Hussein
Obstetrics and Gynecology Department, Cairo University, KasrAlainy St., Garden City, Cairo, Egypt

Mohamed Shehata
Clinical and Chemical Pathology Department, Cairo University, Cairo, Egypt

Estomih R. Mduma
Haydom Lutheran Hospital, Mbulu, Tanzania
Department of Health Science, University of Stavanger, Stavanger, Norway

Paschal Francis Mdoe
Haydom Lutheran Hospital, Mbulu, Tanzania
Department of Health Science, University of Stavanger, Stavanger, Norway
Obstetrics and Gynaecology, Haydom Lutheran Hospital, Haydom, Mbulu, Tanzania

Hege L. Ersdal
Department of Health Science, University of Stavanger, Stavanger, Norway
Department of Anesthesiology and Intensive Care, Stavanger University Hospital, Stavanger, Norway

Jeffrey M. Perlman
Department of Pediatrics, Weill Cornell, New York, USA

Robert Moshiro
Department of Health Science, University of Stavanger, Stavanger, Norway
Muhimbili National Hospital, Dar es Salaam, Tanzania

Peter T. Wangwe
Muhimbili University of Health and Allied Sciences, Dar es Salaam, Tanzania

Hussein Kidanto
Department of Research, Stavanger University Hospital, Stavanger, Norway
Muhimbili University of Health and Allied Sciences, Dar es Salaam, Tanzania

Patricia P. Gomez, Chantelle Allen and Hannah Tappis
Jhpiego/Baltimore, 1615 Thames Street, Baltimore, MD 21232, USA

Allyson R. Nelson
Jhpiego/Liberia, UN Drive, OPP Rock Compound, Mamba Point, Monrovia, Liberia

Amos Asiedu, Etta Addo, Dora Agbodza, Martha Appiagyei, Patience Darko, Julia Duodu and Fred Effah
Jhpiego Ghana, 14 Ollenu Street, East Legon, Accra, Ghana

Cynthia Bannerman
Ghana Health Service, Private Mail Bag, Ministries, Accra, Ghana

Xiao Zhou, Meng Zhang, Zhuang Liu, Meili Duan and Lei Dong
Department of Intensive Care Unit, Beijing Friendship Hospital, Capital Medical University, No. 95 Yong-An Road, Xi Cheng District, Beijing 100050, China

Tessa M. Raams, Joyce L. Browne and Verena J. M. M. Festen-Schrier
Julius Global Health, Julius Center for Health Sciences and Primary Care, University Medical Center Utrecht, Heidelberglaan 100, 3584 Utrecht, The Netherlands

Kerstin Klipstein-Grobusch
Julius Global Health, Julius Center for Health Sciences and Primary Care, University Medical Center Utrecht, Heidelberglaan 100, 3584 Utrecht, The Netherlands
Division of Epidemiology and Biostatistics, School of Public Health, Faculty of Health Sciences, University of the Witwatersrand, Johannesburg, South Africa

Marcus J. Rijken
Julius Global Health, Julius Center for Health Sciences and Primary Care, University Medical Center Utrecht, Heidelberglaan 100, 3584 Utrecht, The Netherlands
Department of Obstetrics and Gynecology, University Medical Center Utrecht, Utrecht, The Netherlands

Index

www.ingramcontent.com/pod-product-compliance
Lightning Source LLC
LaVergne TN
LVHW080733210926
848485LV00003B/552
9781639271641